Medical Education in the Millennium

Medical Education in the Millennium

Edited by

Brian Jolly

Director, Medical Education Unit, University of Leeds, Leeds, UK

and

Lesley Rees

St Bartholomew's and the Royal London School of Medicine and Dentistry,
Queen Mary Westfield College, University of London, UK

OXFORD UNIVERSITY PRESS

OXFORD

UNIVERSITY PRESS

Great Clarendon Street, Oxford OX2 6DP

Oxford University Press is a department of the University of Oxford.
It furthers the University's objective of excellence in research, scholarship,
and education by publishing worldwide in

Oxford New York

Auckland Bangkok Buenos Aires Cape Town Chennai
Dar es Salaam Delhi Hong Kong Istanbul Karachi Kolkata
Kuala Lumpur Madrid Melbourne Mexico City Mumbai Nairobi
São Paulo Shanghai Taipei Tokyo Toronto

Oxford is a registered trade mark of Oxford University Press
in the UK and in certain other countries

Published in the United States
by Oxford University Press Inc., New York

ISBN 0-19-262399-0

Printed in Great Britain by
Antony Rowe Ltd., Eastbourne

Preface

At the time of writing this there are 2 years, 80 days and 14 hours to go before the start of the new millennium. This book has already been a little longer in gestation. When we started, the Internet was something we had all used intermittently and not particularly reliably. Kenneth Calman, the Chief Medical Officer for England and eponymous donor of changes to postgraduate education in the UK, had just commenced the process of reforming the system, and adventurous medical schools in the UK were just starting to adopt problem-based learning as a key strategy, some 30 years after its inception in a medical curriculum in Canada.

This book was initiated by Angela Towle who, upon moving to Vancouver, felt that transatlantic editorial management would be too much on top of a major curriculum renovation and handed over the reins to Lesley Rees. Enormous gratitude goes to her for a great start and for inspiration. This stimulation provided the original goal, which was to comprehensively document and provide a rationale for those ideas and innovations about to appear in medical education that would provide guidance for the next century. As it progressed it became obvious that such a goal was over ambitious. Things were moving too fast and evaluations of those things progressing too slowly to accomplish a wide ranging and well anchored blueprint. Things also, before our eyes as it were, became either less predictable or fully embedded. Many of 'Tomorrow's Doctor's' appeared prematurely. Patients' power and their access to information reached a rapid zenith, on both sides of the Atlantic. The Internet exploded. We moderated our vision.

We have focused on providing a basic description of the enduring trends in western medical education over the last few years, concentrating on established successes. Most of these are UK based, but some involve far reaching developments world-wide. We have done this to provide a stepping stone into the next century for medical educationists. We realize they will need others, but we hope that the reader will find a wealth of experience, valuable references and some basic building blocks for post-millennium developments. We have included two chapters on the change process. They are written from different perspectives, but include much in common. Nevertheless, we took an editorial decision to leave them to speak for themselves rather than attempt what would have been a complex synthesis. We also chose to ignore one of the most rapidly developing topics in the literature – the cognitive processes of doctors. This was largely because the focus of the book was on curriculum and curriculum change, with which all medical teachers frequently impact. By contrast, cognition is a specialized area with a small but important following and we saw it as beyond our scope. Yet a readable, concise account of this area is long overdue and sorely needed, since ultimately how doctors are taught to think should govern, at least partially, how they learn. Our inclusion too of third world developments is not as accomplished as we would have hoped. There remain many useful lessons to be learnt from recent explorations outside North America, Australia, and Europe.

We thank all our contributors for their forbearance, and particularly those who completed early and had to wait for, and subsequently revise their chapters on the basis of our later arrivals. We also thank secretaries Margaret Mirza, Sally Hadden, Carol Icke, and Oxford University Press. We also thank our colleagues who have given us so much insight into the processes of medical education, including, in addition to the contributors to this book, Peter Cull, Annie Cushing, Bill Godolphin, Peter McCrorie, Helen Mullholland, Lesley Southgate, and Richard Wakeford. Dedications are not politically correct in an edited volume, but had they been so we would have made them to Mary Lawson and Gareth Rees as scant reward for putting up with us.

Leeds   B.J.
London   L.R.
December 1997

Contents

Contributors

Peter A.J. Bouhuijs   Associate Professor in Educational Research, University of Maastricht, The Netherlands

Colin Coles   Professor in Medical Education, Bournemouth University

Jane Dacre   Reader in Clinical Skills, Consultant Physician and Rheumatologist, University College London

Thomas H.S. Dent   Consultant in Public Health Medicine, North and Mid Hampshire Health Authority

Lewis Elton   Professor, Centre for Research in Higher Education, University College London

Jenny Field   Senior Lecturer in Primary Medical Care, University of Southampton

Rodney Gale   Fellow in Management, Joint Centre for Education in Medicine

Jonathan H. Gillard   Clinical Lecturer in Radiology, University of Cambridge

Janet Grant   Professor of Education in Medicine, Open University Joint Centre for Education in Medicine

William Howard   Senior Programmer, Centre for Health Informatics and Multiprofessional Education, University College London Medical School, Whittington Campus

David Ingram   Professor of Health Informatics and Director, Centre for Health Informatics and Multiprofessional Education, University College London Medical School, Whittington Campus

Brian Jolly   Director, Medical Education Unit, University of Leeds

Jeannette Murphy   Senior Lecturer in Health Informatics, Centre for Health Informatics and Multiprofessional Education, University College London Medical School, Whittington Campus

David Newble   Associate Professor of Medicine, University of Adelaide, Australia

Julia Neuberger   Chief Executive, The King's Fund. Member General Medical Council and Medical Research Council

Lesley Rees   St Bartholomew's and the Royal London School of Medicine and Dentistry, Queen Mary Westfield College, University of London

Angela Towle   University of British Columbia, Vancouver, Canada

1 Aims of the curriculum

The aims of the curriculum: education for health needs in 2000 and beyond

Angela Towle

The questioning of medical education

In recent years, a variety of sources — government, foundations, educators, the media, and, perhaps most importantly, those who use medical care — have begun to focus on what is required to produce a good physician. Both internal and external forces are encouraging medical schools to alter their curricula and even their basic structure. Accrediting bodies have imposed new standards that call for measuring and evaluating medical school graduates according to a variety of educational outcomes. In some instances, funding has been coupled with the attainment of mandated outcome objectives (Jonas *et al.* 1992).

The biggest questions facing medical education as the twenty-first century approaches are: what will be the roles and responsibilities of a doctor in the next century and how can we prepare young doctors for the future in a world which is rapidly changing? More specifically, what should be the aims of medical education? What should be taught, where, and by whom? And how can we ensure that the curriculum evolves continuously in response to the ever-changing external environment? Medical educators are asking how much change is appropriate and necessary, and whether such changes will indeed better prepare future physicians for practice in the twenty-first century.

These questions are not new and have been addressed repeatedly throughout the twentieth century in a series of major studies (fifteen in the USA alone, Enarson and Burg 1992), but with limited outcomes. Problems with medical education have been identified, recommendations made, but solutions rarely implemented.

> The aim of medical education is to produce doctors who will promote the health of all people, and that aim is not being realized in many places, despite the enormous progress in the biomedical sciences . . . These defects have been identified for a long time, but efforts to introduce greater social awareness into medical schools have not been notably successful. Such facts have led to mounting concern in medical education about equity in health care, the humane delivery of health services, and the overall costs to society. (World Federation for Medical Education 1988).

> Over the last 60 years, most medical schools have done little to correct the major

shortcomings in the ways they educate their students, even though these deficiencies have been documented repeatedly. (Association of American Medical Colleges 1992).

Despite the bold and interesting approaches taken at several institutions, the curriculum at most US medical schools remains quite similar in form to that advocated by Flexner.

Tosteson 1990

The principal features of the Flexnerian system (see also Chapter 7), referred to by Tosteson, are: a clear separation between the basic and clinical sciences with the basic sciences taught in the first year or two and the clinical subjects taught in the last two or three years; the heavy use of didactic instruction in the form of lectures to large groups of students; an emphasis on the teacher's role as an expert source of information; and relatively independent and often poorly coordinated courses (see pp. 179–80), designed and offered by many different teachers during clinical clerkships. It is a model of medical education which has been adopted worldwide. In an international survey of medical education conducted by the American Medical Association in 1990 (Carlson 1991) nearly all the 31 responding countries (92%) described their curricula as typically divided between the basic and clinical sciences. The most common innovative trend, identified by nine countries, was a shift towards curricular integration of the basic and clinical sciences.

In asking why this system has proved so stable and resistant to change, Tosteson (1990) identified both conceptual and organizational reasons. He voiced the concerns of many in stating that 'it is enormously difficult to conceive of the content and form of education that is appropriate to the medicine of the future' and that most medical faculties are not well organized to address such issues. As the World Federation for Medical Education (1988) highlights, medical schools throughout the world have increasingly taken on the spirit and values of the universities of which most are an integral part, resulting in an orientation towards research, both basic and clinical. This evolutionary process throughout the twentieth century has led to remarkable advances in medical research and care, but as medical teachers have become increasingly specialized, following patterns in research and care, so curricula have become increasingly compartmentalized. When devising educational programmes, medical teachers have looked inward to the content of their disciplines rather than outwards to the needs of the community which medical graduates will be expected to serve.

Despite, or perhaps because of, the failure of most earlier attempts at fundamental curriculum re-orientation, the early 1990s have proved to be a time of reappraisal in medical education, with calls for reform being heard throughout the decade. On the international scene, the World Health Organization, the World Federation for Medical Education, and the Network of Community-Oriented Educational Institutions for Health Sciences have widely publicized the need to alter the character of medical education so that it fully meets the defined needs of the society in which it is situated. Even in countries where the traditional Flexnerian curriculum has not been seriously challenged by the majority of medical teachers, a new realization of the need for change has emerged. In the USA, a study of medical educators by the Robert Wood Johnson Foundation in 1989 found that, except for basic sciences faculty, a majority stated that 'fundamental changes' or 'thorough reform' was needed (Cantor *et al.* 1991). This restlessness has led to 'curricular ferment' resulting in attempts to reform the curriculum in the majority of US and Canadian schools. By the academic year 1991–2,

22 schools had completed a major curriculum change within the previous five years, 45 schools had a major change underway, and 32 schools planned major changes within a year (Jonas *et al.* 1992). Similarly, in the UK there has developed a consensus view of the need for change in undergraduate medical education (Towle 1991) and almost all the medical schools in the country are currently reviewing their curricula.

As the next century approaches and the pace of change accelerates, and pressures on medical education from the health care system cannot be ignored, so there appears to be a new urgency to tackle the big questions in medical education. On the one hand, there is an apparent greater commitment to implement current recommendations about which there is general agreement and consensus, and where the problem seems to be one of the effective implementation of curriculum change. On the other hand, forward thinking and influential people are beginning to define a new paradigm for medical education in response to challenges coming from outside the medical profession. Reform of medical education is here seen as part of a larger change: the need to redefine the role of the medical school in terms of its mission to the population which it serves.

The aims of basic medical education in the 1990s: the current consensus

Responding to increasing knowledge

In its recommendations of 1993, the General Medical Council in the UK identified the job of the undergraduate course to be: to produce doctors who have attitudes to medicine and to learning that will fit them for their professional careers and commit them to a lifetime of self-education. They identified as the main challenges facing the undergraduate curriculum the reduction of factual overload and promotion of a capacity for self-education, critical thought, and the evaluation of evidence.

Their ideas are consistent with the many attempts by the medical profession throughout the twentieth century to reform the undergraduate curriculum in response to new knowledge, especially scientific knowledge. The pressure to add more and more into the curriculum (scientific advances and new subjects which have assumed increasing importance in medical practice such as ethics and communication skills) has reached a point of crisis. Not only has the content of the curriculum surpassed students' capacities to learn at anything but a superficial level in order to pass examinations, but it is apparent that the pace of change is so rapid that some of the knowledge and skills that are taught soon become obsolete. As a result there is agreement that the urgent need is to put into practice the often-heard words that the undergraduate curriculum is just the first step in the continuum of a lifelong educational process and that the emphasis should move towards the development of general competencies which will be valid however medical practice develops, and particularly to promote lifelong learning. The former is addressed by defining (and limiting) the content of the curriculum and the latter by changing the process, particularly to a more active style of learning.

In the UK there is a consensus view among those responsible for medical education about the aims of the undergraduate curriculum which is reflected by the recent recommendations from the Education Committee of the GMC (Box 1.1) and the national enquiry by the King's Fund (Box 1.2). Similar recommendations have emerged from thirteen of the fifteen national studies on medical education in the USA since 1910 (Box 1.3). In the Robert Wood

Johnson survey of US medical educators' views (Cantor *et al.* 1991) at least 79% of educators voted support for six specific reforms relating to: evaluating and rewarding teaching excellence; increasing integration; evaluating students' independent problem-solving skills; decreasing didactic teaching and increasing independent learning; moving clinical education from in-patient to ambulatory and community settings; and placing greater emphasis on developing the general medical education of students.

Box 1.1 **The aims of basic medical education**

- The primary aim of the undergraduate course is for the student to acquire an understanding of health and disease, and of the prevention and management of the latter, in the context of the whole individual in his or her place in the family and in society.
- The second main aim is to develop an attitude to learning that is based on curiosity and the exploration of knowledge rather than on its passive acquisition.

Further aims:
- Reduction of the excessive burden of information in the existing undergraduate course;
- Introduction of a substantial component of problem-based learning;
- A clinical component in which students have direct contact with patients and with the analysis of their problems throughout the five years of the course;
- An understanding of research method.

(Adapted from GMC 1993)

Box 1.2 **Aims of the curriculum**

- Reduction in factual information;
- Active learning;
- Principles of medicine (core knowledge, skills, and attitudes);
- Development of general competence (e.g. critical thinking, problem solving, communication, management);
- Integration (vertical and horizontal);
- Early clinical contact;
- Balance between hospital/community; curative/preventive;
- Wider aspects of health care (e.g. medico-legal/ethical issues, health economics, political aspects, medical audit);
- Interprofessional collaboration;
- Methods of learning/teaching to support aims of curriculum;
- Methods of assessment to support aims.

(Towle 1991)

Box 1.3 **Summary of recommendations on curricular content and process from major US studies**

- Medical students should receive a broad general education in both the clinical and basic sciences (1,10).
- The objectives of undergraduate medical education should be clearly defined and curricula designed to meet these objectives (1–3,5,9).
- Schools of medicine must ensure that their educational programmes integrate the sciences of medical practice throughout the entire course of the study (4–6,8).
- The acquisition of lifelong learning skills, values, and attitudes should receive at least as much emphasis as the acquisition of knowledge, i.e. memorization of factual material (4,5,7,9).
- In addition to an understanding of the biological disciplines, physicians must have an understanding of other disciplines critical to the provision of high-quality health care. Therefore, medical education must include the behavioural, social, probabilistic, and information sciences and ethics (6,7).
- The general professional education of physicians should include an emphasis on health and disease prevention (5–7).
- Schools of medicine must expand their educational sites beyond tertiary care hospitals to include, for example, ambulatory care settings, community hospitals, nursing homes, and hospices (6,7).
- Health professions education should be adapted to meet the challenges produced by ongoing changes in the organization, financing, and provision of health care (5,7).

From Enarson and Burg 1992

1. Council on Medical Education (1982); 2. Gastel, B. and Rogers, D.E. (1989); 3. Millis, J.S. (1966); 4. Rappleye, W. (1932); 5. Panel on the General Professional Education of the Physician and College Preparation for Medicine (1984); 6. Robert Wood Johnson Foundation Commission (1992); 7. Shugars, D.A., O'Neill, E.H. and Bader, J.D. (1991); 8. Weiskotten, H.G. (1940); 9. Deitrick, J.E. and Berson, R.C. (1953); 10. Flexner, A. (1910).

These reforms and the aims in Boxes 1.1 to 1.3 reflect an attempt to address the key problems facing the traditional curriculum: factual overload, the stifling of intellectual curiosity, perceived lack of relevance to future practice of much that is taught in the basic sciences, and a restricted view of the practice of clinical medicine. Thus the aims emphasize the acquisition of general competencies and the principles of medicine; the promotion of lifelong, independent learning; integration between basic, social, population, and clinical sciences; early clinical contact; a better balance in the curriculum between curative and preventive medicine; and the inclusion of wider aspects of health care including medico-legal and economic issues, and multiprofessional teamwork. Most of these aims, in the general terms in which they have been presented, have proved relatively uncontroversial, but difficult to implement.

The curricular changes that many schools have instituted to date have addressed the problems in medical education largely through reform of the process rather than the content. They are characterized by fewer intensive didactic-lecture hours, more small-group interactive-learning sessions, increased attention to problem-based learning (see Drop and Post 1990), more integration of basic science and clinical courses, and more interdisciplinary courses (Holsgrove *et al.* 1993), although some have also increased exposure to primary care (Nooman *et al.* 1990) and placed greater emphasis on communication skills, ethics, preventive medicine, and health maintenance.

Defining the content (knowledge, skills, and attitudes)

While reports on the need for change in medical education have broadly defined the aims of the undergraduate curriculum in uncontroversial terms (see above), problems tend to creep in when medical schools attempt to define curriculum aims and objectives more precisely. In the ACME-TRI survey (Association of American Medical Colleges 1992) schools in the USA were asked to respond to the following two recommendations from the 1984 GPEP report (Association of American Medical Colleges 1984).

> Medical faculties should specify the clinical knowledge, skills, values and attitudes that students should develop and acquire during their general professional education.
>
> In the general professional education of physicians, medical faculties should emphasise the acquisition and development of skills, values and attitudes by students at least to the same extent that they do their acquisition of knowledge. To do this, medical faculties must limit the amount of factual information that students are expected to memorise.

The survey found that the 59 schools which replied had been only moderately successful in defining the goals of their students' medical education programme; only two schools had defined the knowledge and skills that students must acquire to graduate. Almost all the schools had focused on defining objectives for specific aspects of the curriculum rather than for the total educational programme; in addition, faculty members could not agree on what should constitute the core knowledge and skills of the medical curriculum. The conclusions drawn from the responses were that 'there is a lack of institutional structure to foster oversight for the curriculum and consequently faculty members and departments independently define their own curriculum agendas and goals'.

This situation is not new and has prevented the translation of the general aims proposed in countless reports into substantial change in curriculum content. Not only do individual departments maintain the right to define their own curriculum in isolation, but medical schools also are reluctant to collaborate in defining common curriculum aims and objectives. One strategy which has been recommended to bring about multidisciplinary discussion and action is to describe the exit objectives that students must achieve in order to graduate (Association of American Medical Colleges 1992). Such objectives could be formulated by having faculty members from each basic science and clinical discipline specifically describe the discipline's graduate objectives and then ask representatives from the other disciplines involved in medical students' education to review and criticize these objectives.

Few institutions have conducted formal surveys of faculty opinion regarding exit objectives and there is very little published. One interesting example of this approach is a paper by Scott *et al.* (1991) which describes the first multi-institutional study of exit objectives. Selected faculties from twelve American and Canadian medical schools were asked about clinical behaviours and skills that students should be expected to demonstrate prior to graduation; 32 of the 77 proposed exit objectives (behaviours and skills) were regarded as essential by 75% or more of the faculty members who responded.

In many ways the definition of skills and behaviours relevant to clinical practice and appropriate for the newly qualified doctor is easier than the definition of knowledge objectives, particularly in relation to the basic sciences. Central to any system of medical education is the question of how much basic science the medical student, as a future physician, will need to know. It has been apparent for some time that it is unreasonable and impractical to continue to assume that a medical student can master six or more fields of basic science in the first two years of medical school. At the same time, it is apparent that the physicians of the future will have to work with more scientific information than ever before: they will have increasingly sophisticated tools that will enable them to 'see' the inner workings of the body, and this information will be used increasingly to make decisions about the care of patients. The question of how much science a medical student should know is not a simple one nor easily answerable in general terms. Medicine is still an incomplete science so the question must continually be reevaluated as both clinical practice and science change (Prockop 1992).

An emerging concern, for example, is the impact of the so-called 'new biology' of molecular genetics, cellular biology, immunology, and neurobiology, which is rapidly providing scientists with a systemic and integrated view of whole structures at molecular through to macroscopic levels. Its focus on the cellular and molecular processes unifies conceptually what had previously been discrete disciplines in the preclinical sciences. Modern science is thus far less a problem of mastery of facts and memorization than it is of principles and methods. It is therefore more important that physicians of the future should develop the skills needed for effective and efficient fact retrieval since they will be dependent on reference sources for the details. The mastery of facts could be greatly reduced in scale to an immutable core which is easily definable and available in standard textbooks (Prockop 1992).

It is commonly believed that the problem of defining such a core arises from the fact that most basic science is taught by non-clinicians who have little idea about the clinical relevance of what they teach and who define the aims of the basic science curriculum in relation to their own interests and priorities rather than the needs of a future practising physician. However, there is some evidence that there is agreement on the basic biomedical concepts that might serve as a focus for the curriculum. In a survey of North American medical schools in 1987, there was considerable agreement between basic science and clinical teachers on the relative importance of a set of 27 biomedical concepts (Dawson-Saunders et al. 1990). Here again, the problem may be one of implementation of the consensus view.

One approach to defining the basic sciences curriculum is to separate out the vocational aims (training in basic science knowledge essential to good clinical practice) and the educational aims (promoting the acquisition of the methods and skills of science). Charlton (1991) suggests that the vocational element constitutes a core curriculum which could be constructed from a consideration of the basic scientific knowledge used by clinicians in their medical practice and which could be prepared and examined on a national basis. The concept of a 'core plus options' curriculum is one that has been espoused by the British General Medical Council (1991) as a way of relieving factual overload and promoting independent learning, but there have been few serious attempts to define the objectives of such a core, and agreement about the detailed knowledge, skills, and attitudes needed by a newly qualified doctor may be elusive. Techniques for determining the content of a core curriculum, such as critical incident analysis, consensus conferences, and expert working groups have been proposed, but there appears to be little collective interest in committing the time and effort which would be involved in such an exercise.

Prockop (1992) favours a different solution: the use of unified basic science–clinical examinations prepared by joint committees of basic scientists and clinicians. In this way the question of how much science the student needs to know would be specifically defined and redefined each year. As the students recognize, the examinations define the curriculum of a medical school far more accurately than the voluminous syllabi now provided for most basic science courses (Newble et al. 1994).

Preparing physicians for the twenty-first century: towards the age of accountability

Until recently, concerns about the aims of medical education were largely the responsibility of the medical profession, and the aims of medical education were defined by medical educators. Medical education responded to advances in knowledge and new technology within the field of medicine and the natural sciences largely by expanding the curriculum. The links between physician education and the health care system that subsequently employed them were often loose, but the signs are that in the future changes occurring outside the medical field will have a greater impact on medical education.

For example, there has been increasing awareness and public expression of the growing discontinuity between medical education and the general health needs of society (e.g. Schroeder et al. 1989; White 1991; Evans 1992; White and Connelly 1992). Concern is being expressed that substantial change in the orientation of medical education towards greater relevance to the needs of society is necessary, unavoidable, and urgent (see Chapter 2). Some within the profession are beginning to say that if changes are not undertaken by those responsible for medical education, they might lose the opportunity to do so and that others would then take the initiative, as a result of public demand (World Federation for Medical Education 1988).

> In the past, physicians' education was formulated and developed by the medical school and the teaching hospital, which together emphasised basic biomedical sciences and supervised clinical experience. In the future, it is more likely that the health needs of the population will be a major factor in determining physicians' education.
> Tarlov 1992

As the twenty-first century approaches it is impossible for those within medical schools to ignore the fact that one of the major challenges facing governments all over the world is how to develop a health care system which meets the demands placed on it but which is affordable. It is clear that health care systems cannot be changed without changing how physicians are educated at all levels (O'Neil 1992; Todd 1992). The public resources that have built educational institutions and the health care system over the past four decades are now severely limited, even in the wealthiest countries.

At three levels the current and future needs of the health care system have begun to act as a stimulus for the re-orientation of medical education. At an international level the agreed policy of 'Health for All by the Year 2000' has led to a worldwide movement towards the community-oriented medical school. In the USA, concerns about the escalating costs and inequality of health care are turning the 1990s into the age of accountability for medical education. In the UK, crisis in the health care system in London has prompted a review of service delivery and a stimulus for long-term strategic planning which has profound implications for medical education.

International perspectives

At the global level, the challenge to medical education has come from, and continues to come from, the World Health Organization's goal of 'Health for All by the Year 2000' established in the 1978 Declaration of Alma-Ata. The adoption of this approach to health care has triggered a worldwide educational and political movement, supported by many governments and regional medical education bodies, towards educational reform for all health professionals. This has led to a reaction against the Flexner-inspired paradigm of medical education and a movement towards community-oriented or community-based education: that is, towards curricula that consider societal needs and the use of different levels of health settings in the community as learning opportunities (WHO 1987).

The most powerful expression of this movement has been through the activities of the Network of Community-Oriented Educational Institutions for Health Sciences, established in 1979 at the instigation of the WHO. Set up as a forum for bringing together like-minded institutions that share the goal of producing graduates whose motivation and competencies are more attuned to community-health needs, network membership has shown a steady increase from the nineteen original members in 1979 to 167 in 1990.

However, although the number of medical schools ostensibly committed to innovative community-oriented models of medical education is growing rapidly, very few meet these demanding requirements. In 1987, no more than 1.5% of medical schools in the world were explicitly concerned with the relevance of their programmes to their communities and with the lifelong capacity of their graduates to cope with the growth and change of necessary knowledge (Kantrowitz et al. 1987). Some of the most successful schools in this regard are relatively new ones, having developed innovative curricula from the outset; some more traditional and long-established schools have developed alternative curriculum tracks in parallel with conventional methods for volunteer cohorts of students (Carvalho 1992).

In reviewing the Network achievements over its first ten years, Schmidt et al. (1991) emphasized that experience had shown that implementing innovative, community-oriented curricula are not enough to achieve the desired goal of producing physicians who will contribute to the health of individuals and communities. Graduates from these programmes had, at least in the short term, less impact on the health of the communities than was hoped or expected. It has become clear that changing medical education alone has a limited impact on the health care system, even though it is also apparent that the health care system cannot be successfully reformed without changing physician education.

The USA

In the USA, ageing of the population, increasing prevalence of chronic and disabling illnesses with multiple social and behavioural risk factors, concern about quality of care, and escalating costs of medical care require fundamental changes in the way that academic health centres discharge their mission.

Tarlov (1992) identifies four health-related changes that will have an impact on medical education: the reconceptualization of the meaning of health; an increase in the number and range of different health-improvement strategies; growing awareness of the relatively low health status of the US population in contrast to high US health care expenditures; and shifts in the causes of illnesses and death.

Todd (1992) recommends a 'Flexner-like study for the 1990s, not because medical education is bad, but because it needs to be different'. He believes that the most difficult task for physicians attempting to reform the health care system will not be to manage new and amazing technologies but to balance the high technology, acute care needs of the population with the management of sickness, disability, and loss of function due to old age. Medical education at all levels will need to prepare increasingly adaptable practitioners. Whatever reforms are ultimately accepted, the physician's role may well change from one of patient advocate, with sole emphasis on the patient's welfare, to one of resource allocator with responsibility for factoring the cost of treatment into decision making. This role will require adding business management, socio-economics, and politics to the curriculum, along with the ethics of limited resources. Furthermore, a key role for medical education in health care reform will be to prepare physicians, their patients, and the members of their communities to accept more realistic expectations, while emphasizing the value of prevention and the elimination of treatments with little or no proven benefit.

A practical attempt to address some of these concerns has been the Health of the Public Program, launched by the Pew Charitable Trusts and the Rockefeller Foundation, to strengthen the population perspective of health care in medical education and encourage health centres to respond to changing health needs (Showstack *et al.* 1992). As part of the programme, the Pew Health Professions Commission, drawn from the health-professional, business, academic, and policy-making communities in the USA, analysed over 90 trends that are likely to impact on the provision of health care over the next two decades. These trends ranged from changes in demography and epidemiology to shifting patterns in cultural values and the nation's economy. The Commission's findings (O'Neil 1991) established nine characteristics that seem to summarize the underlying issues that will drive change in health care in the coming decades (Box 1.4).

Box 1.4   **Characteristics of an effective health care system**

♦ A health care system that is more oriented to health, stressing disease prevention, and health promotion, as well as individual responsibility for health-related behaviours.

♦ Population-based, as more attention is paid to risk factors in the physical and social environments, many of which must be addressed at a community level.

♦ The system will be even more driven by information, using electronic synthesis of complete patient histories and the relevant literature to support providers' diagnostic decisions and treatment recommendations.

♦ Readily available information will facilitate growth of a stronger focus on consumers, as patients become fully informed participants in decisions concerning their own health care.

♦ Decisions will be based largely on expanded knowledge of treatment outcomes in similar circumstances and on the use of integrated and coordinated teams of providers.

♦ This will result in more effective care, more efficiently provided.

♦ A serious concern about balancing technology will intensify as technology's benefits in improving care are weighed against its effects on human values, the interpersonal aspects of provision of care, and an ongoing concern about the costs of care to individuals and society.

♦ Every health care provider will experience an increasing accountability to more interest groups for a wider range of outcomes.

Pew Health Professions Commission (O'Neil 1992)

The UK

In the UK, reform of the National Health Service in 1991, with the introduction of managed competition and the creation of an internal market, has had far-reaching consequences for the delivery of health care. One consequence has been to give a greater sense of urgency to tackling the long-standing problems of health care delivery in London. The King's Fund Commission on London (1992) studied trends and directions in twenty-first century health care in order to develop a vision for the development of London health services over the next thirty years. The Commission called for a rethink of the purposes and funding of acute hospitals and an expansion in the role of primary and community care. It identified trends in the pattern of disease, medical advances (Stocking 1992), and in the social and economic context in which health care takes place. As a result it seems likely that acute hospitals are likely to become smaller and more specialized, while a reasonable proportion of the diagnostic and investigative work that currently takes place in out-patient or other acute hospital settings could be moved to primary and community care, or to patients' own homes.

The implications for the skills and training of the different health professionals involved in such a reorganization have not, as yet, been addressed although there are already signs that the role of doctors is changing. Some traditional tasks are now done by other professionals. Changing work patterns for groups like nurses, pharmacists, social workers, and paramedical technicians have already altered the role of the doctor and in some cases replaced it. Doctors have to work in multidisciplinary teams, but they may not be the automatic leaders. Many members of the public do not remember life before the NHS and there is no longer unquestioning gratitude and acceptance of what the doctor says and does; the medical profession is having to be more accountable for the way in which it spends taxpayers' money (Lowry 1992). In the new-style NHS, the power to make decisions about resource allocation seems to be shifting away from the individual hospital doctor to the managers and a new group, the fund-holding general practitioner.

The consequence of all these changes is a questioning of the role of the teaching hospital in training doctors for the next century, and an interest in moving more medical education into primary care or community settings. At present, such moves are more a change in the location of teaching than a reorientation of the curriculum. However, there are more possibilities of a real shift in the character of medical education than ever before, especially in London, where there is an urgent need to invest in a stronger primary-care service. There are now new opportunities for the integrated development of medical education alongside service development.

Evolution or a new paradigm for medical education?

The implications of these trends for medical education cannot be ignored for much longer. The call for a new doctor is actually a call for fundamental change in medical practice and health care which obviously will profoundly affect the nature of medical education. While the future is always uncertain and predictions may always prove to be way off mark, these difficulties should not be used as excuses for inaction. Changes in the health services can always be made more rapidly than changes in education. The major themes which will shape health care in the future are already clear. Boelen (1992) points out that independently, but with surprising unanimity worldwide, the call has arisen for medical practitioners of the future to be able to do the following:

◆ Assess and improve the quality of care by responding to the patient's total health needs with integrated preventive, curative, and rehabilitative services.
◆ Make optimal use of new technologies, bearing in mind ethical and financial considerations and the consumer's ultimate benefit.
◆ Promote healthy lifestyles by means of communication skills and the empowerment of individuals and groups for their own health protection.
◆ Reconcile individual- and community-health requirements, striking a balance between patients' expectations and those of society at large, both short-term and long-term.
◆ Work efficiently in teams within the health sector and between the health sector and other socio-economic sectors that influence health.

Preparing physicians for the health care system of the future will call for significant change within medical education. The question is, can this be achieved by evolution or does it require a paradigm shift? The evolutionary approach is implicit in the recommendations of the Pew Commission. They identified seventeen competencies for future practitioners (Box 1.5) based on the characteristics of future health care systems (Box 1.4). The general strategies recommended to implement these changes included one on curriculum content and one on process. They suggested a redefinition of the core curriculum directed towards identifying the educational core necessary to develop the competencies desired in graduates who can provide contemporary clinical care as members of health care teams that will function in settings emphasizing cost-effective integrated services. In relation to process, the Commission concurred with the approaches widely recommended by previous studies (see above) and specifically noted that three of the competencies they identified—the ability to manage information, continue to learn, and think critically—are profoundly affected by the educational processes.

Box 1.5   Competencies for future practitioners

- Care for the community's health.
- Expand access to effective care.
- Provide contemporary clinical care.
- Emphasize primary care.
- Participate in coordinated care.
- Ensure cost-effective and appropriate care.
- Practice prevention.
- Involve patients and families in the decision-making process.
- Promote healthy life-styles.
- Assess and use technology appropriately.
- Improve the health care system
- Manage information
- Understand the role of the physical environment
- Provide counselling on ethical issues.
- Accommodate expanded accountability
- Participate in a racially and culturally diverse society.
- Continue to learn.

Pew Health Professions Commission (O'Neil 1992)

The fact that medical schools have such a poor track record in defining core curricula (see above) raises questions about whether this approach is likely to be successful in changing the content of the curriculum to the extent that is required if the needs are truly to be met. The key issue is, to what extent the curriculum can be radically changed unless the entire mission of the medical school, in relation to patient care, research, and education, is redefined. As Bloom (1992) points out, the widespread consensus for educational change cannot succeed if it replaces or undermines the parallel importance of research and service in the medical school. In the absence of any single overriding model for the curriculum of the future, each medical school must plan its own programme. In order to succeed, it must address the structural problems of organization, the sources of authority and allocation of resources, and the power centres of decision making.

References

Association of American Medical Colleges (1984). Physicians for the twenty-first century. Report of the Project Panel on the General Professional Education of the Physician and College Preparation for Medicine. *Journal of Medical Education* **59** (11), Supplement, part 2, 208 pp.

Association of American Medical Colleges (1992). Educating medical students. Assessing change in medical education: the road to implementation. (ACME-TRI report).

Bloom, S.W. (1992). Medical education in transition: paradigm change and organisational stasis. In *Medical education in transition: commission on medical education: the sciences of medical practice*, (ed. R.Q.Marston, and R.M. Jones), pp.15–25, Princeton, NJ. The Robert Wood Johnson Foundation.

Boelen, C. (1992). Medical education reform: the need for global action. *Academic Medicine* **67**, (11), 745–9.

Cantor, J.C., Cohen, A.B., Barker, D.C., Shuster, A.L., and Reynolds, R.C. (1991). Medical educators' views on medical education reform. *Journal of the American Medical Association* **265**, (8), 1002–6.

Carlson, C.A. (1991). International medical education. Common elements in divergent systems. *Journal of the American Medical Association* **266**, (7), 921–3.

Carvalho, A.C.M. (1992). Undergraduate medical education towards Health for All: progress, pitfalls, perspectives. *Health Services Management Research* **5**, (1), 17–31.

Charlton, B.G. (1991). Practical reform of preclinical education: core curriculum and science projects. *Medical Teacher*, **13**, 21–9.

Council on Medical Education. *Future Directions for Medical Education: A Report of the Council on Medical Education*. Chicago, Ill: American Medical Association; 1982.

Dawson-Saunders, B., Feltovich, P.J., Coulson, R.L., Steward, D.E. (1990). A survey of medical school teachers to identify basic biomedical concepts medical students should understand. *Academic Medicine*, **65**, 448–54.

Deitrick JE, Berson RC. *Medical Schools in the United States at Mid-Century*. New York, NY: McGraw-Hill International Book Co; 1953.

Drop, M.J. and Post, G.J. (1990). Perceptions and evaluations by graduates and faculty members of the Maastricht problem-based curriculum. In Medical Education Nooman, Z.M., Schmidt, H. and Ezzat E.S. (eds.). pp.152–64. *Innovation in medical education: an evaluation of its present status*. Springer, New York.

Enarson, C. and Burg, F.D. (1992). An overview of reform initiatives in medical education. 1906 through 1992. *Journal of the American Medical Association*, **268**, (9), 1141–3.

Evans, J.R. (1992). The 'health of the public' approach to medical education. *Academic Medicine* **67**, (11), 719–23.

Flexner A. *Medical Education in the United States and Canada*. New York, NY: Carnegie Foundation for the Advancement of Teaching; 1910.

Gastel B, Rogers DE, eds. *Clinical Education and the Doctor of Tomorrow*. New York, NY: Academy of Medicine; 1989.

General Medical Council (1993). *Tommorow's doctors*. GMC, London.

Holsgrove, G., McCrorie, P., Jolly, B.C., and Bowden, A. (1993). Horizontally integrated assessment within a discipline based faculty. In Harden, R.McG., Hart, I., and Mullholland, H. (ed.), pp. 638–643. *Approaches to the assessment of clinical competence* Proceedings of the fifth Ottawa Conference on Medical Education, Dundee, 1992.

Jonas, H.S., Etzel, S.I. and Barzansky, B. (1992). Education programs in US medical schools. *Journal of the American Medical Association*, **268**, (9), 1083–90.

Kantrowitz, M., Kaufman, A., Mennin, S., Fulop, T. and Guilbert, J.-J. (1987). Innovative tracks at established institutions for the education of health personnel. *WHO Offset Publication No. 101*. World Health Organization.

King's Fund Commission on the Future of London's Acute Health Services (1992). *London health care 2010: changing the future of services in the capital*. King's Fund London Initiative, London.

Lowry, S. (1992). What's wrong with medical education in Britain? *British Medical Journal*, **305**, 1277–80.

Millis, JS. *The Graduate Education of Physicians: The Citizens Commission on Graduate Medical Education*. Chicago, III: American Medical Association; 1966.

Newble, D.I., Jolly, B.C., and Wakeford R.E. (1994). *The certification and recertification of doctors: issues in the assessment of clinical competence*. Cambridge University Press, Cambridge.

Nooman, Z.M., Refaat, A.H., and Ezzat. E.S. (1990). Experience in community-based education at the Faculty of Medicine, Suez Canal University. In Medical Education Nooman Z.M., Schmidt, H. and Ezzat, E.S. (Ed), pp. 279–290. New York: Springer, Innovation in medical education: an evaluation of its present status.

O'Neil, E.H. (1992). Education as part of the health care solution. Strategies from the Pew Health Professions Commission. *Journal of the American Medical Association* **268** (9), 1146–8.

Panel on the General Professional Education of the Physician and College Preparation for Medicine. *Physicians for the Twenty-First Century: The GPEP Report*. Washington, DC: Association of American Medical Colleges; 1984.

Prockop, D.J. (1992). Basic science and clinical practice: how much science will a physician need to know? In *Medical education in transition*, pp. 51–7.

Rappleye W. *Medical Education: Final Report of the Commission on Medical Education*. New York, NY: Office of the Director of the Study; 1932.

Robert Wood Johnson Foundation Commission on Medical Education. *The Sciences of Medical Practice*. Princeton, NJ: Robert Wood Johnson Foundation; 1992.

Schmidt, H.G., Neufeld, V.R., Nooman, Z.M., and Ogunbode, T. (1991). Network of community-oriented institutions for the health sciences. *Academic Medicine*, **66**, 259–63.

Schroeder, S.K., Zones, J.S., and Showstack, J.A. (1989). Academic medicine as a public trust. *Journal of the American Medical Association*, **262**, 803.

Scott, C.S., Barrows, H.S., Brock, D.M., and Hunt, D.D. (1991). Clinical behaviours and skills that faculty from 12 institutions judged were essential for medical students to acquire. *Academic Medicine*, **66**, (2), 106–11.

Showstack, J. *et al.* (1992) Health of the public. The academic response. *Journal of the American Medical Association*, **267**, 2497–502.

Shugars DA, O'Neill EH, Baker JD, eds. *Healthy America: Practitionars for 2005: An Agenda for Action for US Health Professional Schools*. Durham, NC: The Pew Health Professions Commission, 1991.

Stocking, B. (1992). Medical advances. The future shape of acute services. *Working Paper No. 7*. King's Fund London Acute Services Initiative, London.

Tarlov, A.R. (1992). The coming influence of a social sciences perspective on medical education. *Academic Medicine*, **67**, (11), 724–31.

Todd, J.S. (1992). Health care reform and the medical education imperative. *Journal of the American Medical Association*, **268**, (9), 1133–4.

Tosteson, D.C. (1990). New pathways in general medical education. *New England Journal of Medicine*. **322**, (4), 234–8.

Towle, A. (1991). *Critical thinking. The future of undergraduate medical education*. King's Fund Centre London.

Weiskotten HG. *Medical Education in the United States, 1934–1939*. Chicago, Ill: American Medical Association Council on Medical Education and Hospitals; 1940.

White, K.L. (1991). *Healing the schism: epidemiology, medicine and the public's health.* Springer Verlag, New York.

White, K.L. and Connelly, J.E. (Ed.) (1992). The medical school's mission and the population's health. Medical education in Canada, the United Kingdom, the United States and Australia. *Proceedings of a conference sponsored by the Royal Society of Medicine Foundation, Inc. and the Josiah Macy Jr. Foundation. 9–12 December 1990, Turnberry Isle, Florida.* Springer Verlag, New York.

World Federation for Medical Education (1988). *Report of the World Conference on Medical Education, Edinburgh, 7–12 August 1988.*

World Health Organization (1987) Community-based education of health personnel. Report of a WHO Study Group. *WHO Technical Report Series 746.*

2 Curriculum design

2.1 Charting the course: designing a medical curriculum

Brian Jolly

Introduction

In this chapter we shall look at why a curriculum needs to be designed, who should be involved, and different methods and approaches to designing it. We will also look at some of the effects that such decisions have in practice. However, a detailed discussion of course planning is not envisaged here. The title of this sub-chapter is 'charting the course', not 'trimming the sails'. We will take a global approach. A few simple models to help curriculum designers will be presented and the implications of ignoring the interactivity of curriculum decisions discussed. Within each section we will try to identify useful principles for curriculum design in medicine. Finally we will make some remarks on the difficulty of curriculum maintenance in the face of rapid and far-reaching developments in health care.

Why design?

The senior and influential doctors and medical educators of today, charged with developing curricula for the twenty-first century, experienced their own education within the health care systems of the 1950s and early 1960s. At that time the concept of apprenticeship to a master-professional through whom young doctors learnt their craft was not only seen as a clinical necessity, it was deeply ingrained into the medical educational system (see Chapter 7.1 and Field 1970). Such a situation had many advantages, teachers knew their students very well; continuity of patient care was easy; the numbers at the bedside, strictly hierarchical, were manageable; and, as a result, most senior doctors now reflect on those days with affection. However there were disadvantages. Female graduates were uncommon. Patronage was rife, both in selection and in the educational process. For example, one, at least, of the London medical schools gave an automatic entrance interview to children of its own graduates. Notably, this was seen as a positive characteristic by many concerned! During a fairly long period, from about 1920–1960, medical curricula, most founded after the turn of the century, enjoyed a stable and isolated existence, free from interference from government, health service, or educationalists.

Also throughout this period, the concept of curriculum design was virtually unknown. There were very good reasons for this. The notion that certain goals might be achieved through particular approaches was new even in mainstream education. Also there were no reasons to believe that the current system was inadequate. Since science and clinical activity were relatively independent, there were few grounds for questioning the enforced separation between a university-structured, subject-based introduction to scientific method and a patient-oriented, almost totally hospital-based, immersion in clinical practice. It was not uncommon to find the two halves of medical curricula planned and implemented completely independently, often with some denigration of the others' efforts and results. The rationale for such curricula resided in individuals' interests or clinical experience. There was virtually no evaluation, either by students or faculty, of the courses they were receiving/teaching. In the UK a Royal Commission on the state of medical education (Todd 1968), that voiced significant and pervasive criticisms of the status-quo and, uncommonly, was underpinned by a large amount of questionnaire data collected from students, passed with hardly a ripple in the water of British medical education. Medicine had become one of the most active professions with the most passive of pedagogies.

However, the changing social and economic climate (Chapter 1) and attention to patients' rights (Chapter 2.3) have begun to change the tide. In addition, reports on both sides of the Atlantic (AAMC 1984; GMC 1993; ACME-TRI, 1993; SCOPME 1992), some of which echo the criticisms voiced up twenty five years earlier (Todd 1968), together with developing concepts of adult and professional education (Schön 1987), mean that a *rationale* for medical education is both timely and paramount. A systematic approach to curriculum design at least allows a medical school to keep track of its input and output. Although curriculum design is an imprecise and arbitrary rubric, such a code is needed: systematic and arbitrary is somewhat better than capricious.

Who designs?

Traditionally the clinical curriculum was not *designed*, but rather *evolved*, mainly through a system which gave the apprentice time under the wing of physicians, surgeons, or other specialists, who made the curriculum up more or less as they went along out of their day-to-day clinical practice. This was almost entirely opportunistic (see p.180). In contrast, in the basic science curriculum the strategy was founded on *blanket coverage*: everything the doctor was thought to need to know for a thorough understanding of the practice of medicine (as well as many other things not needed) were included. These decisions were frequently made by lecturers or heads of department about a chosen topic within the context of a discipline-oriented course, for example the neuroanatomy of the cerebellum. Scant attention was paid to the eventual tasks of the graduate, or to other disciplines being studied by, or demands made on, the student.

Furthermore, in the UK, a degree in one of the basic science subjects can be taken between the end of the second and beginning of the third year of medical studies, or sometimes later. Since the introduction of these intercalated degrees the notion of coverage has been extended by departments in many schools to ensure that courses taken prior to intercalation include enough of any subject to allow disciplinary-based, single honours degree tracking later, further burdening an already overcrowded curriculum.

Hence the first principle in the planning of medical curricula should be that for a curriculum to be well designed it is important to specify and limit its role and the needs it serves. Too wide a remit will severely compromise significant aspects.

In the twenty-first century these needs are likely to become radically different. Patients (see Chapters 1, 2.1, 2.3 and 4.1) not only require more say, they will become increasingly powerful, largely through the proliferation and use of technology. Economic forces will drive patients to become more self-reliant both in diagnosis and treatment, partly through use of computer and other advanced technology. Many treatments requiring medical expertise are already becoming more technological and dependent on machinery or non-medical personnel to deliver them. Laser, tomographic and magnetic resonance techniques, and minimally invasive surgery were the stuff of science fiction only a few years ago. Recently, especially in the USA, patients have been growing in influence in the learning and assessment processes. Simulated patients (SPs), people with clinically normal or sometimes abnormal findings trained to consistently reproduce patient case-histories (Stillman *et al.* 1983; Barrows 1993), and patient instructors, patients trained to teach examination of particular body systems (Stillman and Sawyer 1992), have been used to introduce more patient-oriented approaches to physical examination and diagnosis. In educational events using SPs there is frequently a potent opportunity for the patient to supplement or supplant the direct role of the physician.

All of this points to another important principle: that medical curricula are now too complex and too powerful to be designed covertly by small, privileged, groups. A curriculum needs to be both explicit and designed by a consensus involving wide representation from interested parties, and taking particular cognisance of the uses to which the skills and knowledge gained in training will be put. As the GPEP report (AAMC 1984) observes, the design and delivery of curricula should be the responsibility of the whole faculty and not franchised out to individual departments to develop self-contained modules or proliferate content uncontrollably.

The management of such an exercise is itself daunting (see Chapter 8) and many curricula have foundered precisely because, while the plan has been collectively designed, the consultations on the basic structure or implementation have not been wide enough, or have ignored important trends and developments. This brings us to the definition of curriculum we will use in this chapter. A curriculum is 'an attempt to communicate the essential principles and features of an educational proposal in such a form that it is open to critical scrutiny and capable of effective translation into practice' (Stenhouse 1975). This is what Coles in Chapter 3 calls the 'curriculum on paper'. Stenhouse also pointed out that a curriculum cannot claim to be ideal or correct, only intelligent, and hence should be judged according to its fitness for purpose in addition to its plausibility. Hence it is important that any plan should match, and be implemented in, the context for which it is designed (see Bridgham 1989). This is what is referred to as 'the curriculum in action' in Chapter 3.

Which designs?

Curriculum change frequently appears cataclysmic, especially so to those involved in the existing curriculum. This is because necessary periodic review has either not occurred or has taken place only when dissatisfaction (from students or teachers) has reached intolerable limits, or when the gap between provision of skills and health care needs (of purchasers) becomes too uncomfortable. Both these factors are operating in the current changes taking place in the USA and Europe. In the early part of this century, Flexner's (1910) revolution was caused primarily by the explosion of scientifically unrespectable medical schools in the USA. Many teachers, and government, wanted to improve or guard the scientific background of medical graduates and were critical of the educational provision of new and unproven schools. Later, both GPEP and GMC reports were partly occasioned by large-scale concern about aspects of physicians' skills—communication, ethics, clinical diagnostic ability, and ability to engage in continual improvement.

Another cause of the ostensibly dramatic alterations in curricula is the imprecision of educational theory. If, for example, curriculum planners knew for certain that a problem-based (PBL) course would lead to the production of more self-directed physicians, or that one hundred hours of clinical experience would result in the development of appropriate skills in the new graduate, courses could be planned accordingly. However this is far from the case. Although some data are now emerging to aid planners (see p. 179) the possibility of curriculum design ever reaching perfection is remote. Even though traditional methods of education are as unproven, except by default, as newer ones, medical schools will tend to opt for the safety of what they know they can do, sheltering from the winds of change behind the request for evidence of positive benefits of proposed revisions. For change to take place, encouragement, funding, and even coercion may all need to be supplied as a matter of principle.

In the remainder of this chapter we will look at tools to help designers think about curricula, and then sketch some of the recent developments in research which might make this process, if not foolproof, then at least more evidence-based. Of the curriculum-design procedures available, none has been developed to the stage where it is totally prescriptive.

Curriculum design: available design tools

There are a number of ways of describing curricula and here we will present just a few to give a flavour of the assistance which they can give. It is too easy sometimes to oversimplify the nature of a medical curriculum, classifying it as PBL or traditional. We have tried to avoid this trap in Chapter 1 by sketching the diversity of aims. In fact, many sub varieties of curricula exist or could be designed, and in this section we will outline how models can be used to think about the required or most appropriate design for the institution's or society's needs. Most curriculum-development models have evolved outside medicine, and therefore have ignored or merely acknowledged the richness of the medical teaching environment (for example see Ramsden 1992; Gibbs 1992). A few relate better to the medical environment and will be discussed here along with the most useful of all, that developed for general use at the University of Sussex.

Curriculum design: the SPICES model

The most comprehensive, but the least prescriptive model, is the scheme developed by Harden and colleagues (Harden *et al.* 1984; Harden 1986). This is useful in categorizing the dimensions of a curriculum so that thinking about their relative weight and importance can proceed. It is not exactly a system or theory for the development of curricula, since the links between aims, objectives, teaching methods, and assessment of students are not discussed in detail. And, although it points towards decisions which need to be made and the conditions favouring one or other end of the continua, it provides little information on precisely what to decide. However, it does supply a specifically health-science framework which can be used to review an existing curriculum and highlights issues which will need addressing. It also acknowledges the fact that no two curricula are alike, largely through recognition of their multifaceted nature. Hence the model is useful in recognizing that a clear division, between a 'PBL' and a 'traditional' curriculum, can be an unhelpful oversimplification.

The model identifies six attributes of curricula, each of which can vary on a continuum. These are detailed in Fig. 2.1 (after Harden *et al.* 1984). Environmental factors or policies can move the institution in either direction on each of the dimensions.

Student centred .... Teacher centred

Problem-based.............................. Information gathering

Integrated...................................... Discipline-based

Community-based .... Hospital-based

Electives.. Standard programme

Systematic.................................... Apprenticeship/Opportunistic

Fig. 2.1 The Spices model (reproduced with permission)

These six dimensions and possible reasons for moving towards one or other end will now be described briefly.

The Student- vs. Teacher- centred dimension relates to the extent to which, in any course, the learners have responsibility for learning and can influence what, how, and when they learn. In a true 'student-centred' course, students may also set themselves assessment targets and judge how well they have reached these, for example by setting up a learning contract with their teachers. While this degree of autonomy is unusual in medicine, it is not uncommon in other subjects (Boud 1988). In contrast, teacher-centred curricula attempt to use the teacher as a role model, repository, selector and communicator of knowledge, assessor, and standard setter. Until recently some basic science curricula epitomized this extremity of the dimension. Vast quantities of knowledge were poured out (see Chapter 3) in lectures to passive students who were expected to absorb and regurgitate it later to prove their readiness for the clinical arena.

Student-centred curricula may be more appropriate when the school wishes to emphaze students' roles in the curricula, to increase motivation, or to prepare for continuous learning. Teacher-centred approaches place fewer demands on teachers, or may be appropriate where students are traditionally passive in their approach to learning.

The problem-based/information gathering dimension refers to the degree to which the curriculum espouses the investigation and resolution of clinical problems by students as opposed to the assimilation of facts, concepts, or principles with a view to their later application. This dimension has certain common features with the first, such as the mode of transmission of knowledge. However the important aspect is that, at one extreme, students tackle patients' problems throughout the course in order to organize their studies of basic and clinical science. At the other, knowledge is organized into boluses about a topic and studied by students in that context. For example, in the 'information gathering' mode, knowledge about disease mechanisms or biochemical configurations provides the building blocks which students acquire to store up against later use, rather than data researched and learnt specifically to understand a patient's problem. PBL has potential (with careful choice of problems) to deal with an overcrowded curriculum, to instil self-reliance, to be more enjoyable, and to build more integrated, clinically related knowledge bases (Norman 1988). Information-gathering models may be more appropriate with strong discipline-oriented departments, teacher inexperience, poor student oriented resources, (e.g. lack of multiple books, computers, background documentation), or where detailed discipline knowledge is needed at an early stage.

The third dimension is the degree of integration vs. the disciplinarity of the course. In other words, the bias of the course towards presenting knowledge in the context of clinical specialties or basic disciplines, as opposed to integration of material. Integration may be horizontal or vertical, or both. Vertical integration is the extent to which clinical information is used to structure, amplify, illuminate, and expand thinking about basic science issues (or vice versa). Horizontal integration relates to the interaction in the curriculum between different academic disciplines or specialties; e.g. medicine and surgery, radiology and cardiology, anatomy and pharmacology. Many precipitative curricular changes in the 1950s and 1960s were based on a move to horizontal integration (i.e. Western Reserve; Ham 1962). Factors/outcomes predisposing to integration include: the potential for an appropriately balanced knowledge-base, students emerging with more contextually relevant, hence better retained, knowledge (see Chapter 3); staff interchangeability and communication through modular design of courses (e.g. the cardiovascular system); and a more focused set of resource materials designed specifically for the course. Disciplinarity may be more acceptable where teachers feel uncomfortable in an integrated setting or are more stimulating in teaching 'their' discipline, and where total coverage is important,

The fourth dimension is the measure of community vs. hospital orientation in the curriculum. Since Harden wrote his SPICES paper in 1984 there has been an explosion of interest in, and extensive pressure towards, community-based medical education in many countries. In particular the developed world, short of resources, is now having to meet the same challenges and problems posed in the 1970s and 1980s by the delivery of health care in developing countries. In this scenario patients largely do not enter hi-technology tertiary-level teaching hospitals, but remain in the community. Although currently politically in vogue, it is not expected that this situation will change much in the future, as the rate of expansion of need seems always likely to outstrip the rate of provision of funding (see Chapter 1). Hence many schools in the UK, USA, and Australia are moving towards a primary health care oriented curriculum, with consequent loss of power to hospital-based specialties. The reshaping of the clinical environment has many advantages to curriculum designers. The hospital-based curriculum remains poorly defined (Jolly 1994). In particular the demarcation and trade off between learning and working are unclear (SCOPME 1994; Salter 1995). A large number of acute conditions and practical procedures are not addressed in the undergraduate curriculum, although the skills associated with them are expected to be in place soon after (Jolly and Macdonald 1989; Gillard, *et al.* 1993; Dacre and Nicol 1996). Thus considerable effort is needed to map out the boundaries between and the requirements of the undergraduate and early postgraduate or internship phases of training. The need for curriculum definition will become even more important as teaching moves out of the hospital ward environment into community activity. Institutional goals, and appropriate means to deliver them, will be necessary features shared between medical schools, hospitals, and general practices. This means dividing and assigning responsibility for certain characteristics of professional development to each sector, and not allowing a *laissez-faire* approach. Community settings may have a greater number of patients but be restricted by their lower level of differentiation and specificity.

The degree of choice is another important dimension of the curriculum. The concept of choice in a medical curriculum, unthinkable to graduates of the 1950s and 1960s, has been forced by the recognition that undergraduate training is part of a lifelong course of learning that cannot be pre-defined too rigidly at an early stage. This is the seed for Harden's dimension of standardization vs. selectivity in a curriculum. This principle has been taken up vigorously by the GMC (1993) in the UK who have recognized the restrictions of a standard course and recommended a rapid move to a 'core + special study modules' approach. Of course it would be wrong to assume that the medical course was ever totally standardized. A large body of evidence collected since rotational models of clinical attachments replaced apprenticeship ones has suggested that no two medical students ever get exactly the same 'course' (Jolly *et al.* 1996; Bennard and Stritter 1989; Mattern *et al.* 1983;). At the basic science level in the UK the intercalated degree (see p.22) is already one option. A choice-based curriculum may be more useful where the current curriculum is overcrowded (c.f. GMC 1993), where independence of students is required, and where career choice would otherwise be based on a 'week only' attachment. A standard programme may be useful where there are few or overloaded staff, where the backup resources are minimal, or where the curriculum is not large, for example in a postgraduate diploma or specific master's programme.

The final dimension in Harden's model is that of systematic preparation vs. opportunistic learning. This is probably the weakest dimension of the model, in the sense that most schools are realizing that in a modern curriculum as little should be left to chance as possible; to do so results in groups of students with very disparate skill bases (Jolly and Macdonald 1989; Hunskaar and Seim 1983). Few would now argue for a serendipitous approach to clinical training. However where ability to select experiences is low, or where service commitments of teachers are high, the opportunistic approach may be the only one possible. Although Harden offers continuity of teaching (attachment to one unit), bringing a sense of professional identity, as another reason why apprenticeship schemes may be preferable, there is no logical reason why it would result in a better medical education. In any case, a structured approach to teaching could be applied just as easily within one rotation as across several.

The main problem with the SPICES model, framed in six 'continua', is that it tends to over support the *status quo*. This is because justifications have to be found for the existence and perpetuation of the 'traditional' end of the continua as if they really existed. In fact since the SPICES model was constructed much has changed in medical education and health care. One might easily add another three or four dimensions. For example, assessment is completely absent from the model, and there is little discussion of teaching methods *per se*. An alternative set of descriptions of curricula, in somewhat more detail, is provided by the Cambridge Conference model.

The Cambridge Conference model

This description of the essential features of medical curricula was developed, with due acknowledgement to Harden, at the Cambridge Conference on Medical Education in Vancouver in 1986. It is again an oversimplification, but is useful in that it relates directly to the main elements of curriculum design (see p.33); aims and objectives, teaching methods, content, and so on.

The Cambridge model (Swanson *et al.* 1989), broadly differentiates between four types of medical curricula, along nine attributes. These attributes are either recognizable aspects of the curriculum itself (e.g. goal, aims, and objectives) or of the way in which a particular institution views the educational process. The model asserts that, although curricula are individual, there is enough in common on these nine dimensions to classify most curricula into four main types: discipline oriented, organ systems, guided-discovery PBL and open-discovery PBL.

These four curriculum types differ on the following nine characteristics, some of which echo those provided by Harden.

1. Institutional context and values—both of the medical school and of the institution and constituency it serves.
2. Educational goals—the knowledge, skills and attitudes that the school seeks to impart to its graduates.
3. Curricular organization—the logical relationships between courses, and the mechanisms used to manage the curriculum.
4. Role of teachers—the institutional view of the responsibilities of staff in curriculum development and teaching students.
5. View of students—the institutional view of the responsibilities of students in the learning process.
6. Content of instruction—the relationship between basic science, clinical material, and emphasis on specific knowledge versus general skills.
7. Teaching methods—the use of different instructional techniques.
8. Assessment—its purpose and style.
9. The role of educational support staff—their responsibilities in curriculum development, management and evaluation.

Interested readers can estimate how close their school is to the resulting four types of curricula described in Table 2.1, and how far they think they will have to change things to be in the next column of the table. It is tempting to think that movement might be made in only one or two attributes. However, because curricular issues are so inter-related (see the subsequent section of this chapter) the implication is that it is very difficult to move only one or two attributes in the appropriate direction (especially left to right) without having sympathetic or conducive conditions in the others. The table is constructed from wide experience of curriculum change in several institutions (Swanson *et al.* 1989) and composed of relatively stable factors in curriculum management.

Two additional comments need to be made in this respect. First the role of assessment is so crucial in any curriculum that change in any attribute must be accompanied by adequate suitable adjustment of the assessment system. Collective approaches in any or all of the domains can be effectively nullified by its wrong choice (Newble and Jaeger 1983; see Chapter 5). The second concerns the difference between plan and context. There may be important differences between staff and students in how they perceive the curriculum. Simply because a curriculum plan, or the educational objectives, espouse certain goals does not mean that the curriculum will be perceived by students as reflecting those goals (see also Chapter 3). For example, trying to develop PBL in tutorials which, perhaps because of faculty skills, actually resemble minilectures will confuse or mislead students. Stating the importance of teaching, but in an institutional framework which rewards only research, will be equally bewildering.

A general curriculum design model

The University of Sussex curriculum model is a generic approach to curriculum design first developed in the early 1970s (Eraut *et al.* 1975). It diverges from the usual approach to curriculum. In most other models the sequence in which decisions are made is an important limiting feature. That is, aims lead to objectives, which lead to methods and so on. In the Sussex model, apart from giving priority to general aims, the other elements in the model are taken as acting together simultaneously as a 'curriculum strategy', (Fig. 2.2). This is useful because it allows considerable variation in curricula, while maintaining strong internal consistency. In Fig. 2.2 single arrows indicate influence and choice, and double arrows interdependency. In the model there is achievement of harmony through directing aims at one or more of the four interacting starting points—Subject Matter, Objectives and Outcomes, Teaching, Learning and Communication Methods, or Assessment. There are some careful distinctions and choices of terminology here. In particular the terms 'subject matter' and 'objectives' are viewed as separate issues. This recognizes that disciplines and related content (knowledge systems developed often over centuries) may have a unique influence on curricular decisions derived from their historical importance. The term 'subject matter' implies organization and structuring of knowledge as well as its selection from a more comprehensive framework. This type of formulation of knowledge concedes that different contexts and orientations might validly be used to structure how this knowledge is to be gained. Hence PBL, body-system, and/or discipline orientations might all be plausible ways of organizing the 'subject matter' of medicine, each with a particular effect on the learner's orientation and use. For example metabolic problems might replace biochemical pathways as the content framework. In contrast the term 'objectives and outcomes' encompasses both explicit and implicit intended and unintended consequences of a curriculum. Recent blueprints for redesigning medical curricula have used the tasks doctors perform after qualification or, from a world health care perspective, the sociopolitical role of the medical school as starting points (AAMC 1984; GMC

Table 2.1 The Cambridge Model of Curriculum: alternative curricular designs compared (Based on Swanson *et al.* 1989)

Dimension	Curriculum design				
	Discipline oriented	Organ systems	Guided discovery PBL	Open discovery PBL
1. Institutional context and values	Elite, research-oriented basic science. Most clinical staff are sub-specialists. Basic science and clinical faculties are separate. Courses departmentally based. Little or no change but changes in courses can be introduced by individuals with departmental sanction.	Elite, research-oriented basic science. Most clinical staff are sub-specialists. Courses are interdisciplinary. Slow changes possible in courses through strong, but cumbersome, multidisciplinary module committees.	Tend to be 'new' schools, sometimes geared to primary-care development in under-served location. Low staff–student numbers; high staff–student ratio. School-wide curriculum committee that selects or constructs problems, linked to defined objectives	Tend to be 'new' schools, sometimes geared to primary-care development in under-served location. Low staff numbers; high staff–student ratio. School-wide curriculum committee that selects or constructs problems.
2. Educational philosophy and curriculum model	Rational practice requires sub-specialization. Student exposure to all specialties to assist career choice. Curative/ medical model of medicine underlies curriculum design. Strong basic science preparation is said to aid future understanding.	Rational practice requires some sub-specialization. Students must be exposed to all specialties to assist career choice. However, pure disciplinary approach viewed as narrow and uses holistic model of medicine for curriculum design.	Emphasis on self-directed learning explicit throughout course, but aimed at specified clinical and related basic-science knowledge objectives. Holistic model of medical care.	Emphasis on self-directed learning explicit throughout course, basic science learnt only as consequence of clinical problem. Holistic model of medical care.
3. Curricular organization	Bottom-up, discipline based. Learning is an accumulation of discipline-oriented knowledge; basic science first. Departmental and faculty hierarchy; no explicit funding for teaching.	Brief modular body-system based course units. Disciplines are correlated rather than integrated. Some early clinical experience. Departmental and faculty hierarchy.	Patient-problem based, supplemented by independent study or group work with a tutor. Problems organized into organ systems. Early clinical experiences and systematic instruction in clinical skills. Matrix organization with teaching funding.	Patient-problem based, supplemented by independent study or group work with a tutor. Early clinical experiences and systematic instruction in clinical skills. Matrix organization with explicit teaching, research, and clinical/administrative funding.

Table 2.1 contd

4. Role of teachers	Are experts who determine educational needs of students.	Are experts who determine educational needs of students. Clinicians may have more say in some modules. Basic scientists asked to justify knowledge inclusion	Tutor small groups in problem-solving and learning exercises. Facilitation more than teaching. Some tutors are expert in area. Tutor assesses group skills.	Tutor small groups in problem-solving and learning exercises. Facilitation more than teaching. Non-expert tutors used. Tutor assesses group skills
5. View of students	Selected on academic ability; raw material to be moulded; should work hard, cover all content, learn what is taught.	Selected on academic ability; however, as consumers of a constructed product, are asked opinion of course function	Selected by many factors. Are viewed as adults who should be responsible for their own learning. Learning critiquing and information retrieval skills is important.	Selected by many factors. Are viewed as adults who should be responsible for their own learning. Learning critiquing and information retrieval skills is important.
6. Content of instruction	Large volume, usually at just below postgraduate level. Follows discipline structure.	Often clinical aspects and basic science taught together. Some prototype diseases taught in depth. No universal coverage attempted. Early clinical exposure.	Process of learning valued as much as content, which is learned problem by problem. Problems are carefully structured by pre-specified learning objectives.	Process of learning valued more than content, defined largely by student picking areas for follow-up.
7. Teaching methods	Lectures, laboratories, content-oriented, same for all students, Teacher centred.	Lectures, laboratories, content-oriented, same for all students. Less teacher centred, with lengthy study guides for each system. Course objectives. Reference material.	Small group discussion follows pattern of problem definition, current knowledge review, identification of gaps, independent study, synthesis of information. Tutor ensures objectives for block are met.	Small group discussion follows pattern of; problem definition, current knowledge review, identification of gaps, independent study, synthesis of information. Students/peers monitor progress.

Table 2.1 contd

Dimension	Discipline oriented	Organ systems	Guided discovery PBL	Open discovery PBL
		Curriculum design		
8. Assessment purposes/ methods	End point written examinations focus on factual information. Little or no use of tests to diagnose problems.	Written but interdisciplinary examinations focus on factual information. Testing can be frequent as courses brief.	Assessment viewed as important. Content and process oriented tests used for all students, heavy peer/ tutor role in grading.	Assessment viewed as important. Process more important. Because not all students are at same stage 'progress testing' replaces testing of precise content. (see v. der Vleuten and van Luyk 1990)
9. The role of educational support staff	Centralized support usually only of audio-visual needs, or test scoring.	Large input in course design, materials development and course evaluation.	Major active roles in all aspects of curriculum development, delivery and monitoring.	Major active roles in all aspects of curriculum development, delivery and monitoring.
Feasible prototypes;	University College London, McGill, Canada, Melbourne, Australia	Case Western Reserve (1970s) Nottingham, UK	Newcastle, NSW Flinders, South Australia	Limburg (Maastricht) McMaster (pre-1980)

1993; Boelen 1994). This has challenged the supremacy of disciplines as the way of organizing knowledge. Hence current curricular objectives will frequently be framed in terms of students' capabilities in certain tasks and roles, for example the diagnosis and management of disease. However such objectives may be informed **both** by the goals of the curriculum **and** by the nature of the subject matter. The Sussex model provides a reminder to deal with the interaction of these two ways of looking at curriculum development.

In addition the organization of subject matter is distinct from learning methods, but frequently influenced by them. For example PBL can be used as a method, but the type of the problems studied constitute the subject matter. The ensuing knowledge structure, inside the head of the learner, would almost certainly be different from that arising had the student studied the problem from a discipline orientation.

The model recognizes two features of real curricula. First it emphasizes the absolute interdependence of the four common elements of curriculum design—a change in any one has immediate effects on the other three. Hence being prescriptive in terms of subject matter (both choice and organization) immediately limits the possibilities in the other areas. This is commonly overlooked in linear or cyclical models and also in the implementation of new curricula where problems arise because of a reluctance to recognize that a design process can bring with it unforeseen design faults. Unlike industrial design, exhaustive trialling of new models to iron out defects is not usually possible in education. It also stresses the importance of having the designers of all aspects interacting frequently and in concert. If those designing the assessment are different people from the methods designers or those choosing objectives then problems will arise.

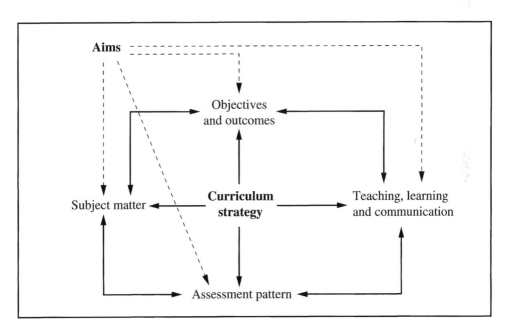

Fig. 2.2 The Sussex curriculum model (Adapted, with permission, from Eraut *et al.*, 1975)

Second, it highlights the fact that the aims of the curriculum designers may actually encompass much more than derivation of, or change to, the objectives of the curriculum (the usual starting point in other linear models). In fact, aims can be expressed through any or all of the components, thus creating the overall framework and mission of the curriculum.

If aims are directed at a particular route into the curriculum this can produce at least four varieties of curriculum.

Content driven

Content driven is frequently the traditional discipline-based curriculum especially in high profile research-based organizations, where the emphasis is on developing comprehensive knowledge systems (Abrahamson 1990). Usually in these content-driven curricula students perceive the curriculum philosophy, of research oriented disciplinary development, as 'learning facts and passing examinations' (Jolly and Rees 1984). But equally a community oriented curriculum might be seen as a content driven curriculum, where the 'content' is equally powerful, but rather more diffuse and dependent on local health care agendas. Such contrasting curricula would tend to emphasize the scientific approach, versus the need to meet the community's needs. The disadvantages of the former include culture shock (especially when moving from a knowledge-based environment into ambulatory and community care), poor real-world preparation, perceived irrelevancy, and a large dispiriting effect (Tosteson 1990). The disadvantages of the latter might include the lack of conceptual structures to organize knowledge in a recognizable or externally validated way, perceived lack of detail and depth, and a totally vocational as opposed to academic orientation. Content-driven remedies for these ills include the 'Core and Options' model (GMC 1993).

Method driven

Method-driven curricula, would include the newer PBL and self-directed curricula (Harvard, Limburg, McMaster). Schools using these newer methods have now become successful and have generated issues that are too important to be ignored by traditionalists. For example the approach is now obviously independent of a number of factors alleged by critics to be crucial to its success. A graduate entry, the existence of national examinations, careful selection of students, and the opportunity to develop on a greenfield site have all been mentioned as key reasons for the success of PBL curricula, but also have all been lacking in one or more recent developments.

PBL courses can be formally structured content-wise around basic science (as at Maastricht) or the clinical domain (as at McMaster). But whatever the approach, most courses espouse the importance of learning in context (see p. 73), early clinical contact, and rational and meaningful assessment. The disadvantages of such curricula are that they may be anxiety provoking, provide an incomplete knowledge base, are arguably resource intensive, require different skills of teachers, and require a multidisciplinary approch (Albanese and Mitchell 1993; Berkson 1993).

Assessment driven

In medicine all curricula are, to some extent, assessment driven. But there is an important distinction to be made between being *intentionally driven* and *unintentionally* driven. In content or method driven curricula, assessment can be an afterthought. For example problem solving skills were seen initially as an important bi-product of the new PBL curricula. However reliable and valid measures do not currently exist for the assessment of these skills (Newble *et al.* 1994), but an attempt at such measurement is usually made. If these measures are inappropriate or given too much prominence the assessments will unintentionally drive the curriculum, perhaps in the wrong direction (Frederikson 1984). On the other hand assessment frequently intentionally drives the curriculum in primary specialty certification (e.g. Royal College, or National or American Board) examinations. There is essentially a 'hidden curriculum' (Snyder 1971) where there are assessments, but no explicit curricula or objectives. Under such conditions learners have to devise their own activities or usurp those provided for other purposes. In the UK the Calman reforms of postgraduate education in hospital specialities are beginning to recognize this problem (Calman 1993) and have encouraged Royal Colleges to describe appropriate aims and objectives, and employers and tutors to provide ring-fenced educational time.

Outcome driven

Outcome-driven objectives incorporate most of the redesigned vocationally-oriented interdisciplinary courses of the last few years (Tresolini and Shugars 1994; Geffen *et al.* 1991; Neufeld and Woodward 1989). These courses also proliferated in the 1960s when the objectives movement swept the USA—the Abraham Lincoln School of Medicine was one extreme example which based much of its curriculum on the job analysis of an intern working under supervision. Such curricula should involve extensive needs assessment and task/job analysis, though many have not done so. Such utilitarian approaches to course design are usually confined to postgraduate or course units of larger curricula. The Advanced Trauma Life Support (ATLS) curriculum is an example in which many objectives are framed in terms of patient outcome or clinical protocols (American College of Surgeons 1995). Used in this way such approaches may be appropriate for current health care problems. However they lack flexibility. In addition it takes a long time from the investigation of need (in health care terms) to curriculum delivery.

The strength of the Sussex model is that it applies to curricula in which any of the four components of curriculum strategy is dominant. Hence most medical courses can be fitted neatly into the scheme, whatever their bias. Naturally the most successful, smoothly running and balanced curricula are likely to be those where the aims inform all four elements and in which the elements themselves are designed to work harmoniously towards the fulfilment of the curricular goals. The components must at least be compatible and certainly not antagonistic. In this context it is easy to see why some newer schools contend that PBL should be used as 'all or nothing' (see Barrows 1986 for an overview of the different approaches), because mixing PBL with traditional course modes undermines the philosophies and values behind PBL.

Using the models for new curricula

We suggest that either of the Harden or Cambridge models can provide the general threads with which to approach the task of curriculum design. Once this has been done for an institution, design teams armed with a sense of the attributes of existing and desired curricula can use the Sussex model to ensure that planning covers all appropriate parts of the strategy and that they harmonize adequately. During the design process several stages will be common to all models (see also Chapter 8).

1) Identify the need for change—by review of the current curriculum or factors in the constituency that have changed.
2) Define aims in terms of philosophy for the curriculum (e.g. a mission statement or charter). Isolate the main areas the aims will address; content, methods, etc.
3) Based on aims, devise strategies within each of the components of the model simultaneously, for example goals and objectives, and assessments.
4) Refine and itemize precisely the curriculum design, paying particular attention to all aspects of the model used.
5) Do it (implement the changes).
6) Look at it (Assess all participants' perspectives on quality, and evaluate these).
7) Fix it (Redesigning may also include a re-evaluation of aims).

Chapter 1 has spent some time identifying needs and clarifying from accumulated reports the current ostensible aims of tomorrow's curricula. Chapters 2.2, 3, 7, and 8 of this book address the implementation, and quality control issues. Evaluation is too large a topic to be included here, but is addressed partly in Chapter 7.4. Below, we sketch some of the issues likely to be prominent or at least provide a further challenge to proposed changes.

The likely curriculum for the twenty-first century

Mission

In addition to those general aims defined in Chapter 1 relating to patient care and the health needs of populations, greater cognisance needs to be taken of the needs and characteristics of learners (see Chapter 3), the context of learning and the potential use of information technology (Chapter 4), and the management of these changes (Chapter 8). It will not be an easy matter to redirect the resources from hospital-based education to a more holistic framework. Many colleagues do not recognize that such changes are possible or even desirable. The capability of non-hospital-based doctors to take major parts in curriculum design and educational delivery has been questioned frequently and many GPs feel themselves to be inadequately prepared for this role (Robinson *et al.* 1994). Hence the mission for the twenty-first century curriculum will involve the mobilization of human resources currently unused to engaging in undergraduate education as well as changing the hearts and minds of those entrenched in an anachronistic view of medical care and professional roles.

Aims and content

The 'core and special study' mode of curriculum delivery advocated in the UK is one way of approaching the problem of curriculum renewal. Unfortunately it suffers from two main problems. First somebody has to define the core; the choice of designers and the frame of reference (what are we aiming to produce?) will be crucial. Usually it will be medical schools, overpopulated with tertiary care specialists, who take on that role. Second, once defined the core cannot be allowed, as happened after the Flexner revolution at the turn of the century, to ossify. Alternatives to the core and option approach include problem-based learning in which the student or student group becomes the integrator, the definer of the depth of knowledge and so on. But this leaves the definition of the content of the curriculum—the choice of problems—as something of an open issue. What problems and how many?

In addition there are a number of topics and issues with apparently legitimate claims for space in the modern course: evidence-based medicine; medical informatics (see Chapter 4.2); population medicine; genetic engineering and molecular biology to name but a few. The task of defining a core is becoming daily more troublesome.

Choosing outcomes and objectives

It seems likely that with the cost of health care under curbs on a world-wide basis one of the major outcomes for newly qualified medical practitioners will be the delivery of cost-effective health care for the highest common denominator with minimal training costs. Even the concept of the way that hospitals are run and personnel used is under fire, and the terminology of health care increasingly is suffused with economic jargon. When the GMC and GPEP documents were constructed both could aim at a house officer/intern with certain defined or characteristic duties. Currently even this view is changing. House officers in the UK are doing less and being trained more. They are being educated to be generalists with fewer opportunities for specialist activity. They are asked to make decisions about specialty choice earlier as undergraduates. For example a one week attachment in urology for all is, in many schools, being replaced by a four-week selective for a few. This ideological clash will need to be addressed in the not too distant future.

Choosing methods

That adults learn differently from children is widely recognized (e.g. Boud 1988). However many medical schools are still wedded to the idea that students can only minimally take responsibility for their own education. The impact of the problem-based schools has been retarded by the near impossibility of clear-cut evaluation data (Albanese and Mitchell 1993) and there is currently much debate about the advantages and disadvantages of PBL, and whether or not it has delivered what it promised (Berkson 1993). Nevertheless it remains true that visitors to PBL schools will, almost without exception, be impressed by the academic milieu, the enthusiasm of the students for learning and the effort expended on study (e.g. Norman 1988). Their achievements cannot be taken lightly. It is therefore likely that in the future much greater thought should be given to the learning methods used by schools in medical curricula, and a considerable move towards PBL and other self-directed methods, such as project work, might be advisable.

Assessment

For the past one hundred years a few essays, a clinical 'long case', a few 'short cases', and latterly a hundred or so MCQs have formed the backbone of assessment in the major medical specialties allowing qualification as a doctor. The paucity of this approach has become evident (see Chapter 5; Wakeford 1985; Newble *et al.* 1994; Nel and Kent 1994). In the UK the Department of Health and the postgraduate deans have also come to realize the importance of assessment during and at the end of postgraduate training (DoH 1996), with a major redesign, along North American lines, of specialty training.

In the future, assessment of competence will become a central issue at undergraduate, postgraduate, and continuing levels. Almost all countries in the western block have recently made major changes to the way medical practitioners are assessed and/or monitored. (Newble and Paget 1996; GMC 1997). Some of these changes will focus on the performance of doctors in actual practice rather than on staged examinations of limited duration (Gabb 1994; Southgate and Jolly 1996). It will be incumbent upon all schools to verse themselves on, and become competent in the use of, the range of technologies now available.

Summary

During the course of this chapter we have identified a number of principles of curriculum design in medicine. It might be useful to distil these out for general use.

1. A rationale for medical education is paramount. A systematic approach to curriculum design at least allows a medical school to keep track of its input and output.
2. For a curriculum to be well designed it is important to specify and limit its role and the needs it serves.
3. Medical curricula are now too complex and too powerful to be designed covertly by small, privileged groups. A curriculum must be both explicit and designed by a consensus involving wide representation from interested parties. As the GPEP report (AAMC 1984) observes, the design and delivery of curricula should be the responsibility of the whole faculty.
4. Each curriculum plan should have features which anchor it in a particular context. It is important that the plan matches, and is practicable within, the context for which it is designed (see Bridgham 1989).
5. All curricular issues are interrelated. Any change will have immediate knock-on effects.
6. Aims can be expressed through any or all of the components, thus creating the overall framework and mission of the curriculum.
7. The role of assessment is so crucial that change in any other attribute must be accompanied by adequate suitable adjustment of the assessment system.

8. Being prescriptive in terms of subject matter (both choice and organization) immediately limits the possibilities of development in the other areas.
9. A curriculum will work best if all the components reflect and are designed to work harmoniously towards the fulfilment of the curricular goals. The components must at least be compatible and certainly not antagonistic.
10. It is important to have the designers of all aspects of a curriculum interacting frequently and in concert.

References

AAMC (Association of American Medical Colleges) (1984). Physicians for the twenty-first century. Report of the panel on the General Professional Education of the Physician (GPEP Report) AAMC: Washington.

Abrahamson, S. (1990). The state of American medical education. *Teaching and Learning in Medicine*, **2**, 120–5.

ACME-TRI (1993). Educating medical students: Achieving change in medical education—the road to implementation. *Academic Medicine*, **68**, (Supplement S1), 1–49.

Albanese, M.A. and Mitchell, S. (1993). Problem-based learning: a review of literature on its outcomes and implementation issues. *Academic Medicine*, **68**, 52–81.

American College of Surgeons (1995). *The advanced trauma life support programme*. American College of Surgeons, Chicago.

Barrows, H.S. (1986). A taxonomy of problem-based learning methods. *Medical Education*, **20**, 481–6.

Barrows, H.S. (1993). An overview of the uses of standardized patients for teaching and evaluating clinical skills. *Academic Medicine*, **68**, 443–51.

Bennard, B.C. and Stritter, F.T. (1989). Teaching medical students in ambulatory clinics: prescribed vs actual practice. *Proceedings of Research in Medical Education* 141–6. Association of American Medical Colleges, Washington.

Berkson, L. (1993). Problem-based learning: have the expectations been met. In *Problem-based learning as an educational strategy* (ed. P. Bouhuijs, H.G. Schmidt and H.J.M. van Berkel), pp.43–65 Network, Maastricht.

Block, S.D., Style, C.B., and Moore, G.T. (1990). *Can we teach humanism?* A randomised controlled trial evaluating the acquisition of humanistic knowledge, attitudes and skills in the new pathway at Harvard Medical School. Harvard Medical School Mimeo, Boston.

Boelen, C. (1994). Interlinking medical practice and medical education: prospects for international action. *Medical Education*, **28**, Supplement, 82–6.

Boud, D. (1988). Moving towards autonomy. In *Developing student autonomy in learning* (ed. D. Boud), pp.17–39 Kogan Page, London.

Bridgham, R. (1989). Theory for curriculum development in medical education. In *Essays on curriculum development and evaluation in medicine: report of the second Cambridge Conference* (ed. G. Page), pp.9–19. Medical School Coordinator of Health Sciences Office, Vancouver.

Calman, K. (1993). Hospital doctors training for the future. The report of the working group on specialist medical training. Department of Health, London.

Dacre, J. and Nicol, M. (1996). *Clinical skills: the learning matrix for students of medicine and nursing*. Radcliffe Medical Press, Oxford.

Department of Health. (1996). *A guide to specialist registrar training*. NHS Executive Leeds.

Eraut, M., Goad, L., and Smith, G. (1975). *The analysis of curriculum materials*. Occasional paper No 2. University of Sussex Education Area, Falmer.

Field, J. (1970). Medical education in the United States: late nineteenth and twentieth centuries. In *The history of medical education* O'Malley, C.D. (ed.), pp.501–30. University of California Press, Los Angeles.

Flexner, A. (1910). *Medical education in the United States and Canada.* Carnegie Foundation, New York.

Frederiksen, N. (1984). The real test bias: influences of testing on teaching and learning. *American Psychologist*, **39**, 193–202.

Gabb, R. (1994). Recertification: an Australian perspective. In *The certification and recertification of doctors: issues in the assessment of clinical competence* (ed. D.I. Newble, B.C. Jolly, and R.E. Wakeford), pp.47–66 Cambridge University Press, Cambridge.

Geffen, L.B., Birkett, D.J., and Alpers, J.H. (1991). The Flinders experiment in medical education revisited. *Medical Journal of Australia*, **155**, 745–50.

General Medical Council. (1993). *Guidelines on undergraduate medical education.* GMC Education Committee, London.

G.M.C. (1997) Performance procedures: a guide to the new arrangements. London: GMC.

Gibbs, G. (1992). Problems and course design strategies. *Polytechnics and Colleges Funding Council Developing Teaching Series No 1.* Oxford Centre for staff development for PCFC.

Gillard, J., Dent, T.H., Aarons, E.J., Smyth-Pigott, P.J., and Nicholls, M.W. (1993). Preregistration house officers in eight English regions: survey of quality of training. *British Medical Journal*, **307**, 1180–4.

Ham, T.H. (1962) Medical Education at Western Reserve University. *New England Journal of Medicine*, **267**, 868–74.

Harden, R. McG. (1984). Educational strategies in curriculum development: the SPICES model. *Medical Education*, **18**, 284–97.

Harden, R. McG. (1986). Approaches to curriculum planning. *Medical Education*, **20**, 458–66.

Hunskaar, S. and Seim, S.H. (1983). Assessment of students' experiences in technical procedures in a medical clerkship. *Medical Education*, **17**, 300–4.

Jolly, B.C. (1994) *Bedside manners: teaching and learning in the hospital setting.* University of Limburg Press, Maastricht.

Jolly, B.C. and Macdonald, M.M. (1989). Education for practice: the role of practical experience in undergraduate and general clinical training. *Medical Education*, **23**, 189–95.

Jolly, B.C. and Rees, L.H. (1984). *Room for improvement: an evaluation of the undergraduate curriculum at St Bartholomew's Hospital Medical College.* Mimeo. SBHMC.

Jolly, B.C., Jones, A., Dacre, J., Elzubeir, M., Hitman, G., and Kopelman, P. (1996). The relationship between clinical experience in introductory clinical courses and performance on an objective structured clinical examination. *Academic Medicine*, **71**, 909–16.

Mattern, W.D., Weinholtz, D., and Friedman, C. (1983). The attending physician as teacher. *New England Journal of Medicine*, **308**, 1129–32.

Nel, C.J. and Kent, A.P. (1994) Maintenance of professional competence, continuing medical education and recertification. *South African Medical Journal*, **84**, 462–84.

Neufeld, V. and Woodward, C.A. (1989). The McMaster MD program: a case study of renewal in medical education. *Academic Medicine*, **64**, 423–34.

Newble, D.I. and Jaeger, K. (1983). The effect of assessment and examinations on the learning of medical students. *Medical Education*, **17**, 165–71.

Newble, D.I. and Paget, N. (1996). The Maintenance of Professional Standards Programme of the Royal Australasian College of Physicians. *Journal of the Royal College of Physicians of London*, **30**, 252–6.

Newble, D.I., Jolly, B.C., and Wakeford, R.E. (Ed.) (1994). The certification and recertification of doctors: issues in the assessment of clinical competence. Cambridge University Press, Cambridge.

Norman, G.R. (1988). Problem-solving skills, solving problems and problem-based learning. Medical Education. **22**, 279–86.

Ramsden, P. (1992). *Learning to teach in higher education*. Routledge, London.

Robinson, L.A., Spencer, J.A., and Jones, R.H. (1994). Contribution of academic departments of general practice to undergraduate teaching and their plans for curriculum development. *British Journal of General Practice*, **44**, 489–91.

Salter, R. (1995). The US residency programme—lessons for preregistration house officer training in the UK. *Postgraduate Medical Journal*, **71**, 273–7.

Schön, D.A. (1987). *Educating the reflective practitioner*. Jossey Bass, San Francisco.

SCOPME. (1994). *Teaching hospital doctors and dentists to teach:* its role in creating a better learning environment. Standing Committee on Postgraduate Medical Education (SCOPME), London.

SCOPME. (1992). *Teaching hospital doctors and dentists to teach:* proposals for consultation. Standing Committee on Postgraduate Medical Education (SCOPME), London.

Snyder, B.R. (1971). *The hidden curriculum* Knopf, New York.

Southgate, L.H. and Jolly, B.C. (1996). The General Medical Council (UK) performance assessment procedure: intended structure and function. Proceedings of *Seventh Ottawa Conference on Medical Education*. (in press)

Stenhouse, L. (1975). *An introduction to curriculum research and development*. Heinemann, London.

Stillman, P.L. and Sawyer, M.A. (1992). New program to enhance the teaching and assessment of clinical skills in the People's Republic of China. *Academic Medicine*, **67**, 495–9.

Stillman, P.L., Burpeau Di Gregorio, M.Y., Nicholson, G.I., Sabers, D.L., Stillman, A.E. (1983). Six years of experience using patient instructors to teach interviewing skills. *Journal of Medical Education*, **58**, 941–6.

Swanson, D., Benbassat, J., Bouhuijs, P., Feletti, G., Fisher, L., Friedman, C., Newble, D., Obenshain, S., and Spooner, H.J. (1989). Alternative approaches to medical school curricula. In *Essays on curriculum development and evaluation in medicine: report of the second Cambridge Conference* (ed. G. Page), pp. 21–34. Medical School Coordinator of Health Sciences Office, Vancouver.

Todd, (ed.) (1968). *Royal Commission on medical education*, HMSO, London.

Tosteson, D.C. (1990) New pathways in general medical education. *New England Journal of Medicine*, **322**, 234–8.

Tresolini, G.P. and Shugars, D.A. (1994). An integrated health care model in medical education: interviews with faculty and administrators. *Academic Medicine*, **69**, 231–6.

van der Vleuten, C.P.M. and van Luyk, S.J. (1990) Evaluating undergraduate training in medical skills. In Nooman, Z.M., Schmidt, H.G. and Ezzat, E.S. (eds) Innovation in Medical Education: an evaluation of its present status. New York: Springer pp. 404–21.

Wakeford, R.E. (ed.) (1985). *Directions in clinical assessment*. Cambridge University Medical School.

2.2 Case studies: recent curriculum designs

Angela Towle and Brian Jolly

Introduction

In this brief chapter we look at some curricula and changes and how they fit into the schemes described in Chapter 2.1. Although many curricula world-wide have undergone recent modification, we confine ourselves here to short descriptions, inevitably over-simplified, of established and large scale changes, that are well reported and relatively permanent. Unfortunately, none are UK-based.

Case 1: The McMaster MD Programme

A true problem-based programme

A new Faculty of Medicine was established at McMaster University in 1965. Intense early discussions among the 'founding fathers' in the late 1960s led to a fundamental decision: to try methods of education, research, health services partnerships, and organizational arrangements that represented clear alternatives to the North American norm prevailing at that time (Spaulding 1991). These goals are still arguably unique in their comprehensiveness. The planners decided that the curriculum would control the structure of the school for both teaching and research. Hence departments were large and multidisciplinary, but did not necessarily encompass *every* discipline.

When the first medical students arrived in 1969 the main elements of the distinctive McMaster approach to medical education were already in place. The key features of the curriculum, which have remained largely unchanged, were: the analysis of health care problems as the main method of acquiring and applying basic and clinical knowledge; the development of independent and lifelong learning skills and learning based around small tutorial groups. Almost one-third of the 33-month programme comprised individual student electives. The problems chosen were wide-ranging and assumed, by faculty, to cover all the necessary objectives by the end of three years. Choosing problems precisely to cover pre-specified objectives was not undertaken initially.

The curriculum structure consisted of a series of interdisciplinary blocks, including the final year of clinical clerkship rotations. Clinical skills, including communication skills, were learned throughout the programme in an integrated parallel course. There were no discipline-specific courses. The programme was considered the responsibility of the

Faculty as a whole with its administration entrusted to a programme committee. Departments and discipline groups supplied the human resources for several defined educational roles within the curriculum.

The assessment system was guided by well-defined principles. These included a balanced emphasis on a range of 'end-product' objectives, although these objectives were not defined in detail as in some other courses (c.f. Newcastle, NSW). In addition, the course involved the use of continuous informal feedback; insisted on shared responsibilities for assessment and feedback by individual students, peers and designated faculty, and used assessment methods designed to be relevant to the objectives. There were no end-of-course (summative) examinations. Assessment of performance occurred continuously, primarily within the informal setting of tutorial discussions. This was supplemented by specially designed individual problem-solving evaluation exercises such as the 'triple-jump exercise' and the Objective Structured Clinical Examination (OSCE). In the 'triple-jump' exercise (Painvin et al. 1979) students are given a problem to work on in the library or on the ward. They formulate and are assessed on their initial approach (Jump 1). They then work on a literature search or further refinement, with guidance from a tutor (Jump 2). Finally they prepare a report or presentation (Jump 3). All three stages are rated.

Curriculum review

In 1981, a major review of the curriculum was undertaken, leading to the approval of three major recommendations:

1. New 'end-product objectives' emphasizing the need for knowledge within three broad perspectives: a) biological, behavioural, and population; b) the introduction of critical appraisal skills as a specific objective; and c) a refinement of objectives related to clinical and learning skills.
2. A rearranged curriculum sequence with Unit 1 as an introduction to all aspects of medical studies, a more integrated combination of organ system blocks, with three systems per twelve-week block, and the introduction of a new block designed around the human life-cycle and with special emphases on community-based experiences and in-depth analysis of the determinants of health. The fifty-two week rotating clerkship block remained relatively unchanged.
3. More flexibility for students both in the duration and in the scope of their studies, with encouragement for the individual student to organize an 'enrichment year' to prepare for a special career in the health field.

McMaster has also recently adopted the 'Progress Test' approach used at the University of Limburg (Verwijnen et al. 1982, van der Vleuten et al., 1996). This is a long, objective-style knowledge test given at frequent intervals throughout the year to **all** students in the school. Each diet of the test is randomly selected from a bank of questions. Each diet is the same for all students, but the notional passmark increases with course year. Students are assessed in terms of their progress, not their absolute score, in the same way that childrens' growth is assessed by Tanner height and weight growth charts. The rationale for the Progress Test is that because each diet of the exam is the same for all students, and because of the frequency of use, individuals can at any time gauge their own progress towards a comprehensive knowledge base and simultaneously compare themselves with their peers. This is the manner in which the test will be used at McMaster. Coincidentally, in Holland, this rationale has been undermined recently by a Dutch government decision that the progress test (along with other tests for all students in the Dutch system, van der Vleuten, personal communication) should become summative (see Chapter 5) and continuation of funding of the student may be contingent upon satisfactory performance in the test. This may have a radical effect on the behaviour of students preparing for the test (see Chapter 5).

Commentary

McMaster was the archetypal SPICES curriculum (see Chapter 2.1). The whole school was student centred, problem-based, integrated, community oriented, elective rich, and moderately systematic. It espoused 'open-discovery' mode, by having few constraints on students in problem groups. In addition the school deliberately set out to harmonize the curriculum strategy with all their aims. Its selection policy was also synergistic. Even though entrants have a lower grade point average than other school's students, they have more PhDs and MAs. Hence not only is the school offering a different curriculum it is teaching cohorts that are atypical of the medical student community in Canada (Ryten 1980, 1981). When student feedback was solicited it was acted upon quickly and the curriculum is still on the lookout for new ideas and operates a 'do it—fix it' policy.

The outcomes have been impressive. Although the school as a whole does not usually feature in the top rank on knowledge tests of the Canadian licensing examinations, it has by no means crumbled or reverted to a traditional curriculum as predicted by early sceptics. Moreover it produces graduates who consistently enter general practice or academic medical posts, and are sought after by employers (Ferrier and Woodward 1987, Woodward and Ferrier 1982). The school has achieved most of its goals; more and better community oriented doctors, a more enjoyable curriculum and one which offered choice, early clinical contact and a humanistic approach to its students.

The main problems, in the early years, have been with the extraordinary amount of anxiety produced by the lack of examinations, which excluded much potentially objective feedback (now being remedied with the Progress Test), and the perceived inadequacy (or subjectivity) of the tutor's feedback, and the difficulties experienced by entering non-scientists.

Case 2: University of Newcastle, Australia

Curriculum design based on content (objectives) and process (problem-based learning)

The original curriculum

The new medical school at Newcastle took its first students in 1978. The Dean and a small number of foundation professors first attempted to answer the question, 'what constitutes a general preparation for further study?' by defining the competencies that students should demonstrate prior to graduation (Engel and Clarke 1979). The programme objectives were a set of forty-five general statements of aims (Faculty of Medicine 1976, 1980, 1983, 1986; Hamilton 1992). The planners for each segment of the course were required to generate more specific objectives, consistent with the Programme Objectives, which described the competence of the student at the end of that segment in terms of observable behaviours. This enormous task was undertaken by faculty members with assistance from visiting colleagues from Britain, Canada, and the USA. The programme objectives emphasized not only the content to be mastered but also the process by which students should be assisted towards the stipulated goals. The foundations of the educational process were: integration of basic and clinical sciences; problem-based learning; small group learning; progressive independence of learning; acquisition of professional skills.

The consideration of issues pertaining to groups or communities was included in the range of problems. The chosen problems, unlike those of McMaster, were all tied to specific objectives. For first year students the problems were usually paper, audiotape, or videotape simulations, but with increasing student confidence and competence, their contact with patients was allowed to increase.

The curriculum was constructed by inviting a wide range of medical and health professional and lay people to list the clinical problems they expected newly qualified doctors to be able to cope with, and by consulting statistical data on hospital and community morbidity and mortality (Clarke 1979). Problems were included only if they were common (incidence or prevalence) and/or serious (life- or health-threatening) and amenable to action by the doctor, and/or preventable.

Suggested problems fell into two main categories: the undifferentiated problem as it is presented to the doctor (e.g. a man complaining of chest pain) and a diagnosis or underlying cause for the problem (e.g. coronary thrombosis). The presenting problem was the one given to the students, while the underlying condition or diagnosis (undergraduate condition) was the one used for curriculum planning. The combination of a particular presenting problem with its undergraduate condition which the students studied was called a 'working problem'. The working problem was underpinned by the development of learning units—discrete boluses of prescribed knowledge, clinical experiences (which might be in the form of videotapes), and/or laboratory exercises. These units had very precise criteria for their construction. Hence the same underlying condition could be studied at different levels of complexity at different stages of the curriculum by altering its presenting features. Students studied about one per week during the first year, spending up to 15 hours a week in scheduled small group activities; the rest of the time was devoted to individual or informal group study, work with patients and informal contact with staff. There were almost no formal lectures and no independently scheduled laboratory classes.

The first term, Phase I, constituted an introduction to the university and to medicine. In Phase II (8 terms) students considered a series of problems that appear only in the adult, arranged on a body-system basis, and proceeding from simple, single-system problems in the first few terms to complex, multi-system problems by the end. The adult was chosen as the 'steady-stage' baseline on which to build knowledge and understanding of human structure, function and abnormality, and as a stage in the human life cycle with which students could easily identify. Phase III (one year) focused on the problems of growing up and growing old. Phase IV was a year in which students took increasing clinical responsibility under supervision, while continuing to learn through the study of clinical problems posed by the faculty.

Students had two elective terms to undertake study in greater depth in a field of their own choice. There were also brief mini-electives at the end of most terms for those students who had demonstrated their competence in the assessment of the term's activities. Elective time consisted of about 20% of total curricular time.

Initially 10–15% of time in the first year was allocated to the longitudinal strand of Group or Population Medicine. Groups of eight students were each allocated a district in Newcastle about which they had to obtain general information. They then identified a community group with special health needs, worked out strategies to attempt to meet those needs and tried to implement one or more of their strategies. Many problems were encountered in implementing this part of the curriculum and students were hostile, so that in later years the community project was replaced by a smaller community-oriented but disease-based research project.

Review and revision

The curriculum was reviewed in 1982 using a Delphi survey (for a description of the Delphi technique see Towle 1991) and wide discussion. The original curriculum was organized by both content and types of learning but it was now considered preferable to organize it primarily by distinct domains of learning, which run in parallel through each year. Five domains were defined and the educational objectives were rearranged, but not substantially changed, to match them.

Domain I: Professional skills—students who are studying clinical problems in a tutorial must see real patients and learn appropriate clinical skills, beginning in the first months of the course. It is geared in its content to Domain III and includes communication skills and continuing contact with families experiencing chronic illness or disability.

Domain II: Critical reasoning—the main items of study are published papers and students are assessed on their ability to critique papers and apply the conclusions to the rest of their work.

Domain III: Identification, prevention, and management of illness—the learning is around individual problems, some of which are those used in the original curriculum.

Domain IV: Population medicine—students are led through a series of concepts as they undertake their own research studies, either from the literature or within the community.

Domain V: Self-directed learning—students learn by study tasks with open access to the library and staff. It includes an elective programme in the final two months of Year 3 and Year 5 when students arrange their own elective, its objectives and supervision.

Commentary

Newcastle was a typical guided-discovery curriculum, more or less at the SPICES end of the continua, with curriculum design being very strongly led by objectives. In fact for its first few years the aim of the curriculum group was to find problems that covered a myriad of, albeit carefully selected, objectives. The original construction of problems was constrained, not only by morbidity criteria, but by the subject matter/objectives and outcomes dimensions, organized by body system. In part this was because Newcastle commenced with a small and overburdened cohort planning the curriculum, with a start-up time of only three years. The resulting curriculum was actually fairly mechanistic and fragmented even though problem-based, and highly dependent on specially constructed resources for the learning units.

The curriculum review altered the balance towards a range of skills which included educational approaches as well as content. Important threads could now be traced through the curriculum.

Newcastle had paid attention to all aspects of the design process; mission, content, subject matter organization, teaching methods and assessment, by setting up working parties for each of these, with good communication between the groups. But the heavy emphasis on objectives restricted the initial curriculum strategy and the early clinical contact of students. The guiding hand had a vice-like grip.

Case 3: University of New Mexico

The primary care curriculum

The experimental parallel track called the Primary Care Curriculum (PCC) accepted its first students in 1979 (Kaufman *et al.* 1989). The track was devised to meet the needs of producing primary care doctors able to assume responsibility for their future learning, who could co-operate with one another. Several of the educational ideas for the PCC emerged from a series of small curricular experiments conducted in the early 1970s by the Department of Family and Community Medicine, and the faculty was subsequently influenced by the McMaster curriculum. A core group decided to introduce their new ideas in the form of a very small parallel experimental track (ten students per year out of a fixed admitted class of 73).

The PCC programme subsequently took 20 students during the first two years of medical school and offered small group, problem-based learning with early sustained introduction of clinical skills and community health care experience. Tutorial groups of five students met with one tutor three times per week during the first year and twice weekly in the second. The tutorials functioned to provide a forum for students to exercise and refine their clinical reasoning as they applied the basic medical sciences to real-life, biomedical problems.

The first year of the PCC (Phase I) comprised an on-campus phase (IA) during the first six and a half months and an off-campus phase (IB) for the last four to five months. In Phase IA the curriculum was divided into three eight-week units, each emphasizing a different theme: a large part of each week was left unscheduled for students to pursue issues raised in the tutorial groups and for clinical electives. The first fifteen weeks included a problem-based clinical skills session one morning per week and students were able to put these skills into immediate use during the clinical electives.

In Phase IB students relocated to rural, medically under-served areas of New Mexico. Working in teams and under supervision of primary care physician preceptors, their goal was to extend and apply their self-directed problem-based learning skills (acquired in Phase 1A) in a real-life setting. Instead of the simulations and paper problems used in Phase 1A, students used actual patients in the office or health problems in the community. Half the day was spent caring for clinic patients and the other half was devoted to study and a community health project.

In Phase II, case problems were grouped according to the basic organ systems, and at the end students took the first of the National Board Examinations. Most of the remaining two years took place in a tertiary care hospital setting. Students from both the PCC and conventional tracks progressed together through the traditional clinical rotations (medicine, obstetrics/gynaecology, paediatrics, psychiatry, surgery and surgical specialities). During the fourth year PCC students were required to do a two-month primary care subinternship in a medically under-served area of the State.

The conventional track

The conventional track programme emphasized the acquisition of an expanding body of knowledge and skills. The first year was devoted to study of the basic principles and concepts of normal structure, function and behaviour. The second year focused on abnormal and pathological processes. In the latter part of the second year there was an 'Introduction to clinical medicine' course which introduced students to history taking and physical examination. Clinical electives, in which students interacted with patients were available throughout the first two years. About half the courses were taught interdepartmentally and the other half by discipline. The lecture remained the main method of teaching, although different courses offered a mixture of approaches, including small groups, conferences, laboratories, and self-directed study. In the third year, students completed the clinical clerkships and in the fourth year they were able to pursue a curriculum developed on a more individual basis as they continued their learning in the context of patient care.

To facilitate the diffusion of ideas, all faculty who taught in PCC also taught in the conventional track.

Evaluation of and comparison between the two tracks has revealed no differences in performance on national examinations, a higher motivation and lower levels of distress in the PCC, and a positive change towards family medicine as a career (Baca *et al.* 1990). There are no differences in cost between the two tracks, although staff contact is higher and preparation time much lower in the PCC. The new track has also been highly successful in attracting educational research and development grants.

The unified curriculum

In 1992 a five-year grant was received from the Robert Wood Johnson Foundation under their 'Preparing physicians for the future' programme to support the implementation of a planned new, integrated four-year curriculum for all students. The new curriculum was to achieve two objectives:

1. It was to incorporate and extend successful aspects of the school's prior educational innovations including the PCC, particularly through the use of problem-based and

student-centred learning, early clinical skills learning, coupled with sustained community-based learning; the incorporation of a population and behavioural perspective into the clinical years; peer teaching; computer-aided instruction; bi-weekly seminars on professional responsibility.

2. It was to address the historically unmet as well as changing health care needs of the population and learning needs of future physicians.

Key features of the new curriculum include a fully integrated basic and clinical science approach built around organ systems, incorporating biological, behavioural, and population perspectives. In the first two years learning methods feature a variety of approaches, with approximately half the time reserved for self-selected student learning. In addition students will serve and learn in a continuity clinic held one day per week in all four years of the curriculum. At the end of the first year, each student is assigned a mentor in either a clinical or laboratory setting. The mentor provides time to explore further the basic sciences in a manner that addresses the students' individual learning needs in a setting that permits exploration of career options.

In the second two years, problem-based tutorial learning in both in-patient and ambulatory setting continues with additional features, for example continued reinforcement of basic and clinical science integration, development of basic science learning resources adapted for ready use of clinical services; and establishment of two, three-month ambulatory blocks in the third year in primary care clinics and off campus.

In addition, socialization into the profession and mentoring of students in a caring humanistic environment will be fostered by creating vertically integrated 'learning families', in which small groups of students from each year will meet frequently with house officers, faculty, community physicians, and other health professionals who will serve curricular, advisory, supportive, and social functions.

Commentary

New Mexico is one of the schools to have tried parallel tracks—one at the left hand end of the SPICES continuum and the other more to the right. In general, parallel tracks tend to be methods driven, while the traditional courses are content driven. This is probably why they can be merged successfully, as most have done; there are not too many competing or unadaptable philosophies. The first ever parallel track was devised by Professor William Chew at the Medical College of Georgia in the late sixties. He was forced by student pressure to give up the experiment as conventional track students perceived the experimental ones as having a favoured existence. This seems to be a fairly standard outcome in such experiments (c.f. Harvard; Armstrong 1991); students enjoy the alternative much more than their traditional counterparts who then become active in forcing changes.

The PCC curriculum at New Mexico was also one of the more radical in terms of its dedication to rural and deprived areas, and in allowing students a great deal of flexibility in what and how they learnt. The aims were to give students much greater autonomy, and this was reflected in the curriculum strategy.

Case 4: Sherbrooke, Canada

The new problem-based curriculum

Beginning in 1986, a curriculum reform group comprising 25 clinicians, basic scientists, students, and resource persons convened by the Dean decided upon the characteristics that would underpin the new curriculum. In addition to preparing students to pass the national licensing examinations and making them eligible for residency programmes, the undergraduate curriculum was reformed to attain three new goals: to promote independent learning, to elicit concern for community problems, and to foster humanistic behaviour. It was therefore agreed that the curriculum would focus on patients (community-oriented, centred on human values) and students (problem-based and autonomous learning).

A conscious effort was made to develop learning activities that were consonant with the reform's three goals in a student-centred, community-oriented philosophy. The content was defined more precisely by multidisciplinary working groups for the seven four-week organ/system units of the first new year. They were asked to select problems that were relevant to clinical practice or best illustrated basic concepts. The same mechanism was used to define the new second-year content. Another task force planned the students' learning assessment system for the entire preclinical years. The new and old curricula at Sherbrooke are compared in Table 2.2 (Des Marchais 1991).

Table 2.2 Characteristics of the first 2½ years at Sherbrooke

Aspect	Old curriculum	PBL curriculum
Basic sciences	First year	11 week biomedical units integrated in 14 units throughout two years
Curriculum design	Organ-system	Organ-system
Participation by departments	Many	Many
Lectures	1645 hours	1 hour/week
Small group tutorials	None	Throughout (5364 hours total teaching time)
Clinical skills	From the first year but not integrated	From the first year and integrated with the PBL units
Summative assessment	Every 4–6 weeks	3 times per year
Formative assessment	Rare	Regular

Des Marchais, J.E. From traditional to problem-based curriculum: how the switch was made at Sherbrooke, Canada. **33** 234–7, © by The Lancet Ltd, 1991.

Problem based learning

The new curriculum keeps as close as possible to the previous calendar based on a four-year undergraduate programme. The first two and a half pre-clerkship years begin with a semester in which students are introduced to both the medical curriculum and the profession. In the first two weeks students work on learning skills, small group dynamics and problem-based learning which they practice with community health problems in small group tutorials. The course continues with a series of 13 four-week organ/system units. The concluding four-month unit is devoted to integration of previous material by analyses of complex multidisciplinary problems. Throughout these two and a half years, students attend a clinical skills course half a day a week. In December of the first term they spend three weeks in community hospitals. Students receive six hours of tutorials and three hours of clinical skills instruction per week; the remaining time is left for their own self-directed study.

The preclinical philosophy is continued in the 18-month clerkship phase during which time students rotate through the regular disciplines: medicine, surgery, psychiatry, paediatrics, and obstetrics and gynaecology. The emphasis is on the specific clinical problems which are encountered. There are bi-weekly two-hour sessions on clinical reasoning for small groups when one of the students works up a clinical case and then acts as a data resource, answering questions from the other group members. There is a three-month community-based rotation in family medicine comprising four weeks in community health centres and eight in family medicine settings, walk-in clinics, and emergency rooms. Even during the busy clinical clerkships the aim is for 20% of normal working hours to be 'protected' free time for learning, although this is not always achieved.

In the preclinical phase, summative examinations are limited to three a year. Marks for factual recall comprise only 25% of the total and two new types of testing have been introduced: the short open-ended question (weighted 35%) and problem-analysis questions (25%). In addition tutors assess individual contributions to problem-analysis, participation in small group work and mastery of self-directed learning (25%). The remaining 15% of marks are allocated to clinical skills. At the end of the first and second years students progress onto the next phase of the course if they have performed satisfactorily in the three examinations. During the middle of the third year similar decisions are made before they enter the clerkship phase. At the end of the clerkship there is a final provincial (public) examination which counts for 30% of the total marks; the remaining 70% are derived from the various clerkships through which they have rotated.

Commentary

Sherbrooke is one of the few schools to have changed from a traditional to a problem-based curriculum. In doing so it recognized that new methods required new approaches to assessment, and a vast programme of staff development. In fact the proportion of staff involved in development was very high for a traditional school.

Essentially it grafted new aims onto more traditional ones and rounded up its curriculum. It started slowly and gained momentum later.

Notably the faculty at Sherbrooke have made some substantial rebuttals of the common criticisms of PBL approaches:

> The majority of 20 year-old students are capable of adjusting to autonomous PBL learning, despite no previous university experience, . . . The small group tutorial is a force driven by peers . . . They all admit that the PBL is quite demanding but stimulating . . . Tutors have expressed surprise at how much young medical students can learn 'on their own' and at the level of excitement and motivation not seen in the previous traditional curriculum.
> *Des Marchais et al.* 1992.

Discussion

All the examples of curriculum change cited here show the impossibility of 'getting it right' first time, either for the organization or for the curriculum. However they do demonstrate that radical and substantial change is both feasible and robust. The challenge to traditional modes of education of medical students provided by these examples cannot be ignored by governments and health departments, nor by universities and medical schools for much longer. For the first time schools in the UK are responding to this challenge. More than thirty five years after McMaster threw down the gauntlet, Liverpool, Manchester and Glasgow have picked it up. It is too early to say what problems they are facing. In rapidly changing economic and social circumstances models of appropriate medicine are changing almost yearly. The development of information resources and rethinking about the distribution of health care also presages a new era of health care professionalism. In this general trend the definition and control of the constituency of medicine, and consequently the nature of medical training, is indeed problematic. For the last half of the twentieth century medical schools have been running to catch up. The degree of vision, change and development needed for the next phase may be beyond our current grasp. Possibly a totally new paradigm is needed— perhaps one based on the generic health professional with subsequent specialization. The probability with which this can be realized is significantly increased by the audacity and imagination of the changes these schools have made in the last ten years.

References

Armstrong, E.G. (1991). A hybrid model of problem-based learning. In *The challenge of problem-based learning*, (ed. D. Boud and G. Feletti), pp.137–49. Kogan Page, London.

Baca, E., Mennin, S.P., Kaufman, A., Moore-West, M. (1990). Comparison between a problem-based, community oriented track and a traditional track within one medical school. In *Innovation in Medical Education: an evaluation of its present status* (ed. Z.M. Nooman, H. Schmidt and E.S. Ezzat), pp.9–26. Springer, New York.

Clarke, R.M. (1979). Design and implementation of the curriculum in a new medical school. *Programmed Learning and Educational Technology*, **16**, 288–95.

Des Marchais, J.E. (1991). From traditional to problem-based curriculum: how the switch was made at Sherbrooke, Canada. *Lancet*, **388**, 234–7.

Des Marchais, J.E., Bureau, M.A., Dumai, B. and Pigeon, G. (1992). From traditional to problem-based learning; a case report of complete curriculum reform. *Medical Education*, **26**, 190–9.

Engel, C.E. and Clarke, R.M. (1979). Medical education with a difference. *Programmed learning and Educational Technology*, **16**, 70–87.

Faculty of Medicine (1976). *Working Paper VI: Undergraduate Programme Objectives*. University of Newcastle, Newcastle NSW.

Faculty of Medicine (1980). *The undergraduate programme: Volume 1*. University of Newcastle, Newcastle NSW.

Faculty of Medicine (1983). *The undergraduate programme: Volume 2*. University of Newcastle. Newcastle NSW.

Faculty of Medicine (1986). *The undergraduate programme: Volume 3*. University of Newcastle. Newcastle NSW.

Ferrier, B.M. and Woodward, C.A. (1987). Comparison of the career choices of McMaster medical graduates and contemporary Canadian medical graduates: A secondary analysis of physician manpower data. *Canadian Medical Association Journal*, **136**, 39–44.

Hamilton, J.D. (1992). A community and population-oriented medical school. Newcastle, Australia. In *The medical school's mission and the population's health*, (ed. K.L. White and J.E. Connelly), pp.164–202. Springer-Verlag, New York.

Kaufman, A., Mennin, S., Waterman, R., Duban, S., Hansbarger, C., Silverblatt, H., *et al.* (1989). The new Mexico experiment: Educational innovation and institutional change. *Academic Medicine*, **64**, 285–94.

Mennin, S.P., Woodside, W.F., Bernstein, E., Kantrowitz, M. and Kaufman, A. (1987). University of New Mexico USA. In *Innovative tracks at established institutions for the education of health personnel*, (ed. M. Kantrowitz, Kaufman, A., Mennin, S., Fulop, T. and Guilbert, J.-J. *et al.*) pp.149–76. World Health Organization.

Neufeld, V.R., Woodward, C.A. and MacLeod, S.M. (1989). The McMaster MD Program: a case study of renewal in medical education. *Academic Medicine*, **64**, 423–32.

Painvin, C., Neufeld, V.R., Norman, G.R., Walker, I. and Whelan, G. (1979). The triple jump exercise: a structured measure of problem solving and self-directed learning. *RIME Proceedings of the Eighteenth Conference Association of American Medical Colleges*, pp.73–7. AAMC, Washington DC.

Ryten, E. (1980). *Canadian Medical Education Statistics 1979/80*. Research Division. Association of Canadian Medical Colleges, August 1980, p.26, table 26.

Ryten, E. (1981). *Canadian Medical Education Statistics 1980/81*. Research Division. Association of Canadian Medical Colleges, August 1981, p.37, table 35.

Spaulding, W.B. (1991). *Revitalising medical education: McMaster Medical School the Early Years 1965–74*. BC Decker, Hamilton.

Towle, A. (1991). *Critical thinking. The future of undergraduate medical education*. King's Fund Centre, London.

van der Vleuten, C.P.M., Verwijnen, E.M. and Wijnen, W. (1996). Fifteen years of experience with progress testing in a problem-based learning curriculum. *Medical Teacher*, **18**, 103–9.

Verwijnen, G.M., Imbos, T.J., Snellen, H., Stalenhoef, B., Pollemans, M., Luyk, S. van, Sprooten, M., Leeuwen, Y. van, and Vleuten, C. van der. (1982). The evaluation system at the Medical School of Maastricht. *Assessment and Evaluation in Higher Education*, **3**, 225–44.

Woodward, C.A. and Ferrier, B.M. (1982). Perspectives of graduates two and five years after graduation from a 3 year medical school. *Journal of Medical Education*, **57**, 294–302.

2.3 The patient's perspective: a challenge for medical education

Julia Neuberger

The public view

When the public examines the way young doctors are trained, they gasp in admiration at the hours students and house officers put in on the wards. They see a medical student going through her preclinical and clinical training, spending some of the time on the wards on the 'firm' of a senior doctor, a consultant, who is often treated like God. It often seems that on the impression that student makes on that consultant, her future reputation rests. If she wants to please, then she must imitate the behaviour of that consultant. She must act as the apprentice, learn from the man on the job, stay silent very often, and then practise in the same way.

Now that in itself is not necessarily the recipe for a progressive profession, with close attention being given to the needs of the client—the patient. Indeed, it has all the makings of a conservative one, with its emphasis on imitation, rather than independent thought, and with little opportunity being given for students to examine the ways that other young professionals in training are taught to communicate with their clients, and see whether those are better than the medical model. Meanwhile, most senior consultants are still male, leading to a decidedly male chauvinist profession, especially in some fields, such as surgery, where studies have demonstrated that women have made little impact on senior posts, even after a generation of roughly equal numbers of men and women studying and qualifying as doctors (Department of Health 1988; NHS Management Executive 1992; Dillner 1993). To add to that even now after considerable numbers of reforms (see Chapter 6.1), junior doctors, house officers, spend long hours on the job. The explanations for this vary from: 'It's the only way of learning the job.' 'I did it, and it was the making of me . . .' to: 'If you can't take the heat, then you must get out . . .' 'It sorts out the *men* from the *boys* . . .'.

Whenever one hears such comments, it seems that this has a remarkable similarity to the initiation rites that used to take place for boys in public schools, roasted over the fire until they died, or did not, in eighteenth and nineteenth century England. It has all the marks of a male initiation rite into a peculiarly male world, and nothing to do with those whom the profession is, after all, there to serve, the patients. Indeed, it can only be said to be harmful to the patients to have young doctors in charge who are exhausted, unable to think straight, and there to be initiated. And one might argue that the later stages of medical training are ripe for reform—not least because they actually convey to those undergoing it precisely the wrong impression of the values of the profession.

If that is so, it is even more cause for concern at a time when there is major change in health service provision in the UK, with a move away from hospitals into the community, and teaching hospitals being for referral, specialist needs, and difficult cases. Medical education does not only seem old-fashioned in pedagogic terms, imitative rather than educative, but also wrongly placed, with too much emphasis on the hospital, and too little on the community, and on how ordinary people live their lives. It seems as if recent medical education, with its late nineteenth and early twentieth century feel, addresses neither the needs of the students nor the needs of the patients—nor, indeed, the wider social concerns of either group.

The role of the health professional

The modern health professional needs to fulfil a myriad of different roles. Downie and Calman (1987) suggest that,

> the following list gives an idea of the wide variety of roles that any health care professional might adopt:
> *Healer*: The primary function here is one of caring and healing. All professional health care groups have this as a basic function.
> *Technician*: There is a technical role in almost all professional activities, whether it is in performing an operation, dressing a wound, massaging a leg, pulling a tooth, or knowing the relevant section of welfare legislation.
> *Counsellor*: Much of the routine work of health care workers is dealing with the psychological and social problems of patients and their families. In some instances, this may even overlap with the spiritual area.

They also include educator, scientist, friend, politician, and campaigner. These are some aspects of the role of the professional doctor; confused roles in many cases, with conflicting values. The conflict between values is often all too clear to patients. They see a doctor's care for a particular patient at a particular time set against the medical profession's, and the individual doctor's, wider concern for the welfare of society as a whole. They also see that doctors have some doubt as to whether expenditure on treatment will make an enormous difference to outcome, a perfectly reasonable doubt but not necessarily comforting to the individual patient. Such wider concerns can make a doctor pay less attention to the patient's desires, because she is thinking as a campaigner for health service resources, or because she wishes to be a counsellor to the patient and his family, when all he wants is a prescription for tranquillizers. Her professional concerns include a worry about his addiction to these tranquillizers, and a concern for the National Health Service drugs bill, in direct conflict with his simply expressed desires.

Science and healing

Similarly, there are conflicts over the scientific process. A good scientist has a real curiosity about conditions and causes. Scientific values are about finding out truths, experimenting in order to further human knowledge. A doctor may well be conducting some form of research, satisfying that natural curiosity which may be one element of what involved him or her in medicine in the first place. But it is psychologically remarkably difficult for both doctor and patient to include a patient in any randomized controlled trial. The whole point of such a trial is that neither the patient nor the doctor should know which arm of the trial the patient is in. For a doctor with a close personal relationship with a patient, such as the general practitioner or specialist who has cared for a patient with a chronic condition for years, entering the patient into such a blind study goes against the comforting and supportive values of real patient care, and can be destructive of trust. All the theorizing in the world about how it may be therapeutic, because the patient may end up in the arm of the trial that has the most beneficial treatment, does not help in explaining to a patient that no-one knows the best treatment. Nor does it help a patient accept it, particularly as some aspects of the conduct of trials, such as the financial benefit to the researcher and his department, are hidden from patients. (Neuberger 1992)

These are conflicts which young health care professionals must think about, beyond the four principles of medical ethics which are normally cited, of beneficence, of non-maleficence, of justice and respect for autonomy (Beauchamp and Childress 1989). The friend scientist conflict is only one of the many possible ones. The individual versus society is another. Which, as the doctor, do you have in mind with the patient before you? The individual? Or the sense of the public good, the totality of the patient population? Do you spend your budget on treatment with a poor success rate, but something, right now, for this patient, or save the money for the next patient, who may or may not come, with a condition where the treatment is expensive, but more successful? And do you tell the patients the truth, about what treatments cost, about likely outcomes, and about how you make your decisions?

The patient and medical education

Medical education has, thus far, signally failed to take these issues on board. Yet patients are beginning to expect young doctors to have thought about these matters. The Patient's Charter makes it clear that doctors have to ask for consent to treatment. But that consent does not necessarily include details of cost and resource allocation, of public concern versus the individual concern for the patient facing you right now. The Patient's Charter merely requires that the patient 'be given a clear explanation of any treatment proposed, including any risks and any alternatives, before (you) decide whether you will agree to the treatment.' The American form of fully informed consent, with all the possible side-effects and risks explained, is not really known in the UK. Nor are the added complications of cost and outcome analysis properly put into the equation. But if there is no real informed consent, if patients are not even used, because of the way medicine has been taught and practised in the UK thus far, to consenting fully to treatment, how is it going to be possible to share with them the difficult decisions?

Gradually patients will come to realize that there are questions they can ask about whether they are getting the best treatment available, or merely the best that the GP fund-holder can afford. As they do that, explicit measures of outcomes of certain procedures will become commonplace, and a large patient input into the calculation should have been made. Patients will need to understand, and doctors be taught to explain, the evidence that many standard procedures are of little benefit. The implications for communications-skills training for medical students are enormous. At the same time, medical students could be taught something about evoking a patient response, about the use of focus groups where selected patient groups focus on issues which matter to them within a general practice setting, and about different ways of measuring health outcomes to take full account of patients' views.

To the patient, it seems as if there is no accurate match between professional and medical school curriculum concerns and patient concerns at all, other than over rationing of resources. That mismatch makes complete openness with patients essential. To be true to the values of respecting autonomy, and acting both beneficently and non-maleficently, decisions must be made explicit, and patients must know the basis on which they are made. But that kind of explicitness has considerable difficulties for patients coping with a less clearly powerful and all-providing health care professional, as well as taking away some of the perceived professional power of the health care professionals.

These issues, of disclosure, consent, respect for autonomy, beneficence, non-maleficence, justice, are all there within the stated professional values of doctors. Yet few young health care professionals in training or recently out of medical school, could even begin to go through them. Despite the insistence on the four principles, the majority of medical students cover very little medical ethics in their training even now. Their ability to argue through these puzzles, and work out for themselves their beliefs about what is right and wrong, is decidedly weak. Their training is largely as technicians and scientists, wholly within an apprenticeship model.

Other countries, especially the US and Canada, have gone further than the UK, though not without much agonizing. They have adapted to criticism both from patients and from those who have gone through the medical education process themselves, such as Perri Klass, who described Harvard's traditional approach in unforgettable terms in a book aptly entitled '*A not entirely benign procedure*' (Klass 1987). The attempt that Harvard has made to change its medical school teaching has been of great interest. The drive has been to emphasize in the idealism that is inherent in medicine, an ideal of service to the public, rather than what is effectively a technique, a series of skills, a discipline, which is how it has been taught in recent years with the Flexnerian, scientific, model in medical schools, ignoring the human element, as Charles Odegaard put it in his cry to American doctors to think again about medical practice and medical education '*Dear doctor*' (Odegaard 1988).

At Harvard, the whole curriculum has been overturned in order to provide a more humanistic framework for medical teaching. Entitled '*The new pathway*', this system values education as paramount, in order to produce more thoughtful, less aggressive, more 'humane' young doctors. Harvard has had clear success in its professional schools in getting its students, largely postgraduate, thinking in a different way about moral problems, such as many other professional schools have not yet begun to approach (Ethics at Harvard 1992).

The human element has been writ large in the New Pathway at Harvard. Central to the programme is the course entitled 'Patient doctor', taught in small seminar groups with two or three faculty. The course, in its earliest stages, encourages first-year medical students to think about the medical interview, to take a history, to practise in a group, with a well-primed patient volunteer, and then to go out in pairs to talk to patients. Unlike the old system, and the European system at the preclinical stage, the idea is to get students talking with patients as early as possible. But that encounter is in the context of extremely disciplined analysis of what the talking is about. Students are taught to interview, to interpret interviews, to watch for signs of nervousness, of terror, of depression, and then to reconstruct the interview in order to begin to inform a diagnosis.

Patient volunteers were clear in their own minds what they were doing, and had been well briefed to help the students by dramatizing their responses in some cases. The relationship between patients in this kind of teaching setting and the doctors who had asked them to take part was clearly one of equals. Secondly, patients were quick to give consent for students to come to talk to them. Thirdly, the thinking behind this teaching was entirely to do with relationships. The emphasis in the first year was on making good relationships, on working on that relationship, on understanding elements which made up that relationship. As a result, basic communications skills were valued very highly, and questions about the nature of pain and suffering were addressed early on in the course.

This was not formal medical ethics, as we now see in a very small way in the UK. Medical ethics as a separate subject is taught as an elective at Harvard Medical School, not central to the programme as 'Patient doctor' is. The ethics course is largely case-based, rather than theoretical, as well as providing encounters with people who have a particular view or experience, such as a Jehovah's Witness on the subject of the use of blood products, or a recently bereaved wife on the subject of suffering, knowledge, and what to tell the patient. This was mirrored in the ethics and literature elective, featuring discussion of literary descriptions of illness, training students to notice signs of stress, and to watch for conflict.

One can imagine parallels to all this in other more traditional settings. Patients could be brought in to teach the students in a quite different way from simply being used as 'teaching subjects' as the firm gathers round the bed and talks over the patient's recumbent body. They could enter into debates about hard choices, and set the agenda by stating their views, along the lines of Carolyn Faulder's *Whose body is it?* where the patient's agenda is clearly set out (Faulder 1985). They could talk about the quality of care they expect, at all stages of their lives, whether as very sick children and their carers, who begin to dispute the value, and the riskiness, of hi-tech interventions (Alderson 1990), or other patients who wonder whether the issue of the quality of their lives has been taken into account, and may have strong views themselves about what is tolerable and what is not (Fallowfield 1990). And they could talk about the different expectations they have of life and health at different stages of their lives. Similarly, teaching in the community will require students going out into people's homes from early in their training, and knowing something about different cultural and religious attitudes and beliefs, rarely taught to doctors, but of central concern to patients (Neuberger 1987; Sampson 1982; Locke 1992).

Patients would also value young medical students being more versed in human suffering. Being young, they are less likely to have experienced much suffering. But they could learn from literature, if properly taught, and a course which included reading the works of Robert Coles (Coles 1990) on people's spiritual ideas, or Rosemary Dinnage (1990), whose anthology of accounts of how people faced their own deaths is both moving and enlightening, might help them. The works of Eric Cassell, a doctor who has examined ideas about suffering over a lifetime (Cassell 1991) might help students come somewhere near patients' expectations that doctors' should understand something of what they go through.

If doctors and patients were prepared to look at new alliances and new relationships, better communication and a strong sense of openness and explicitness about decision-making, we could see some very exciting changes. If all the participating groups in health care are honest enough to define their values, ambitions, and desires, it should be possible to come to new types of decisions, taking account of all the interest groups. But that would require training young doctors to think about their values, those of their patients, and those of society as a whole.

References

Alderson, P. (1990). *Choosing for children—parents' consent to surgery*. Oxford University Press, Oxford.

Beauchamp, T.L. and Childress, J.F. (1989). *Principles of biomedical ethics* (3rd edn). Oxford University Press, New York.

Cassell, E. (1991). *The nature of suffering and the goals of medicine*. Oxford University Press, New York.

Coles, R. (1990). *The spiritual lives of children*. Houghton Mifflin, Boston.

Department of Health (1988). *Health and Personal Social Service Statistics for England*. HMSO, London.

Dillner, L. (1993). Why are there not more women consultants? *British Medical Journal*, **307**, 949–50.

Dinnage, R. (1990). *The ruffian on the stir—reflections on death*. Viking, London.

Downie, R.S. and Calman, K.C. (1987). *Healthy respect—ethics in health care*, pp.159–60. London.

Ethics at Harvard (1992). Five years of the program in ethics and the professions 1987–1992 *Program in Ethics and the professions*. Kennedy School of Government, Harvard University, Cambridge.

Fallowfield, L. (1990). *The quality of life—the missing measurement in health care*. Souvenir Press, London.

Faulder, C. (1985). *Whose body is it?* The troubling issue of informed consent. Virago, London.

Klass, P. (1987). *A not entirely benign procedure—four years as a medical student*. Signet, New York.

Locke, D.C. (1992). *Increasing multicultural understanding—a comprehensive model*, Sage Publications, Newbury Park, California.

Neuberger, J. (1987). *Caring for dying people of different faiths*. Lisa Sainsbury Foundation, London.

Neuberger, J. (1992). *Ethics and health care*. Research Ethics Committees in the UK, King's Fund Institute, London.

NHS Management Executive. (1992). *Women in the NHS*. Department of Health, London.

Odegaard, C. (1988). *Dear doctor*. Henry Kaiser Foundation, Menlo Park.

Sampson, C. (1982). *The neglected ethic: religious and cultural factors in the care of patients*. McGraw-Hill, Maidenhead.

3   How students learn

3　How students learn: the process of learning

Colin Coles

Introduction

In this chapter we will look at how people learn. Drawing on theories of learning, we will explore the practical implications for educators, and address the following questions: How do medical students learn? What makes them learn the way they do? How should they be learning? What can educators do to help? In what ways should educational events be arranged so that learners can learn as they should?

The chapter is arranged as follows: first, there is a review of studies on how medical students learn, and then a discussion of the mechanisms that link the curriculum arrangement and learning outcomes. Following this, we shall examine educational theories, and establish a number of principles. Out of this we will derive and explain a model of learning, and finally discuss some of the implications for medical educators.

Throughout the chapter we shall see that learning is something that only learners can do. Teachers cannot do it for them. Teachers are there to help it happen as effectively as possible. In short, we shall look at what it means to be 'learner-' or 'student centred'.

Medical student learning

Marton and his colleagues in Sweden showed twenty years ago (Marton and Saljo 1976a,b) that university students approach learning in one of two ways, either with a deep approach, which means they attempt to understand the meaning of what they are studying, or a surface approach, that is they merely reproduce what they learn. They found that deep rather than surface approaches were associated with success in a subsequent test of knowledge, and students with a deep approach changed to a surface approach when told they would be tested on their factual knowledge but surface approaches did not become deep when people were tested for understanding. In other words, deep approaches are desirable, and although you can shift people quite easily towards a surface approach it is much more difficult to persuade people to adopt a deep one.

These findings were incorporated by Entwistle (1983) into an inventory which made it possible to test large numbers of people. Using this inventory (Coles 1985a), medical students were shown to enter medical school with apparently highly desirable ways of approaching their studying, that is high deep scores and low surface scores, but after just a few months their deep scores decreased and their surface scores increased significantly. In short, their learning approaches deteriorated. This finding has been replicated elsewhere (Newble and Clarke 1986).

Earlier observational research with medical students had anticipated these inventory findings (Becker *et al.* 1961; Maddison 1978; Simpson 1972). Students felt overloaded with content, lost their motivation, became somewhat cynical about their work, failed to see the relevance of much of what they studied especially in the early years, committed vast amounts of knowledge to memory, and quickly forgot what they had learnt. Then, when they entered the clinical phase of the curriculum, many students found they were unable to retrieve and use the knowledge they had acquired to pass earlier examinations. This made the task of their teachers much more difficult than it might be, and some of them, frustrated at this, resorted to teaching by humiliation.

Clearly then, medical students are not inherently poor learners but rather they adopt inappropriate ways of studying because of the way they are taught. The curriculum can, and often does, have a negative effect on their learning.

Knowledge and elaboration

More positively, research also shows that under particular curricular conditions medical students can adopt highly appropriate ways of learning. In one piece of research it was found that students' approaches to studying in a problem-based curriculum did not deteriorate compared with a traditional one (Coles 1985*a*), and in another study they even improved (De Volder and de Grave 1989). In a further study, students tested on their basic science knowledge after, rather than before, their first clinical attachments (Coles 1990*a*), were found to make more sense of the basic science information they were revising because they could see it in the context of their clinical experiences. These students 'elaborated' their knowledge, that is, they saw 'things fitting together', had intuitive insights into what they were studying, and found that knowledge gained in one area could be applied in others. They felt that their studying led to a qualitative change in their knowledge rather than merely a quantitative one. They also believed that they could remember and apply more of what they learnt this way than previously.

Similarly, at a Canadian medical school where basic science subjects were taught as an option for students to choose in their final clinical year (Patel and Dauphinee 1984), students found the basic sciences making much more sense than they had when they were previously taught during the preclinical phase, and these students too elaborated their knowledge. Other researches have demonstrated similar findings when university students study for their final examinations (Entwistle and Entwistle 1992).

These various studies show that the curriculum can have either a positive or a negative effect on student learning. The way it does this will be examined shortly but before that a number of issues about approaches to studying and the processes of learning need to be clarified.

Approaches to study and student learning

First, a distinction needs to be made between study *approaches* and student *learning*. Study approaches are, by definition, intentional. On the whole, students set out to study in a particular way. The learning that occurs, on the other hand, refers to the mental processes that go on. Given this, deep and surface approaches are ways of studying consciously adopted by students. Elaboration, however, is something that occurs in a student's mind. We will look again at this distinction later.

Next the relationship between deep approaches and elaboration needs clarifying. Students adopting deep approaches to studying attempt to understand the meaning of what they are learning. Elaboration on the other hand occurs when students discover how the things they are learning relate to other topics, and especially how theory links with practice. It is perfectly possible for students to learn deeply without elaborating their knowledge. They can, as many do, adopt an academic or scholastic approach to their studying. This occurs particularly in the early years of the curriculum when many of their courses are highly theoretical and abstract, and where the curriculum gives little insight into the setting in which students are likely to need the information they are having to learn. But while these students may be using deep approaches they do not necessarily elaborate their knowledge, that is they do not seek the links between one subject or another, or gain insight into how to use their knowledge in an applied setting.

This then raises the question as to whether deep approaches are sufficient, or if elaboration is needed as well. It was noted earlier that university students perform best with deep approaches and least well with surface ones. Interestingly, this finding has not been replicated with medical students. While surface approaches do indeed correlate significantly with poor examination grades in medicine, deep approaches do not seem to correlate with high performance (Coles 1985*b*; Newble *et al*. 1988). Elaboration though does correlate significantly with academic success in medical examinations (Coles 1990*a*). It seems that although deep approaches might pay off in a strictly academic setting such as studying for a university degree, elaboration is needed in an applied one such as studying medicine.

Elaboration, then, is different from deep processing. It involves increasing the depth and breadth of one's knowledge. Indeed, other research has shown that this is the very kind of knowledge one needs to be able to explain and solve clinical problems, and to engage effectively in the process of clinical diagnosis (Bordage and Zacks 1984; Grant and Marsden 1987; Norman 1988; Patel *et al* 1990, see Chapter 2.1).

What links the curriculum arrangement and learning outcomes?

As we have already seen the curriculum arrangement strongly influences the kind of learning that occurs. How does it do this? What are the mechanisms involved? On the face of it (Fig. 3.1) the curriculum causes learning to occur. Teachers teach and learners learn. That is what education is all about. But it is not as simple as that. Despite their teachers' efforts, some students never seem to learn appropriately. Even more challenging, other students appear to learn very well despite rather poor teaching.

Curriculum - - - - - - - - - - - - - - -► Learning

Fig. 3.1 A simplistic view of the curriculum and learning model

To begin with we should turn to the curriculum itself, and address the question what is a curriculum? The curriculum can be thought of as comprising at least three elements

(Fig 3.2). One is 'the curriculum on paper'—its aims and intentions. Sometimes it comprises a set of national recommendations (GMC 1991; GPEP report 1984) or what the people most closely concerned with the curriculum say should be in it. Although 'the curriculum on paper' implies it is written down, it is not always explicit, and you might have to extract it from committee minutes, reports, and other documents relating to the curriculum. In short, the curriculum on paper is what people hope it will achieve.

However, when the curriculum is implemented, things don't always go as they were planned. What was intended might never actually happen, and things happen that were never actually intended. Hence the second circle in Fig 3.2 'the curriculum in action'. This comprises lectures, seminars, tutorials, ward rounds, laboratory classes, examinations, etc. It is the events that occur from day to day in the lives of teachers and students. Interestingly, this second circle does not entirely overlap with the first. Some of the intentions are missed out when the curriculum is implemented, and others that were never intended are included or simply just 'happen'.

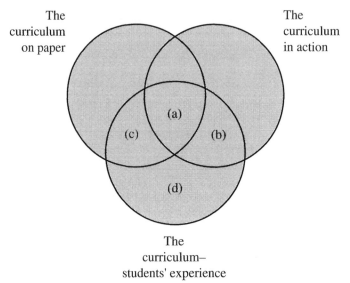

The
curriculum
on paper

The
curriculum
in action

(a)

(c)

(b)

(d)

The
curriculum–
students' experience

Fig. 3.2 The curriculum

The third aspect of a curriculum is 'the curriculum students experience' (Fig 3.2), and can be rather different from what was intended *and* what actually happened. In this circle there is an area (a) in the middle which appears rather small. This is those curriculum intentions which became actions which students experience. Perhaps it should be larger than this! There is also an overlap with the curriculum in action (area b). Students might for example believe that biochemistry is simply a matter of learning 'cycles' by rote. This may never have been intended by the curriculum planners but could have been suggested by some teachers or perhaps previous students. There is too an overlap between the first and the third circles (area c). Students 'pick up' from their teachers what the curriculum intentions really are even though these are not made explicit by the curriculum in action, for example that the students should be linking together preclinical and clinical subjects. The final area (d) is enigmatic. It is a part of the curriculum which was never intended nor became the curriculum in action yet nevertheless it forms a large part of the students' experience, sometimes called the 'hidden curriculum' (Snyder 1971). It can be much more powerful in determining what students actually do than many teachers or curriculum planners imagine, for example when students decide not to study a particular subject because it never comes up in the examinations. Students very quickly learn to 'play the system', and they learn a great deal about how to cope through the 'student grapevine'.

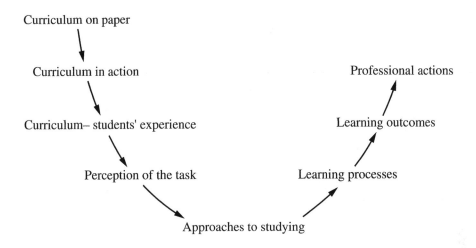

Fig. 3.3 An expanded view of curriculum teaching and learning

These hidden messages then determine the students' perception of their task (Fig 3.3). This is a crucial factor in understanding how curriculum and learning are linked. It is what students see themselves as having to do. When we ask students what they see as their job the answers are sometimes surprising and often illuminating. They tell you a great deal about what is going on in the students' mind and why, and they also give you hints as to the causes and likely outcome. This is so important in understanding the dynamics of a curriculum that some examples might be helpful here.

Curriculum and students' tasks

In the early part of an undergraduate medical curriculum, particularly in the preclinical years, it is not uncommon for students to see their task as a passive one: they sit and listen to their teachers, and they learn what they are taught, often by attempting to memorize what they are studying. This is very much a description of a 'surface approach'.

Alternatively they might see their preclinical task as requiring a deep approach, and they will tend to look for the meaning of what they are studying and the internal logic of the subjects they are taught. They will probably still see the courses they are studying as separate from one another and not greatly related to the practice of medicine but they will almost certainly achieve a high degree of examination success because they are doing a very competent academic job.

Some preclinical students, though, perceive their task as seeing how the basic principles they are learning help explain clinical conditions. Lectures provide a framework, and their studying is driven by questions they themselves are posing: Why is this happening? What does that mean? In what ways does this link with what we were taught last week? These students perceive their task as elaborating their knowledge.

These perceptions of the task can be seen in the clinical years too. Students performing poorly have a very unclear perception of what to do. Indeed, they feel in the way. They do not know why they are there or what they should be doing. Other students see their clinical task more deeply. They read a lot, and focus on clinical management and therapeutics. They are likely to be interested in clinical trials and research studies, but often fail to see patients as more than diagnoses, and frequently miss the wider implications of someone's illness. They might know a great deal about medical science but very little about people.

Clinical students who see their task as elaboration use their clinical experiences as opportunities for directing their own study, and of generating questions in their mind for which they will seek answers. They use any resource available to them such as journals and text books, and they reprocess their notes from preclinical courses. They are interested in the mechanism of disease, and in seeing how unique each case is. They make connections and see how things fit together.

The next part of the chain linking curriculum and learning (Fig. 3.3) concerns students' approaches to studying. The way they perceive their task makes them study in particular ways. Paradoxically, the dozens of books suggesting various study methods have had little impact on improving student learning (Becher and Kogan 1980; Ford 1980; Hartley 1986). The reason is clear. The student's intention is central to the quality of the learning that occurs. Study methods are directly related to what you see yourself as having to do. Merely learning new study skills does not address the fundamental problem regarding the students' perception of their task.

Summary of how students learn

So far we have looked at learning from the students' perspective, and have drawn on research into how they study, or at least are constrained to, by the curriculum arrangement. The learning processes that occur greatly influence the learning outcomes. In short, information which has merely been rote learnt is liable to be forgotten or remembered inaccurately. Information that has been understood but not elaborated will be sound but possibly narrow and unconnected. Also, learning is enhanced by knowing how well we are doing. We need feedback to learn effectively, but this must be constructive. Negative feedback weakens a response (we tend *not* to do it again) but tells us little about what we should be doing.

Learning and educational theories

We will now review briefly some more general educational theories, partly to see how they have influenced current thinking but also to examine their value in guiding medical educators. In general, educational theories describe what might be done *to* students to make them learn more effectively. In doing this most start with some consideration of how students learn, or at least process, information. Theories which start from the information processing perspective are called cognitive theories.

Cognitive theories

It is well established that learning involves the processing of information (Broadbent 1975; Klatsky 1980), and some important principles need revisiting here. First, what we learn is greatly influenced by what we already know. New information is processed in the light of existing information. Second the quality of the resulting knowledge rests on the degree of restructuring that occurs. The more complex the restructuring the more versatile the memory store. Information which has been built into an elaborate knowledge structure is much more likely to be retrieved and used in novel settings because 'multiple routes of access' to it will have been created in our minds (Broadbent 1975).

An important contribution here comes from the work of Ausubel (*et al.* 1978), 'The most important single factor influencing learning is what the learner already knows. Ascertain this and teach him accordingly'. Indeed, Ausubel went further to propose a way in which one could manipulate the learning situation educationally so as to ensure that learners have the necessary prior knowledge to allow them to process new information. He suggested people need an 'advanced organizer' to act as a bridge between what the learner already knows and needs to know before successfully learning the task in hand. An advance organizer might be some kind of framework for understanding complex concepts, or as we shall see some clinical experience to illuminate abstract principles.

Others have taken the notion of advance organizers further. Grotelueschen (1979) showed that people who had little prior knowledge benefited most from advanced organizers that were concrete examples, whilst people who had a high level of prior knowledge found abstract advanced organizers useful. Mayer (1979) suggested that when the things you are learning will not be used until much later, you will learn best if concrete information is presented first. He showed that when the material to be learnt was conceptual but unorganized or unfamiliar to the learner, where the learner lacked relevant prior knowledge, and where the information to be learnt was to be applied subsequently in areas that were unknown to the learner at the time the learning took place, then a concrete-to-abstract sequence of information was needed. There seems a clear message here for medical education. Students enter medical schools with some prior knowledge and are then expected to learn considerable amounts of new information. Not just this, they must acquire this knowledge in one setting and apply it in a very different one. Under these circumstances students can be helped to learn abstract material with the aid of concrete advance organizers. Put another way examples and illustrations should form the initial input for teaching theoretical principles.

Action and reflection theories

Kolb (1984) makes a similar point. He suggests that learning occurs best when it is based on the learner's *own* experience, and proposes what he calls an experiential learning cycle (Fig. 3.4). When people reflect on their experience they can derive a theoretical understanding of it, which if applied to new situations, can provide opportunities for further experience and reflection. By proceeding round this cycle, learners build up deeper theoretical knowledge about their practical experiences. One central feature of this cycle is that, experience *precedes* abstract studying. This of course is in complete contrast to the traditional curricular pattern in medical education where the preclinical subjects, which are theoretical and abstract, precede the clinical experiences which are concrete and practical. Perhaps medicine should be taught 'upside down' (Kriel and Hewson 1986), that is with clinical experience coming before (and thus providing a context for understanding) the basic sciences.

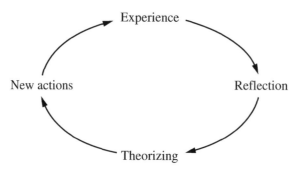

Fig. 3.4 Experiential learning (after Kolb 1984)

Schon's (1983) theory of professional development goes even further. Professional practice, he suggests, involves acting on the basis of what he calls theories of action which are often unrecognized by the practitioner. Indeed, professional education (Schon 1987), whether in its initial stages which prepare professionals for practice or during continuing professional education once qualified, rarely teaches people about these theories. Certainly this is true of medical education. It often fails to acknowledge the intuitive nature of medical practice. On the contrary, the educational process presents students with clear cut certainties about what doctors do. Students are taught orthodoxy, and rarely allowed the opportunity to reflect on their own or other people's practice. Yet Schon argues that when professionals reflect on their practice their otherwise hidden theories of action emerge, and by putting these into words professionals can be helped to see more clearly for themselves the mechanisms underpinning what they do, and thus pass this knowledge on to others.

Adult learning theories

Knowles (1990) proposes a theory of adult learning. He emphasizes that the subject matter must be seen as relevant to the learner who should be able to relate the knowledge and skills being acquired to what he or she intends to do. Education for adults should build on the individual's day-to-day experience, and any new knowledge should be appropriate to the learner's current level of knowledge and skills. Again, these ideas seem in contrast to much medical education where the learner is treated more like a child than an adult. What knowledge the student brings to the learning situation is rarely utilized, and little attention is paid to helping students develop sound learning strategies.

Knowles' views have led to the development of what has been called 'self directed learning' (1988), where students take control of the learning process and establish a kind of 'learning contract' (Knowles 1986) with the teacher in which both parties agree what should be learnt, set targets, and agree how these will be met.

Perry suggests (1970) a developmental view of learning, and shows that when people learn something new they pass through certain stages. Initially they have a 'dualistic' view of education. They think that what they have to learn is either right or wrong, and the teacher is there to tell them everything they need to know. This stage can give way to 'relativism' where the learner sees that knowledge is not necessarily absolutely true, but its 'correctness' depends on the situation you are in. At this stage you can even debate topics with your teachers, perhaps as a 'devil's advocate', that is by arguing a case you do not believe yourself. However, prolonged relativism is uncomfortable, and leads ultimately to what Perry calls a position of 'commitment' where the learner adopts a personal view of the world. Perry suggests that teachers have an important role in encouraging the move from dualism, through relativism, to commitment. They must not intervene too strongly but be supportive and encourage the learner to develop personal insights. Inevitably, this process can lead to misunderstanding and even distrust between teachers and learners. Learners may feel the teacher is playing some kind of game with them, and teachers can become frustrated at the lack of vision on the part of the learner. In Perry's terms, much medical education is dualistic, reinforcing a right/wrong view of knowledge, and few medical teachers know how to mediate the sometimes painful shift to commitment.

A developmental view of learning raises a further issue: the learner's emotional state. Maslow (1970) suggested that there is a hierarchy of learning needs (Fig. 3.5). At the very basic levels, the learner's physiological and physical needs must be met: the environment should be conducive to learning. Next, the learner's emotional needs are important. If the learner's emotional state is impaired, learning is unlikely to take place. For this reason alone teaching by humiliation is undesirable. After this, the learner's social needs must be met. The learner should feel a sense of belonging to a social group and not isolated or alone. Only when all of these needs have been met, can higher order needs such as learning and problem solving begin to be addressed. Again there is a contrast here with much medical education which often fails to consider the learner's emotional needs, and is frequently competitive rather than cooperative. Most medical learning is solitary rather than social, and the educational climate often unsatisfactory.

Rogers sees learning as a 'self actualizing tendency' (1961, 1983). He believes that if the conditions for learning are right then learning will occur automatically. These conditions are that learners should be presented with 'the relevant problems of their existence so that they perceive problems and issues which they wish to resolve . . . Students who are in real contact with life's problems wish to learn, want to grow, seek to find out, hope to master, desire to create' (Rogers 1961). The teacher's role in all of this is to develop 'such a personal relationship with his students, and such a climate in his classroom' (Rogers 1961) that learning occurs quite naturally. The implication for medical education is that students will automatically learn what they need to know if exposed to medicine's problems, provided they receive the support they need from their teachers.

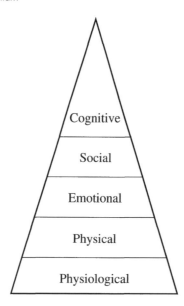

Fig. 3.5 Hierarchy of needs (after Maslow 1970)

The principles of effective learning

Out of this discussion of student learning and educational theories it is possible to distil a number of principles that underpin effective learning.

1. It is essential to start where the learner is, and in particular for learners to discover where they are. However, some learners may not know where they are at the start and should be helped to do so. They should be allowed the opportunity to identify what they already know and don't know about a subject.
2. Professional education should begin in a concrete manner rather than in the traditional abstract way that many undergraduate medical courses do. This is essential when learners have no relevant prior experience, or only poorly formed conceptual ideas concerning the knowledge to be acquired, or have little idea of the situations in which that knowledge will be needed. Starting in a concrete manner means providing learners with first hand experiences of relevant examples and illustrations prior to the presentation of conceptual information. In this way, learners are much more likely to be motivated to learn.
3. Learners will only learn what they see themselves as having to learn. They should be closely involved in determining their learning objectives. However, their perception of what they have to learn (their learning *wants*) may differ from what the teacher sees as their learning *needs*. Teachers must ensure that there is no gap between these wants and needs. They must learn how to articulate and negotiate any differences between them, and know how to get students to agree what they have to learn.
4. An essential feature of effective learning is that the learner is an active participant in it. Learning requires the processing of information by the learner to build up more and more complex networks of knowledge, that is elaborate what they know. Learners should attempt to put into words what they are learning. This helps them

to clarify for themselves their growing understanding. The very act of articulation helps the learning process.

5. Teachers are there to ensure that learning takes place. Teaching is an activity that should focus on facilitating learning rather than providing learners with information. Not only this: teaching should be carried out in a supportive manner, thus addressing the learner's social, emotional, and physical needs.

6. Learners must be able to assess their own performance and progress. Knowing how you are doing is essential to effective learning. So too is an insight into your own strengths and weaknesses. Much of the feedback from teachers, and most examinations, do not help this process. Traditionally, teachers assess the students. As a result, learning is restricted to what students believe is needed to pass the exam rather than to elaborate their knowledge. In medical education, there is a conflict between examinations which act as some form of certification, and assessment which facilitates learning, that is between so called 'summative' and 'formative' assessment. This conflict needs to be resolved.

In summary, people learn best when they are helped to define their own problems, acknowledge and accept their strengths and weaknesses, decide on a course of action, and evaluate the consequence of their decisions. The teacher's role in this process is to facilitate, that is to arrange educational experiences, and to create a constructive and supportive environment so that elaboration will occur.

A model for promoting effective learning

In order to apply these educational principles we need to construct a model for promoting effective learning. Such a model is shown in Fig 3.6. It emphasizes three features of any educational situation: (a) the context, (b) information, and (c) opportunities for elaboration. Each of these will now be described more fully.

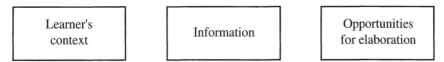

Fig. 3.6 Contextual learning model

The learner's context

The learner's context is by far the most important feature of the learning model and we will deal with it in more detail than the other two. If as educators we can get their learning context right, students will stand a good chance of directing their own learning.

What is meant by the learner's context? It is not just the environment in which learning takes place, important though it is to see that the physical, emotional, and social setting is conducive. In this discussion the learner's context will mean *what is going on in the learner's mind*. We know that the learner must ask the right questions, must see that there is a problem to be solved, must want to learn what the teacher believes he or she needs to learn, and must have understood, agreed, and have some ownership of the learning objectives. So how can such a context for learning be established? How can teachers create circumstances in which the learner's context will become established in an appropriate way? Merely *telling* students what the learning objectives are, or demonstrating a clinical problem, will not necessarily achieve this. Learners must have the motivation to learn. How can this be achieved? There are three elements to this, the use of concrete examples, establishing a 'set' or readiness to learn, and reflection.

Concrete examples

When a learner comes fresh to a topic, his or her context for learning can best be established through being presented with a concrete example or illustration that relates to the learner's purpose in learning. Having said this, the level of concreteness of any example or illustration needs to be considered (Fig. 3.7). The highest level of concreteness is personal experience of a situation, such as seeing and clerking a patient, contemplating the patient's problem, formulating differential diagnoses, tentatively establishing a clinical management plan, etc. A simulation involving the learner, as in the case of an actor patient or role play, would be at the next level of concreteness. Slightly lower in concreteness would be a demonstration in the presence of the learner. Lower still would be a video recording of the example or illustration, and slightly lower than this an audio recording. A paper-and-pencil example comes lower than all of these. Lower still on the scale of concreteness would come a reported description of a case. Below that one is in the realms of diagrammatically represented concepts such as biochemical cycles and pharmacological pathways, and lowest of all would be abstract concepts such as homeostasis.

Highest

Actual experience

Simulated experience

Role play

Demonstration

Video recording

Audio recording

Paper-and-pencil case

Reported case

Diagrams

Concepts

Lowest

Fig. 3.7 Levels of concreteness of examples and illustrations

The level of concreteness of any example or illustration should be carefully considered in terms of the learner's level of development regarding the subject being taught. As a rule-of-thumb, the newer the learner to a subject, the higher on this scale of concreteness should be the presentation of any example or illustration. Learners more familiar with a particular topic can probably cope with examples which are more conceptual than concrete. Interestingly, as people become familiar with conceptual material it often takes on a concrete quality for them. Thus a concept such as homeostasis will, to someone conversant with it, appear almost tangible.

Learning set

A further consideration regarding the presentation of examples and illustrations is the way the learner responds to them. People can be shown things but not observe them, and observe but not reflect upon them, such as a student watching a clinician in an out-patient clinic but not quite knowing what to look for. Whether or not the student perceives the situation in the same way as the clinician depends on his or her learning 'set'—a term which refers to the learner's frame of reference or readiness to carry out the task. Put another way, we see what we are expecting to see. Educationally, set is concerned with what the learner sees as the objectives of a learning episode, and how he or she perceives his or her role with regard to them. As far as the out-patient clinic is concerned, what is the student there for? What is his or her task in observing the clinician? Has this been discussed before the patient arrives?

Reflection

Even if the learner has a 'set' to observe, what does it mean to reflect on the observation? The student in the clinic might 'see' what happens but is there much 'reflection' occurring? Reflection is more than merely looking: it involves the processes of analysis and synthesis. Analysis would mean the student dissecting the consultation into its constituent parts. Who said what and why? What was the outcome? How was this arrived at? Synthesis, on the other hand would mean recognizing the general principles involved, and appreciating how they could be applied to other situations. What principles of history taking and physical examination were used and how did the clinician's knowledge of pathophysiology and clinical management help to form a diagnosis and management plan?

Schon's notion of professionals understanding their theories of action relates to this ability to reflect effectively on practice. We should not assume that learners automatically have the skills to do this effectively, and should recognize that teachers may need to help them learn to reflect in an active rather than a passive way. Similarly, teachers need to be able to reflect on their own practice, and to learn to identify their theories of action.

Reflecting on one's own performance rather than someone else's requires, in addition to the skills of analysis and synthesis, personal insight, the skills of self assessment, and often the ability to act upon feedback from one's peers. A protocol (Fig. 3.8) has been described to achieve this. This has proved valuable when groups of general practitioners reflect on video recordings of their consultations with patients (Coles 1989), and when hospital consultants discuss with one another their teaching of junior doctors. Rather than discussing the whole scheme here, we will look at how the early stages establish the learning context.

First, someone observes an example of his or her practice, then identifies the strengths and weaknesses in it. For example, in a piece of one-to-one teaching with a junior doctor a consultant might say 'I felt I had good rapport but the junior didn't seem to open up very much'. His colleagues would add their positive and negative comments too. Then the consultant would say what he would want to do differently next time, for example 'I would like to be able to get the junior to say more in tutorials'. Next, the group say what they believe the consultant needs to do differently, for example 'The consultant should ask open rather than closed questions'. Negotiation of any difference in views might lead to the consultant asking for clarification about the distinction between open and closed questions. As a result of this process the consultant establishes some learning objectives.

Once defined, objectives can be dealt with, and the remainder of the scheme shown in Fig. 3.8 completes the process. Suffice it to say here, by agreeing the learning objectives the consultant's learning context has been established, and learning is likely to occur in a self-directed manner.

Experience using this protocol suggests that negotiating and agreeing a set of learning objectives takes longer than might be thought necessary, yet perhaps this is the best use of contact time between teachers and learners. Rather than teachers spending their time telling learners what they should know or do, they should help them sort out their learning objectives, and then let them get on with achieving them.

1. Observe the learner's practice

2. What went well? (learner first)

3. What didn't go well? (learner first)

4. What would the learner want to do differently?

5. What does the teacher think the learner needs to do differently?

6. Negotiate the learner's 'wants' and 'needs'

7. Agree the educational objectives

8. Meet these objectives

9. Articulate the educational outcomes (learner first)

10. Set new educational task as a result

Fig. 3.8 Protocol for reflecting on practice

Information

Once the learner's context has been established, information can be provided. The presentation (or at least the making available to learners) of information is a vexed educational question, and there are several issues to discuss. First, we should look at the timing of information. Much of the information presented to medical students is relevant to the task of medicine but often hardly relevant to the learner at the stage at which it is presented. Teachers often talk about students needing to learn what they call 'the basics' prior to its application in the clinical field. This confuses two meanings of the term 'basics'. Much (though by no means all) of what is taught is basic in the sense that it underpins medical practice but we also use the term 'basic' to mean 'coming first'. Our discussion in this chapter has established that information needs to be presented in the learner's context. A lot of the information teachers give students is out of context, or rather is in the teacher's rather than the learner's context.

The next consideration is how the content is determined. In conventional teaching, especially in the preclinical years, lecturers decide the content, often guided by what they see as relevant or perhaps the internal logic of their discipline (or worse the staffing of their department) rather than the practical applications of the information they want to present. The content needs to be determined by some conversation between preclinical and clinical teachers, with its application being paramount (Barnett et al. 1987). Teachers do indeed often include clinical examples and illustrations as part of their lectures but frequently do so in order to illuminate the content rather than using the content to explain their examples. In curricula which have been reorganized along problem based lines, students study information in relation to clinical cases presented to them (Walton and Matthews 1989). In other words, the problems chosen determine the content that is learnt.

Next, how should the content be presented? One way is of course through lectures, and we need to look at how possible it is to lecture in a learner centred way (Gibbs et al. 1992). Again, the overriding educational principle is that learners must first have established an appropriate learning context. They should (through some means) have identified (or been helped to identify) for themselves the gaps in their own knowledge and clearly see why they need to learn what they are to be taught. Once this has happened information can be presented to help make sense of the examples and to fill gaps in the learner's knowledge (Coles 1993a).

A rather different way of dealing with information is for learners to work in groups to seek out and pool their knowledge. The group's total fund of knowledge is likely to be greater than that of any one individual, and can often surpass what the teacher and the group imagined they knew (Walton 1973). Moreover, the very act of putting into words what you have found out in order to explain it to others helps you to understand it and your own misconceptions of it more clearly. Tutors have a clear role in helping students learn effectively through the tutorial process (Barrows 1988). Here, though, the task is to facilitate learning rather than give information. This means encouraging students to say what they know and clarify their understanding rather than adding new knowledge.

Private study is also a highly appropriate way of obtaining information but it needs to be 'self directed' which means people being purposeful in their study. Partly this requires resource materials—texts, notes, study guides, reading lists, etc—but fundamentally it needs a clear perception of the task. Why am I studying this? What do I want to find out? What questions am I addressing? What are the problems to be solved? The so-called SQ3R method of reading rests on the same principles. Readers should first scan (S) the piece, next pose questions (Q) they want answers for by reading the piece, then read (R) it, try to recall (R) what they have read, and finally revise (R) the piece once more.

Opportunities for elaborating knowledge

As already emphasized, the kind of learning that needs to take place is for learners to incorporate new information into what they already know, and thereby to restructure or elaborate what they know into more and more complex networks of knowledge (Coles 1990*a*). Educationally this means helping learners to 'fit things together' in their minds.

Elaboration means, in part, relating theory and practice. In medicine, there is often a separation between the preclinical and the clinical phases. Even postgraduates studying for higher examinations often see their 'book work' quite separately from their day-to-day clinical work. Learners should be encouraged to make the links between the two, for example by using clinical experiences as a basis for academic work.

We have looked at how lectures can be more learner centred. Elaboration can also be encouraged. Lecturers could stop at key points to get students to discuss a topic amongst themselves or to summarize in their own words what the lecturer has said. At the close, lecturers might suggest what students could do on their own to make links and connections. Sadly, many students come to the end of a lecture with pages of notes but no idea what to do with them. A few hints from the lecturer would help enormously. Elaboration occurs especially when learners see how knowledge acquired in one situation can be applied in another, for example that acid–base balance is relevant to understanding acidosis. Students and postgraduates should be encouraged to 'cross refer' what they are learning, that is to link one piece of teaching with another.

The role of the teacher in encouraging elaboration is important. No longer should teachers see themselves as the fount of all knowledge, nor should good teaching be seen simply as the clear presentation of information. Rather the teacher should be facilitating learning, and encouraging learners to make links and interconnections between the topics they are studying. The teacher is there to support learning, to provide a conducive educational environment in which effective learning can take place.

Sometimes, this facilitating teaching role becomes almost that of a counsellor. For example, students and trainee doctors are deeply engaged in learning at a stage in their lives when lots of other things are going on. They are striving to establish a career, and experiencing enormous changes in their social and domestic life. Inevitably some of this will affect their work. Unless these 'external' events are satisfactorily addressed it is unlikely that effective learning will occur (BMA 1992). The teacher's counselling role is to help learners cope with these situations and to see their education in perspective. There are implications here for staff development: teachers may not have these skills, and may need to be helped to develop new roles and educational approaches (Coles 1993*b*; SCOPME 1992).

The curriculum structure, too, can provide opportunities for elaboration through the kinds of tasks that students are set. Traditionally these have included essays and project work, case reports, and laboratory write-ups. Increasingly, use is being made of computer assisted learning, though whether or not this achieves elaboration is debateable since computer assisted learning can all too easily involve students merely in answering multi-choice tests on information presented to them. This does not necessarily encourage them to interconnect their knowledge or to restructure it in an elaborated manner. Exactly the same criticism was made of programmed learning when it was in vogue in the 1970s.

The examination arrangements also need consideration regarding elaboration because revision time is a golden opportunity, often sadly missed, for effective self study. Exams exert considerable pressure on students and can affect the quality of their learning. Certainly examinations that merely test factual knowledge encourage a surface approach. This has led some writers (Newble and Jaeger 1983) to suggest that deeper approaches would be encouraged if curriculum planners devised examinations which test understanding and problem solving. However, this view is too simplistic. We saw earlier that you can easily turn students' deep approaches to surface ones but not vice versa. The issue is not so much the examination's format but its timing. Elaboration has been found to occur when the examination, despite testing factual knowledge, comes *after* students have had some clinical experience, that is when they are in a position to link theory and practice. Put another way, surface approaches occur if examinations are held when students are not in a position to apply their knowledge. When they are, students can elaborate their knowledge (Coles 1987), even without radically altering the nature of the examinations.

Applying the contextual learning model

This model with its three elements—the learner's context, information, and opportunities for elaboration—can be applied in medical education in a number of different ways. It is not possible to explore these in detail here, but some brief speculative examples might illustrate how this could occur.

The model can be used to plan the entire curriculum. Problem based learning (Barrows and Tamblyn 1980) may well be one application. The context is provided through the problem, information is made available either through lectures (Armstrong 1991) or through self study and group work (Barrows 1988), and opportunities for elaboration happen when students solve the problem they have been presented with.

But curriculum planners need not go to the extreme, redeveloping their courses along problem based lines. Existing curricula would become much more appropriate if they were to adopt the three phase model outlined above. At the start of any learning sequence, such as a week's work, students could be presented with examples of clinical situations carefully chosen to suit the topics being taught. Through these examples students should be encouraged to set some learning objectives—what do they want to learn in relation to the cases they are seeing? Some negotiation may of course be needed to ensure that their learning wants are what their teachers see to be their learning needs, and their teachers might need training in the skills required to bring this about. Then, resource material should be made available to learners to provide information for them to fill the educational gaps they have recognized. Lectures could be a highly efficient way of doing this. The tasks students take on as a result should then be carefully chosen and clearly set, and will largely involve private study, together perhaps with group work and tutorials with their teachers. Again, staff development is likely to be necessary. The students themselves, too, will need help to develop their own skills of self learning and self assessment in order to learn effectively and to be able to judge their own performance and evaluate their own progress.

The model can also be used for individual educational events. As already suggested, lectures could be greatly improved, perhaps by starting with a presentation of clinical examples and illustrations, and by clearly establishing the lecture's objectives. Then, information presented should be relevant to the objectives and examples posed, and opportunities for elaboration need to occur during and after the lecture to ensure that active learning takes place.

At the individual level, learners too can use the model as a basis for their own private work. In the early years of the curriculum they will need to find ways of making sense of all they are being taught. Above all, they should come to see that any educational event, whether lecture, tutorial, or ward round, is an opportunity for elaboration. In the clinical years they can begin with their own clinical examples, and use these to drive their own studying, having elaboration clearly in mind as their perception of their task. Above all, their tutors should help them to study in this way (Coles 1990b), and they in their turn will need to learn the skills of doing this. What for example is the difference between telling and facilitating? How can we encourage students to want to learn what they need to learn? How can we deal with the difficult student? This shift of emphasis may be particularly difficult for clinicians. Their clinical role is largely to solve other people's problems for them. Their educational role, on the other hand, is to help people identify their own problem and solve it for themselves. This is the essence of learner-centred teaching.

Perhaps most important of all, as curriculum planners and teachers we need to be able to trust our students and trainees more than perhaps we do. They are adults. We must recognize them as such. Our efforts should be directed towards creating the conditions needed for effective learning, that is by contextualizing the educational events we arrange and by supporting our learners in their learning. Nothing more is needed. Nothing less will do.

References

Armstrong, E.G. (1991). A hybrid model of problem-based learning, in *The challenge of problem based learning*, (ed. D. Boud and G. Feletti), pp.137–49. Kogan Page, London.

Ausubel, D.P., Novak, J.S., and Hanesian, H. (1978). *Educational psychology: a cognitive view*, 2nd Ed. Holt, Rinehart and Winston, New York.

Barnett, R.A., Becher, R.A., and Cork, N.M. (1987). Models of professional preparation: pharmacy, nursing and teacher education. *Studies in Higher Education*, **12**, 51–63.

Barrows, H.S. (1988). *The tutorial process*. Southern Illinois University School of Medicine, Springfield.

Barrows, H.S., and Tamblyn, R.M. (1980). *Problem based learning. An approach to medical education*. Springer, New York.

Becher, T. and Kogan, M. (1980). *Process and structure in higher education*. Heinemann, London.

Becker, H.S., Geer, B., Hughes, E.C., and Strauss, A. (1961). *Boys in white*. University of Chicago Press, Chicago.

BMA (1992). *Stress and the medical profession*. British Medical Association, London.

Bordage, G. and Zacks, R. (1984). The structure of medical knowledge in the memories of medical students and general practitioners, categories and prototypes. *Medical Education*, **18**, 406–16.

Broadbent, D.E. (1975). Cognitive psychology and education. *British Journal of Educational Psychology*, **45**, 2, 162–76.

Coles, C.R. (1985a). Differences between conventional and problem-based curricula in their students' approaches to studying. *Medical Education*, **19**, 4.

Coles, C.R. (1985b). *A study of the relationships between curriculum and learning in undergraduate medical education*. PhD thesis, University of Southampton.

Coles, C.R. (1987). The actual effects of examinations on medical student learning. *Assessment and Evaluation in Higher Education*, **12**, 209–19.

Coles, C.R. (1989). Self assessment and medical audit: an educational approach. *British Medical Journal*, **299**, 807–8.

Coles, C.R. (1990a). Elaborated learning in undergraduate medical education. *Medical Education*, **24**, 14–22.

Coles, C.R. (1990b). *Helping students with learning difficulties in medical and health care education*. ASME Medical Education Research Booklet 24, Association for the Study of Medical Education, Dundee.

Coles, C.R. (1993a). Developing medical education. *Postgraduate Medical Journal*, **69**, 807, 57–63.

Coles, C.R. (1993b). Education in Practice: Teaching Medical Teachers to Teach. In *Learning in Medicine*. (ed. C.R. Coles and H.A. Holm), pp.45–65. Oxford University Press, Oxford.

De Volder, M.L. and De Grave, W.S. (1989). Approaches to studying in a problem based-medical programme: a developmental study. *Medical Education*, **23**, 262–4.

Entwistle, N. (1983). *Styles of learning and teaching*. John Wiley and Sons, Chichester.

Entwistle, A. and Entwistle, N. (1992). Experiences of understanding in revising for degree examinations. *Learning and Instruction*, **2**, 1–22.

Ford, N. (1980). Teaching study skills to teachers: a reappraisal. *British Journal of Teacher Education*, **6**, 71–8.

Gibbs, G., Habeshaw, S., and Habeshaw, T. (1992) *53 interesting things to do in your lectures*. Technical and Educational Services Ltd, Bristol.

GMC (1991). *Undergraduate medical education*. Discussion document by the Working Party of the GMC Education Committee, May 1991.

GPEP (1984). Report of the Project Panel of the General Professional Education of the Physician and College Preparation for Medicine. Physicians for the twenty-first century. *Journal of Medical Education* **59**, 11 part 2, 1–31.

Grant, J. and Marsden, P. (1987). The structure of memorized knowledge in students and clinicians: an explanation for diagnostic expertise. *Medical Education*, **21**, 92–8.

Grotelueschen, A.D. (1979). Introductory material structure and prior knowledge effects on adult learning. *Adult Learning*, **29**, 2, 75–82.

Hartley, J. (1986). Improving study-skills. *British Education Research Journal*, **12**, 111–23.

Klatsky, R. (1980). *Human memory: structures and processes*, 2nd edn. W.H. Freeman & Co, San Francisco.

Knowles, M.S. (1986). *Using learning contracts*. Jossey-Bass, London.

Knowles, M.S. (1988). *Self directed learning: a guide for learners and teachers*. Jossey-Bass, London.

Knowles, M.S. (1990). *The adult learner: a neglected species*. Gulf, Houston.

Kolb, D.A. (1984). *Experiential learning: experience as a source of learning and development*. Prentice Hall, Englewood Cliffs, New Jersey.

Kriel, J. and Hewson, M. (1986). Conceptual frameworks in preclinical and clinical textbooks. *Medical Education*, **20**, 94–101.

Maddison, D.C. (1978). What's wrong with medical education? *Medical Education*, **12**, 97–106.

Marton, F. and Saljo, R. (1976*a*). On qualitative differences in learning I—outcome and process. *British Journal of Educational Psychology*, **46**, 4–11.

Marton, F. and Saljo, R. (1976*b*). On qualitative differences in learning II—outcome as a function of the learner's conception of the task. *British Journal of Educational Psychology*, **46**, 115–127.

Maslow, A.H. (1970). *Motivation and personality*. Harper & Row, New York.

Mayer, R.E. (1979). Can advance organisers influence meaningful learning? *Review of Educational Research*, **49**, 371–83.

Newble, D. and Clarke, R.M. (1986). The approaches to learning of students in a traditional and in an innovative problem based medical school. *Medical Education*, **20**, 267–73.

Newble, D. and Jaeger, K. (1983). The effect of assessment and examinations on the learning of medical students. *Medical Education*, **17**, 165–171.

Newble, D., Entwistle, N.J., Hejka, E.J., Jolly, B., and Whelan, G. (1988). Towards the identification of student learning problems: the development of a diagnostic inventory. *Medical Education*, **22**, 518–26.

Norman, G.R. (1988). Problem-solving skills, solving problems and problem-based learning. *Medical Education*, **22**, 279–86.

Patel, V.L. and Dauphinee, W.D. (1984). Return to basic sciences after clinical experience in undergraduate medical training. *Medical Education*, **18**, 244–8.

Patel, V.L., Evans, D.A., and Kaufman, D.R. (1990). Reasoning strategies and the use of biomedical knowledge by medical students. *Medical Education*, **24**, 129–36.

Perry, W.G. (1970). *Forms of intellectual and ethical development in the college years: a scheme*. Holt Rinehart and Winston, New York.

Rogers, C. (1961). *On becoming a person*. Constable and Co Ltd, London.

Rogers, C. (1983). *Freedom to learn for the eighties*. Charles E Merrill, Columbus Ohio.

Schon, D.A. (1983). *The reflective practitioner: how practitioners think in action*. Jossey-Bass, San Francisco.

Schon, D.A. (1987). *Educating the reflective practitioner: towards a new design for teaching and learning in the professions*. Jossey Bass, San Francisco.

SCOPME (1992). *Teaching hospital doctors and dentists to teach: its role in creating a better learning environment*. Standing Committee on Postgraduate Medical Education, London.

Simpson, M.A. (1972). *Medical education: a critical approach*. Butterworth, London.

Snyder, B.R. (1971). *The hidden curriculum*. Knopf, New York.

Walton, H.J. (1973). *Small group methods in medical teaching*. Medical Education Booklet 1, Association for the Study of Medical Education, Dundee.

Walton, H.J. and Matthews, M.B. (1989). *Essentials of problem-based learning*. ASME Medical Education Research Booklet 23, Association for the Study of Medical Education, Dundee.

4   Where students can learn

4.1 Opportunities outside hospitals

Jenny Field

Doctors of the future must provide health care which is responsive to the needs of all the people in the region which they serve. Medical students, who will become those doctors, are traditionally trained in hospitals, concentrating on the needs of a much smaller and sicker part of this population. The tension created here has been most clearly recognized in parts of the world where there is a major disparity between the provision of high technology care in hospitals and the priority health care needs of much of the population, which may lie mainly in primary care. In the United Kingdom appreciation of this same tension has been precipitated by recent changes in the delivery of health care. The revolution in the provision of care, involving minimally invasive surgery and investigations, shorter hospital stays for acute disease, and the transfer of care for many chronic diseases into general practice means that patients in hospital are even fewer and sicker than before. In order to deliver a curriculum which can prepare doctors to care for the health needs of all, students must be given opportunities to learn where all types and severity of disease present and are managed, that is, both inside and outside hospitals.

Learning outside hospitals is frequently and somewhat loosely termed *community based teaching*. In this chapter I consider the use of the terms *community, community oriented medical education*, and *community based teaching* and some of the difficulties associated with their use. This is followed by a discussion of how the content of a medical curriculum may be defined, and therefore how we might determine where students should learn. I will describe some ways in which students are learning outside hospital settings in the United Kingdom, the factors influencing the development of teaching programmes outside hospitals, and what a vision of the future might be.

The 'community' in medical education

In the context of medical education, the term *community* has been used extensively, but with differing meanings and implications.

The community as the whole population

The term can be used to define the total population of the region in which doctors are being trained. For example the WHO (1987) suggested a definition for use in this context: the *community* is 'a group of individuals and families living together in a defined geographical area, usually comprising a village, town, or city'. This group would require primary, secondary, and tertiary care services.

Using the term in a similar way, the WHO (1987) defined *community oriented medical education* as 'an education which is focused on population groups and individual persons taking into account the health needs of the community concerned'. The value of this term is dependent on the way in which the community is defined (usually geographical) and the methods by which its health needs are assessed, and is open to a wide range of interpretations. It is usually taken to include learning about health care services both inside and outside hospital, though with a focus on the latter.

There is an implication in the use of the term that the *community* has one voice as far as its health care needs are concerned. In fact, any geographical group is not likely to be homogeneous, but is a complex web of individuals, associations, and interest groups with variable status and conflicting views. Agreeing on the health care needs and priorities of such a group is a complex task, with political and ethical implications as well as medical ones, and there is a risk that the use of the word *community*, with its somewhat cosy associations, may obscure this.

The community as the world outside hospital

However, the term is also in common use to mean only that section of the population outside the hospital, so that *'teaching in the community'* (McCrorie *et al.* 1993; Field and Kinmonth 1995) comes to mean only teaching outside hospitals, mainly relating to primary care services. The term *community based teaching* has assumed this meaning of *community*, and is now used to describe any teaching activities occurring outside traditional hospital settings (Towle 1992; McCrorie *et al.* 1993; Murray *et al.* 1995).

With this potential source of confusion, for the purposes of this chapter, I shall avoid using the word *community* except when referring to other writers' use of the word. If we accept that medical education should enable future doctors to cater for the health care needs of the local population, addressing these needs for a western population will require learning about the delivery of primary, secondary, and some aspects of tertiary care. The question 'Where should students learn?' is therefore about the appropriate balance of learning activities in different sites. It is important that the present bandwagon to provide more teaching outside hospitals does not deflect thought on how to determine the ideal balance of environments in which students can learn.

What determines where students should learn?

In order to decide on appropriate educational methods and locations which will enable medical education to cater for the health needs of all, it is necessary to define the content of the curriculum. The ways in which this is commonly done have important implications for the choice of sites for learning.

The curriculum pie

As Oswald (1989) points out, it is traditional to look at the medical curriculum as a pie, divided according to the contribution of medical disciplines in terms of time. Students learn in the base location of each specialty, usually a hospital. In most cases there is historical rather than educational justification for the relative contributions of different disciplines to the pie, and certainly there is a tendency for specialists to see any suggestion of a reduction in their contribution as a reflection on their professional status, and to resist this fiercely.

In addition, in the United Kingdom the changes in the structure of the National Health Service have promoted demarcation and competition between budgetary groups, which are also discipline based. The situation is now being further exacerbated by the perceived threat of reallocation of funding from SIFT, which is the Service Increment for Teaching: a major source of National Health Service income in teaching hospitals, which may in part be moved around depending on teaching load. These factors make it difficult to focus clearly on educational factors when agreeing on a curriculum that is defined by disciplines.

Health care needs

An alternative way of defining what students should learn is to base the decision not on doctors and their disciplines but on patients and their health care needs. This requires serious consideration of the relative importance for medical students of rare but serious diseases compared with common illnesses, with important but less urgent consequences. Assignation of priorities to topics in medical education raises the same political and ethical difficulties as assigning health care priorities for a population, but methods to carry out this latter task are now being developed, for example in the well known Oregon experiment (Kitzhaber 1993), in Sweden (McKee and Figueras 1996), and in local health authorities in the United Kingdom (Honigsbaum *et al.* 1995). Although the methods used have limitations, a common aspect is wide consultation, which would seem equally appropriate in medical education. Final decisions about curriculum content are likely to be made by consensus agreement of a small group of planners, but the preceding consultation and debate must take place if these are to be determined by educational need rather than the status of disciplines.

A result of considering a curriculum based on patients' health care needs is a clearer idea of where students might learn. Learning about health care is likely to be most effective if related to the context in which it will be used (Coles 1990 and see Chapter 3). Acute life threatening disease is cared for mainly in hospital and the management of emergencies must remain part of every medical student's experience. Chronic illness, which is the main health burden for our society, is now more likely to be managed within primary care, with secondary care support for specialist investigations and treatments. A person with non-insulin dependent diabetes may be diagnosed and treated in general practice and have her first visit to a hospital twenty years later for treatment of an ischaemic toe. Most minor illnesses will, as before, be dealt with entirely in primary care. How an individual school assigns educational priorities will determine the balance of sites for learning.

Relationship to problem-based learning

Problem-based learning and community orientation have often been associated as desirable features of modern medical curricula (WHO 1987). In schools using problem based learning as the principal learning method (Barrows and Tamblyn 1980) agreement must be reached on the important 'problems' which define the curriculum content and it might be assumed that this would result in a curriculum responsive to local health needs. However, Richards and Fulop (1987) studied ten innovative medical schools, and showed that five were using problem-based learning and the other five were community oriented, that is, addressing the health needs of the local population. By the criteria used, there was no overlap. Glick (1991) has subsequently pointed out that problem-based learning may on occasions be a hindrance to this type of community orientation, as the exaggerated focus on introducing a new teaching method may divert energies from the primary goal of identifying a curriculum content which relates to local needs. Influential individuals may determine the curriculum content whatever learning method is used, and this finding should not rule out problem based learning, but emphasize the need for wide consultation.

Even allowing for the inertia produced by the enforcement of disciplinary boundaries, and differing views of influential individuals involved in curriculum planning, it seems likely that with the continuing changes in the delivery of health care, students in the future will spend more time learning outside hospitals. As Silver wrote in 1983, 'Medical education is a reflection of medical practice; it is not the education that will change the practitioners, but reformed practice that will redesign medical education'.

How can students learn outside hospital?

Experience world-wide

In the twentieth century there has been an enormous advance and expansion in the provision of high technology curative health care, based mainly in hospitals. Over the last twenty years this has been followed by the realization that there has not, in most countries, been an equivalent expansion in the availability and quality of primary health care. This resulted in the Alma Ata declaration of 1978, declaring the strategy of 'Health for all by the year 2000', promoting primary health care and confirming the need to reform manpower development programmes (WHO 1978). The consequence of this was a corresponding need to reform the education of health care professionals, and, in the following year, ten schools of health care education, already attempting to reform their curricula in a community oriented direction (using the WHO (1987) definition), founded the Network of Community-Oriented Educational Institutions for Health Sciences. In 1995 this organization had 57 full member institutions and 118 associate member institutions. The World Health Organisation has published reports both of new schools world-wide (Richards and Fulop 1987) and of innovative tracks within established institutions (Kantrowitz et al. 1987), all of which have made a commitment to relating medical education to local needs. The programmes implemented outside hospitals in these schools are many and various and by definition, the content of a curriculum which relates to the health care needs of the local population will be quite different in different parts of the world. This may create difficulties if doctors train in regions demographically different from where they wish to practice, or if they choose to practice in areas different from where they train, but it seems reasonable for schools to prepare doctors for their local health care situation.

Experience in the United Kingdom

Prior to the development of academic departments of general practice over the last twenty-five years, most medical students' only learning experience outside hospital, if provided at all, was a two week attachment to a general practitioner. The student would have observed the doctor at work, and might, with luck, have been able to discuss some of the contrasts with hospital practice with the teacher. Lacking in academic co-ordination, these two weeks did not have any clear educational aims, were certainly not assessed, and were usually seen as an 'aside' from the rest of the course. The Todd report (Royal Commission on Medical Education 1968) encouraged the concept of learning in general practice, and with the increasing support of academic departments which have developed since that time (Fraser and Preston-Whyte 1988), medical students of the 1990s have almost universally had attachments to general practice with clear aims, formal assessment, and a slice of the curriculum pie of variable size, alongside other disciplines. Departments of general practice have also taken on additional educational responsibilities: they have been involved in early patient contact (Metcalfe *et al.* 1983) and family placement schemes (Pill and Tapper-Jones 1993) in the early years of the course, and such departments in many schools are responsible for training in communication skills (Whitehouse 1991). However, teaching in general practice has been closely related to the development of general practice as a discipline in its own right without a change in the overall orientation of the rest of the curriculum, and until recently learning outside hospital in settings other than general practice has been relatively rare.

A new incentive for the development of teaching programmes outside hospitals has been a crisis. With the changes in the delivery of health care, resulting in patients spending less time in hospital, some hospital based disciplines have found that they are no longer able to provide adequate clinical experience for students. This situation has been particularly acute in London (Schamroth and Haines 1992) where there has in addition been an acute reduction in the number of hospital beds. One response to this has been to maintain the traditional general medical firm, but to locate the firm in a general practice setting. This approach has been used by both King's College Hospital Medical School (Seabrook *et al.* 1994) and the University College of London Medical School (Murray *et al.* 1995) whose departments of general practice have set up innovative programmes (see Boxes 4.3 and 4.4).

Over the last five years, in response both to educational pressures and the pragmatic need for change, a number of other UK schools have also arranged new learning opportunities outside hospitals. The General Medical Council's recommendations for undergraduate medical education (1993) have now given clear advice that, owing to the changes in the pattern of health care delivery, students must spend more time in out-patient clinics and in primary care settings, and have given added weight to the changes that were already occurring.

Features of innovative courses outside hospital

The major reason why students must spend time learning outside hospital is that they will have better opportunities for learning if they have contact with the whole range of patients and people who have the problems about which they must learn. In practice, the innovative courses that have been set up have used the opportunity to address other difficulties of traditional medical education. Examples of recent courses developed for medical students in the United Kingdom to learn outside hospital are given in Boxes 4.1–4.6, and may illustrate some of these features. The term *community* is used where it has been used in the literature relating to the courses.

Box 4.1   **City and East London Confederation**

The community module (Wykurz 1992)

This course, initiated in 1990, was devised specifically with the aim of involving the community in the development of the curriculum to ensure that it reflected local health issues. It incorporated two elements, one in the first year and one in the second year during a predominantly lecture based preclinical course. In the first year students spent twelve half days in small groups, each attached to a specific neighbourhood minority group in East London. Tutors from community organizations and the medical school generated programmes for each student so that they could meet local people, contact workers in health care and community organizations, and do anything else that would enable them to reflect on the issues of concern to the local people. This part of the course was assessed by means of an essay and a presentation.

In the second year students again had twelve half days in which they were encouraged to build on their experiences from the first year and carry out a project on a specific issue in the community. The projects were identified by both community organizations and health care providers and the students again worked in small groups with tutors. Students were assessed by means of a group report and an individual report.

Widening the range of clinical experience

All the examples given enable the students to meet people and patients outside the hospital setting, extending the range of their experience. This has been done in various different ways. Students can be introduced to a wide variety of social, cultural, and health related groups in the locality, as described in Box 4.1, giving them a broader view of the place of health care in society. Using a focus more closely related to health care, Box 4.2 describes how students can be based in a general practice and follow patients into hospital, turning the traditional teaching arrangement on its head. Both these arrangements use the health care issues arising in the local population to determine the content of the learning, although in Cambridge (Box 4.2) there is also a core curriculum, defined by discipline, for guidance.

The other examples show how, even with a predetermined content for learning, time spent outside hospital will extend the students' experience. A general practice population can provide students with a wide range of clinical contacts within one hospital discipline, as with general medicine in Boxes 4.3 and 4.4. In a curriculum using problem based learning (Box 4.5), students can be given the opportunity to meet patients with the problem under

Box 4.2   **Cambridge University**

The community based clinical course (Oswald *et al.* 1995)

This is an experimental parallel clinical course offered to a self selected group of four to six students annually which has been running since 1994. The students spend fifteen months at the beginning of their clinical course based in general practice, covering the same content of general medicine, general surgery, obstetrics, gynaecology and some minor specialties as the hospital based students.

In order to cover the agreed curriculum content, a written curriculum has been prepared, divided by specialty and illustrated by key conditions. The key conditions are those which students are likely to encounter while at the practice, and which can be used to trigger learning about other related conditions. By means of sophisti-cated information technology, students are able to track patients through the process of referral to out-patient and sometimes in-patient care. They are thus able to see illnesses from early stages through to resolution, and can accompany patients to hospital where they receive teaching from consultants and hospital doctors.

By the end of this course students are expected to pass the final examination in pathology, obstetrics, and gynaecology and to be on a par with students in the rest of the year. It is hoped that the students will additionally acquire skills in self directed learning and will have a person-centred approach to medicine.

discussion in both hospital and general practice settings, and this is the only example in which learning about the basic sciences is currently related. Box 4.6 shows how students can learn the same clinical skills in a variety of settings, although general practice offers a different range of contacts from those in any hospital discipline, with a generally healthier population base.

Collaboration between disciplines

In recognition of the way in which medical teaching has been traditionally divided by discipline, the General Medical Council (1993) specifically recommended interdisciplin-ary collaboration in order to achieve an integrated approach towards common goals. One major advantage of this approach is the resulting balance between a focus on patients as people, which gains priority in general practice and where patients are less seriously ill, compared with a focus on their individual organs, as in an organ based discipline, such as cardiology or gynaecology. Collaboration in teaching between generalists and specialists is occurring to varying degrees in most of these examples. In Boxes 4.3 and 4.4 it is occurring within general medicine. In Box 4.5 the problem based learning programme requires collaboration in both planning and implementation, and the teaching method requires the students to integrate their learning in the basic sciences with both primary and secondary clinical care. In Box 4.2 the patient rather than the problem is the link, as students may accompany them in visits to both generalists and specialists. In Box 4.4, and to a lesser extent in Box 4.6, the staff development programme gives the opportunity for coherence of aims, if not for direct collaboration.

Box 4.3   **Kings College Hospital Medical School**

The Kings medical firm in the community (Seabrook *et al.* 1994)

In 1990, Kings College Hospital produced a Kings 2000 plan, a scheme to develop the teaching hospital in a more community oriented direction, as a response to the increasing pressure on a reduced number of beds within hospitals. As part of this plan an agreement was reached that some of the students could undertake a medical firm based in general practice. During this eight week firm, students are attached in ones or twos to a general practice. The aim is to teach general medicine, not general practice, and other intentions include teaching whole person medicine, a team approach to health care and encouraging self directed learning. Teaching methods used include opportunistic learning, planned encounters, self directed learning and feedback from tutors, and an OSCE (Objective Structured Clinical Examination) arranged in one of the practices is used as the means of assessment.

*   Particular efforts have been made for this course to develop resources for self directed learning and a series of structured learning packs have been produced (Graham and Seabrook 1994, 1995). These have been developed with the help of students and tutors and provide a range of activities for students to carry out on their own or with patients. The packs, including guidance notes for tutors, have been published and are available for general use.*

Encouraging responsibility for learning

There is increasing evidence from the literature on adult education for the importance of self-directed learning (Brookfield 1986; Knowles 1975), and this has been reinforced by the United Kingdom General Medical Council (1993). Many innovative courses claim to encourage this process, and problem based learning in particular aims to enable students to set their own learning objectives and then achieve them. However, there is a limit to the degree of freedom available to medical students to determine their own goals, and it may be more appropriate to help students take responsibility for their own learning within given boundaries. It is notable that the example of problem based learning described (Box 4.5) uses the term 'directed self learning' for this purpose. The example in Box 4.3 provides specific resources in order to help students learn alone, and those in Boxes 4.1 and 4.2 encourage them to use unstructured time efficiently.

Rational choice of sites for learning?

In only two of the examples given (Boxes 4.2 and 4.5), is it clear that the choice of a learning site outside hospital has been made on the basis of an overview of the whole curriculum. In Cambridge (Box 4.2) there is a firm intention to offer the students opportunities to learn in sites appropriate to the health care needs of a general practice population, while covering the traditional curriculum content, but at present this is only possible for a small group of students, and it would require major curriculum change if it were to be

Box 4.4   **University College London Medical School**

The community based medical firm (Murray *et al.* 1995) and the CeMENT professional development programme (Jolly, personal communication)
University College London Medical School has explored two models of community based medical firms since 1991, and has developed one in which students are attached to a teaching general practice for six weeks. During this time they spend two days a week at the surgery, seeing about six patients a week with whom they can spend time taking a full history and performing a physical examination: the traditional 'clerking' carried out in hospital attachments. They also sit in on one general practice surgery weekly, attend a seminar in the Department of Primary Health Care and attend traditional hospital based teaching for the rest of the time.

The CeMENT professional development programme is a joint initiative of the University College London Medical School, the Royal Free School of Medicine, St Mary's Hospital Medical School, and St Bartholomew's and the London Hospital Medical College, that started in October 1995. It aims to develop and evaluate a comprehensive programme of community based education in the four schools. General practitioner tutors, hospital specialists, and educationalists will collaborate to agree on clinical and educational standards for teaching general medicine, to train and support GP tutors to teach clinical skills and assess clinical competence, and to evaluate the effectiveness of the scheme.

offered to all. In Liverpool (Box 4.5) major curriculum change has occurred, and a decision has been made, presumably based on the curriculum content, that students should spend around half their clinical time outside hospitals. It will be some time before the primary care teaching units necessary to support this will be fully active.

In the other examples, rational choices have been made within the confines of the traditional curriculum pie, with slices allocated by discipline. Box 4.1 is effectively gaining a slice of the pie for a population perspective, but there is a risk that without links with the rest of the curriculum, such a course may become marginalized. Box 4.4 is an example of a reasonable division of learning sites within one slice of the pie (the discipline of general medicine), and Boxes 4.3 and 4.6 offer the same slice of the pie to different students in different sites, which may result in an accusation by the students of injustice if the learning opportunities are unequal.

Influences on the development of teaching programmes outside hospitals

As the examples given have shown, students are now learning outside hospitals in a diverse range of teaching programmes. Innovations bring new problems, and although there would appear to be good reasons why students should have more opportunities to learn in a wide range of sites, there are also barriers to change in this direction. The choice of new learning sites is not always underpinned by clear principles, a number of the stakeholders affected by change have strong views and there are practical difficulties to consider.

Box 4.5 **Liverpool**

The new curriculum (University of Liverpool 1995)

In the UK, Manchester was the first medical school to institute a new curriculum using problem based learning as the main teaching method in September 1994. Glasgow and Liverpool Medical Schools followed in September 1996. In Liverpool, the new course is planned to be problem based and community oriented. Students will spend more time learning in small groups during the theoretical part of the course. The problems, around which the course is built, have been developed by multidisciplinary teams, and will be backed up by separate threads of clinical skills and communication skills. The students will spend up to half their clinical time outside hospitals, and, to provide this, a number of health centres in the region will be converted into primary care teaching units. Didactic teaching should be reduced, 'directed self learning' increased, and assessment will focus on providing feedback on strengths and weaknesses.

Principles underlying the choice of sites for learning

The ideal situation

In order to base the choice of sites on educational need, it is necessary first to agree on what students should learn, and this in turn should be based on agreement about the health care needs of the population these future doctors will serve. Prioritizing these needs is difficult, and has both political and ethical implications, but should at least be based on wide consultation. This process should contribute to a set of principles to guide the choice of curriculum content and sites for learning. Without them changes, including new courses outside hospitals, are likely to be haphazard, and ineffective in directing students' learning.

Coherence with hospital based teaching

If the new courses are seen as isolated islands off the shore from the mainland of a traditional curriculum, collaboration with teachers from other disciplines will be more difficult and there will be a real risk of marginalization, as reported in the course described in Box 4.1 (Wykurz 1992). Coherence with the aims and principles of the rest of the educational programme will aid both students and teachers. Courses undertaken by only some students away from the hospital base (Boxes 4.2, 4.3, and 4.6) have inherent problems, as the choice of learning site is unlikely to have been based on educational need alone.

Assessment

Ideally the overall goals of an educational programme should determine both the nature of the courses provided and the assessment of their achievement. Unless these links are

Box 4.6	**Southampton**

The clinical foundation course

A new course introducing students to clinical skills at the beginning of the first clinical year was introduced in Southampton in 1992, these skills having previously been taught in a hospital based introductory course. Students are attached in groups of three to a tutor, and tutors are chosen from consultants, senior registrars, and increasingly, general practitioners. Hospital doctors come from a wide variety of specialties (including general medicine, surgery, paediatrics, psychogeriatrics, and palliative care) and the number of general practitioner tutors has increased from one to five over the last four years following positive evaluation by the students. The aims of the course in all locations are to enable the students to feel comfortable talking to patients, to learn how to take a full medical history and to perform a full physical examination. All the tutors are offered the opportunity of attending a workshop on the use of video and feedback to teach communication skills, run by tutors from general practice and psychiatry. The aim is to offer a consistent approach to teaching clinical method across a wide variety of disciplines. Assessment is formative and variable depending on the tutor.

clear, it is difficult to develop appropriate assessment procedures. Assessment has been shown to be a major influence on learning (Rowntree 1987), and in spite of recent changes in medical education, final examinations have changed very little. In the example in Box 4.2, students on the community based clinical course are expected to pass the examination set for the traditional hospital based course. A failure to adapt the assessment procedures to altered educational goals carries the risk of leaving the student confused about the relevance of the new programmes.

Links with postgraduate education

Even with clear principles underlying the planning of the undergraduate curriculum, one part of the educational programme in the UK that may be particularly resistant to change in response to changes in the delivery of care is the preregistration year. Pilot programmes have taken place offering a preregistration attachment to general practice (Freeman and Coles 1982; Wilton 1995). Although these are attractive educationally, they raise problems of funding, as preregistration house officers in general practice need considerable supervision, especially as they are not permitted to sign prescriptions. There is already disquiet about the unsatisfactory nature of hospital preregistration posts (where adequate supervision is also a problem) as part of medical education, and the need for them to be coherent with an undergraduate curriculum based partly outside hospital must now be added to that debate. Links with postgraduate education beyond the preregistration year must also be considered.

Evaluation

Evaluation of the new programmes is also dependent on clear statements about the overall aims of the curriculum. These must then be translated into appropriate assessments of outcome and there are a whole range of issues relating to appropriate evaluation methods to be addressed. Even then it will take some years for evaluation to provide even partial answers to the questions of feasibility and outcome of courses in which students are less hospital based, and it seems likely that uncertainty and disagreement will remain. However recent studies are encouraging (Murray *et al.*, 1997).

Views of the stakeholders

The success or failure of implementing change will depend on the attitudes of those who will be affected by it. Spiegal *et al.* (1991) point out the importance of identifying these groups, providing clear information about proposed changes and eliciting their views. They suggest that many changes fall foul of the wrecking power of individuals who were unaware of the effect of their actions, due to poor communication by those directing the change. Similarly, where those involved have other pressing and conflicting priorities, it is helpful to know these early on.

The Dean

Cohen and colleagues (1994) have shown that in six medical schools in the USA two major facilitators of curriculum change were the support of the Dean or equivalent and centralization of curriculum planning. In keeping with this, a major barrier to change was a departmental structure contributing to territorial management of the curriculum. This may be associated with the advantage of having a set of principles to support the choice of learning sites in the whole curriculum.

General practitioner teachers and primary care teams

If students are to learn outside hospitals, general practice teachers are likely to carry an increased load of teaching and supervising students. Academic departments of general practice, which co-ordinate most teaching programmes outside hospitals, give under-graduate education high priority (Fraser and Preston-Whyte 1988), and have shown some enthusiasm about taking on an increased proportion of the curriculum (Iliffe 1992; Oswald 1989). However, the majority of teaching is carried out not by academic departments but by full time general practitioners. Fine (1994) interviewed a small group of general practitioners in depth, and showed that these teachers had a real interest in teaching, based on an enjoyment of the process of learning, seeing teaching as being associated with personal learning and development, a way of giving value to one's work, and a natural part of general practice. They also enjoyed the personal aspects of the teacher/student relationship. However, there was major concern about the lack of time and financial resources for teaching, the need for training and support for teachers and worry about the impact of more teaching on their practices and patients.

As well as general practitioners, other health professionals and community workers may be involved in teaching. Jee (1994) has reported on discussion groups on this topic held with a variety of health workers in the community. All groups were enthusiastic about the extension of undergraduate medical education into community settings and saw it as an opportunity to break down barriers between professional groups that would bring benefits to patients as well as students. However, there were also some realistic concerns expressed about practical difficulties of time, space, and funding, the risk of compromising the teaching of their own students and the need for clear learning objectives and efficient co-ordination of teaching programmes.

Hospital based teaching staff

Medical teachers within hospitals are reported to have considerable concerns about students spending more time outside the hospital base, although there is at present little systematic information on this. There may be reasonable concern on the students' behalf that the teaching, especially of clinical skills, will not be of a consistently high standard, and that it will be difficult to maintain quality control of teachers' clinical skills. Some may be anxious that teachers will be unable to relate their teaching to the basic sciences and will not be familiar with up to date clinical research. On their own behalf they may feel that students are being deprived of adequate time to acquire the appropriate knowledge and experience of their specialty, and in the United Kingdom there is also likely to be serious anxiety about the implications for clinical care in teaching hospitals of the reallocation of funding related to teaching load out of hospitals into community settings.

Students

Students are the group most affected by curriculum change. However, it may be difficult for them to consider a major change in curriculum direction at a stage in their own careers when they have only experienced traditional hospital based teaching. Students at Kings College Hospital, London (Charles et al. 1994) attended a debate on the motion 'that it is both desirable and practical that the bulk of medical education should be taught in the community'. Relatively small numbers attended and although most students realized that a greater role for the community was necessary they felt that it was unacceptable that the bulk of medical education should be taught outside hospitals. They were anxious about losing their student identity and protected environment, about the knowledge and skills of the general practitioner teachers and about the cost and time involved in travel between sites. However, they also saw the advantage of learning a whole person approach to medicine and of working with other health professionals in a team.

Patients

Although patients attending general practitioners have become increasingly familiar with finding a student in the surgery over the last twenty years, it is still not a frequent occurrence. While in hospital a patient may have to be fairly assertive to avoid seeing students, it remains possible to offer patients in general practice genuine choice about seeing students, as there is at present no shortage of willing patients. The exceptions to this are patients with gynaecological problems, whose reluctance was described by Towle (1992) and possibly those with psychological problems. A change in the balance of teaching would create greater pressures on patients and their support for change and involvement in it, where this is possible, would be important. Pill and Tapper-Jones (1993) showed that most patients welcomed visits of students on a family attachment. Seabrook *et al.* (1994) held discussions with two patient groups and individual interviews with a small number of patients in order to assess the range of views. Patients were in general positive about seeing students, and felt that it ensured that the doctor was on their best behaviour. Other advantages of seeing a student included having someone to talk to, feeling that they were contributing to medical education and in particular giving students an opportunity to learn about how the experience of illness had affected them. They felt that it was important that they were given a real choice about whether or not to have a student in the consultation and were concerned about the risk that students could be used instead of doctors, resulting in a second class service.

Practical difficulties

In the United Kingdom these have been considered in some detail by Higgs and Jones (1995) and Towle (1992) covering the following common range of issues.

Funding

The most fundamental limiting factor to extending teaching outside hospitals at present is the availability of funding. The issues relating to this differ world-wide. In the UK the costs of teaching within teaching hospitals are currently borne by SIFT (Service Increment For Teaching) of which 80% is considered to pay for 'facilities' and 20% 'clinical placements'. Facilities costs are those which do not change when the number of students change, for example additional space, accommodation, reception staff, and equipment. Clinical placement costs refer to the opportunity costs of teaching due to carrying out this clinical work. In 1996, clinical placement funding became available for teaching outside hospital for the first time. If students spend more time learning outside hospital, it seems unlikely that they will cease to need the facilities provided within hospitals, but on the other hand, learning sites in the community need resources to provide an infrastructure for a high quality learning environment. Total facilities costs are likely to rise with a larger number of sites for learning, so to implement change without new funding, savings may have to be made in other areas.

Recruitment of teachers

The majority of teachers outside hospitals are likely to come from general or family practice. In the United Kingdom they have been paid a meagre sum for teaching, but have therefore been a self selected group of enthusiasts. With the changes in the general practitioners' contract, and increasing pressures on their time alongside higher expectations of teachers, recruitment even of these enthusiasts has become more difficult. It is clear that proper remuneration and contracts with practices to enable long term planning will be necessary to provide enough high quality teachers.

Quality of teaching

Although staff development is an area which has been variably addressed within hospital teaching, if students are to learn at a variety of different sites, the need for good programmes and continuous evaluation of teaching will intensify. Combined staff development workshops between hospital and community based teachers, as carried out in London recently (Hoffman, 1997, personal communication) have the enormous advantage of encouraging a consistent approach to teaching across a variety of learning sites. These programmes have paid attention to both clinical and educational skills, but have been implemented in a situation of adequate remuneration for teachers to ensure recruitment.

Distance from teaching hospital base

Solutions need to be found to students' anxieties about being away from the main hospital base, most of which would require additional resources. Practice bases would benefit from additional space, networked computers for students to maintain contact and good arrangements for student travel. The costs of travel for students are increasing at the same time as their financial situation is deteriorating with the current reduction in government grants and increases in direct payment of fees. Support for this is a necessity, especially if there is inequity between students.

Administration

Increasing numbers of sites for teaching will create difficulties for those who arrange timetables, co-ordinate visits to practices and other community groups, and arrange payments to teachers. Without good organization any development will fall into disrepute. Already some academic departments of general practice in the United Kingdom employ teaching co-ordinators, and they have recently formed a network to support each other (Schmedlin, personal communication).

Safety and insurance

Students may be at risk in some hospital based teaching attachments, but are not likely to be alone. Away from the hospital base they may need guidance on how to avoid and cope with potentially dangerous situations, and the legal and insurance consequences of any injury will need to be considered.

The way forward

In the light of the experience of innovative programmes outside hospitals in the United Kingdom, and some of the influences on the success or failure of these, some general recommendations can be made to aid the planning of opportunities for students to learn in a wider range of sites.

Learning sites determined by content

There should be agreement about the principles which underlie the core curriculum content, which should then be used to determine where students should learn. Learning outside hospitals would then become an integral part of the curriculum, avoiding marginalization.

Leadership and inter-disciplinary collaboration

Curriculum change requires leadership, as does the process of reaching agreement on curriculum content mentioned above. The Dean or equivalent is central to this, in providing both personal leadership and recognition for others involved, without which continued development will be impossible. Collaboration between disciplines rather than competition will avoid the spectre of teaching outside hospitals being seen as an attempt by general practice to grasp a larger slice of the curriculum pie. Collaborators should include basic scientists and social scientists as well as clinicians, to help students relate their basic science and social science education to clinical contexts, and to integrate learning in primary and secondary care. Funding arrangements may need rearrangement to allow this.

Continuity throughout medical education

Students will benefit from opportunities to learn in appropriate sites throughout their medical training, from the first year (traditionally 'preclinical') into their preregistration year in the United Kingdom or internship in the USA. This would allow maximal benefit to be gained from interdisciplinary collaboration.

Local ownership

In response to some of the concerns expressed by stakeholders as mentioned above, involvement of as many groups as possible in consultation will improve the chances of success (Grant and Gale 1989). Seabrook and colleagues (1994) pointed out that 'telling is selling': the process of engaging stakeholder groups in discussion actually increased support for curriculum change. Local ownership will enable the development of courses appropriate to local circumstances.

Staff development and assessment

In order to support such programmes, teaching should be a valued activity and staff development programmes an integral part of curriculum planning. Assessment procedures which relate directly to the content and aims of the revised programme will direct the students' learning most effectively.

Provision of appropriate sites for learning outside hospitals

Although schools are likely to move in different directions depending on local opportunities and pressures, one solution to a number of the practical difficulties of teaching and learning outside hospitals is the establishment of a number of academic primary care bases around each medical school (Royal College of General Practitioners 1994; Field and Kinmonth 1995). The example in Box 5 above is moving towards this approach. Contracts over several years could be arranged with these general or family practice bases, allowing for the provision of extra medical, nursing, and administrative staff thus encouraging recruitment. Teachers working in these practices would have a major commitment to education, and would thus be motivated to attend staff development sessions and be involved in curriculum development and the evaluation of their teaching, alongside hospital based teachers. Students attached to these large practice bases would be in greater numbers than at present, overcoming the problem of isolation. If additional space and computing facilities are to be provided, it would be appropriate to install these in major practice bases rather than spread them thinly across the region. Students could have subsidiary attachments to other practices and local community groups in the area. Collaborative teaching programmes, administration and travel, while still problems, would be easier to arrange if restricted to fewer larger sites.

This vision may gain additional strength in the United Kingdom from the concurrent moves to provide infrastructure for research in a chosen number of general practices (Pereira Gray 1995). Already some practices are offering preregistration house officer posts (Wilton 1995) and offering to host general practice registrars who are undergoing academic training (Field *et al.* unpublished report to Nuffield Provincial Hospitals' Trust 1996). Education of other health professionals might appropriately be arranged at the same sites, giving opportunities for multiprofessional education. It makes little sense for all these ventures to be set up in different practices when they have the same need for space, administrative support, and a critical mass of educators and researchers within primary care.

Conclusion

Medical students of the future, instead of having a single teaching hospital base, may rotate around a number of well equipped teaching bases, including university departments, primary care academic practices, secondary care district hospitals, and tertiary care referral centres, while also visiting people in a variety of other places. The range of sites for learning could offer a curriculum based on wide local consultation about the health care needs of the population. Collaboration between teachers could allow learning in the basic and social sciences to be related to the context in which it will be used, and could help students to understand individual patients' health care needs in both primary and secondary care, integrating their education in and out of hospital. Only if such a range of opportunities for learning can be provided can future doctors hope to be prepared to care for all of us.

References

Barrows, H.S., and Tamblyn, R.M. (1980). *Problem-based learning*. Springer, New York.

Brookfield, S. (1986). *Understanding and facilitating adult learning: a comprehensive analysis of principles and effective practices*. Open University Press, Milton Keynes.

Charles T., Hassan, S., and Scott, R. (1994). Students' attitudes towards increased community-based teaching. In *Widening the horizons of medical education*, (eds M., Seabrook, P., Booton and T., Evans), pp.00–00 Kings Fund, London.

Cohen, J., Dannefer, E.F., Seidel, H.M., Weisman, C.S., Wexler, P., Brown, T.M. *et al.* (1994). Medical education change: a detailed study of six medical schools. *Medical Education*, **28**, 350–60.

Coles, C.R. (1990). Elaborated learning in undergraduate medical education. *Medical Education*, **24**, 14–22.

Field, J., and Kinmonth, A.L. (1995). Learning medicine in the community. *British Medical Journal*, **310**, 343–4.

Fine, B. (1994). GP's attitudes towards CBME (sic) In *Widening the horizons of medical education*, (ed. M., Seabrook, P., Booton and T., Evans). pp.66–75 Kings Fund, London.

Fraser, R.C. and Preston-Whyte, M.E. (1988). *The contribution of academic general practice to undergraduate medical education*. Royal College of General Practitioners, London. (Occasional Paper 42).

Freeman, G.K. and Coles, C.R. (1982). The preregistration houseman in general practice. *British Medical Journal*, **310**, 369–71.

General Medical Council (1993). *Recommendations on undergraduate medical education*. General Medical Council, London.

Glick, S.M. (1991). Problem-based learning and community oriented medical education. *Medical Education*, **25**, 542–5.

Graham, H.J. and Seabrook, M. (1994). *Structured learning packs for medical students*. King's College School of Medicine and Dentistry, London.

Graham, H.J. and Seabrook, M. (1995). Structured packs for independent learning in the community. *Medical Education*, **29**, 61–5.

Grant, J. and Gale, R. (1989). Changing medical education. *Medical Education*, **23**, 252–7.

Higgs, R. and Jones, R. (1995). The impacts of increased general practice teaching in the undergraduate medical curriculum. *Education for General Practice*, **6**, 218–25.

Honigsbaum F., Richards, J. and Lockett, T. (1995). Priority setting in action: purchasing dilemmas. Radcliffe, Oxford.

Iliffe, S. (1992). All that is solid melts into air: the implications of community based undergraduate medical education. *British Journal of General Practice*, **42**, 390–3.

Jee, M. (1994). The implications for community health services and the primary care team. In: *Widening the horizons of medical education*, (ed. M. Seabrook, P. Booton and T. Evans). pp.75–83. Kings Fund, London.

Kantrowitz, M., Kaufmann A., Mennin S., Fulop T., and Guilbert, J.-J., (1987). *Innovative tracks at established institutions for the education of health personnel*. WHO Offset Publications No 101, Geneva.

Kitzhaber, J.A. (1993). Prioritising health services in an era of limits: the Oregon experience. In *Rationing in action*. (ed. R. Smith). BMA publishing group, London.

Knowles, M.S. (1975). Self-directed learning: a guide for learners and teachers. Cambridge Books, New York.

McCrorie P., Lefford F., and Perrin F. (1993). Medical undergraduate comminuty-based teaching: a survey for ASME on current and proposed teaching in the community and in general practice in UK Universities. ASME Occasional Publication No 3, ASME, Dundee.

McKee, M. and Figueras, J. (1996). Setting priorities: can Britain learn from Sweden? *British Medical Journal*, **312**, 691–4.

Metcalfe, G.C., Bain, D.J.G., Freeman, G.K., and Rowe, L.J. (1983). Teaching primary medical care in Southampton: the first decade. *Lancet*, **i**, 697–9.

Murray, E., Jenks, V., and Modell, M. (1995). Community based medical education: feasibility and cost. *Medical Education*, **29**, 66–71.

Murray, E., Jolly, B.C. and Modell, M. (1997) Can students learn clinical method in general practice: a randomised cross-over trial. *British Medical Journal*, **31**, 920–23.

Oswald, N. (1989). Why not base clinical education in general practice? *Lancet*, **2**, 148–9.

Oswald, N., Jones, S., Date, J., and Hinds, D. (1995). Long term community attachments: the Cambridge course. *Medical Education*, **29**, 72–6.

Pereira Gray, D. (1995). Research general practices. *British Journal of General Practice*, **45**, 516–17.

Pill, R. and Tapper-Jones, L.M. (1993). An unwelcome visitor? The opinions of mothers involved in a community-based teaching project. *Medical Education*, **27**, 238–44.

Richards R. and Fulop T. (1987). *Innovative schools for health personnel*. WHO Offset Publication no 102, Geneva.

Rowntree D. (1987). *Assessing students: how shall we know them?* Kogan Page, London.

Royal College of General Practitioners (1994). Conference of academic organizations in general practice. Research and general practice. RCGP, London.

Royal Commission on Medical Education (1968). HM Stationery Office, London.

Schamroth, A., and Haines, A.P. (1992). Student assessment of clinical experience in general surgery. *Medical Teacher*, **14**, 355–62.

Seabrook, M., Booton, P., and Evans, T. (ed) (1994). *Widening the horizons of medical education*. King's Fund, London.

Silver, G.A. (1983). Victim or villain. *Lancet*, **ii**, 960.

Spiegal, N., Murphy, E., Kinmonth, A-L., Ross, F., Bain, J., and Coates, R. (1991). Managing change in general practice: a step by step guide. *British Medical Journal*, **304**, 231–4.

Towle, A. (ed.) (1992). *Community based teaching*. King's Fund, London.

University of Liverpool (1995). *New undergraduate medical curriculum 1996*. University Medical Education Unit, Liverpool.

Whitehouse, C.R. (1991). The teaching of communication skills in UK Medical Schools. *Medical Education*, **25**, 311–18.

Wilton, J. (1995). Preregistration house officers in general practice. *British Medical Journal*, **310**, 369–71.

World Health Organization (1978). *Alma-Ata 1978: primary health care*. WHO, Geneva.

World Health Organization (1987). *Community-based education of health personnel*. Report of a WHO Study Group. WHO Technical Report Series 746.

Wykurz, G. (1992). In Community based teaching, (ed. A. Towle), pp. 9–11. King's Fund, London.

4.2 The Internet ward round

Jeannette Murphy, David Ingram, and William Howard

Introduction

The end of the twentieth century will doubtless be remembered as the age of the Internet. In a few short years, the Net has gone from being a vehicle for scientific communication, to a playground for the many. Phrases such as 'information superhighway', 'surfing the Net', and 'navigating through cyberspace' have become part of everyday vocabulary. Those who are not connected feel that they are not part of the modern world. Faced with this rapidly expanding information warehouse, educationalists are trying to decide whether the Internet is in fact a cornucopia of new learning resources. And if it is, how do we tap into this resource? How do we integrate it into the curriculum?

This chapter seeks to explore these questions and to achieve three outcomes. First, it sets out to explain the Internet to medical educationalists; secondly, it considers ways in which the Internet can deliver new resources and new learning opportunities to medical students. The final goal is to suggest what needs to be done to make effective use of Internet resources.

After a brief look at the way in which the Internet has evolved, the chapter reviews some general issues relating to the place of electronic learning resources such as Medline, databases, and computer-assisted learning packages (CAL) in the curriculum. Having established a framework for thinking about digital tools and resources, we move on to survey Internet sites which provide useful material for medical students and clinical tutors. Discussion groups and mailing lists are also covered. The subsequent section suggests what actions educationalists must take in order to harness the Internet to their curriculum objectives. Since the Net offers the opportunity to be both information users *and* information providers, the chapter also considers what is involved in providing information. The penultimate section looks at the problems associated with the Internet. The chapter ends with a brief consideration of technological developments which have implications for medical education.

Throughout the chapter the emphasis is on how to *use* the Internet as an educational resource; coverage of technical issues have been omitted. Readers wanting coverage of *technical matters* should consult *Medicine and the Internet* by Bruce McKenzie (1996).

The Internet and the World Wide Web

What exactly is the Internet? Essentially the Internet is a vast number of world-wide INTERconnected computer NETworks which all communicate with each other. This network of networks makes it possible for information to be exchanged freely through a complex Web of computers located throughout the world. A fundamental consequence of this decentralization is that no one agency, corporation or country owns it. However, a common communication language, Transmission Control Protocol/Internet Protocol (*TCP/IP*), ensures that different computers are able to exchange information.

The Internet began as one computer network in 1969, designed to link the US Department of Defense to researchers, contractors, and universities. As independent and private networks were established, they were added to the world-wide hook-up of smaller networks called the Internet. In the early 1980s, the US National Science Foundation decided to create a system of five national supercomputer centres to serve the research community and to link the centres to all the American campuses via a long-distance network. Although the initial idea was that the network would allow research-ers to gain access to supercomputers from a distance, it soon became apparent that the network could be a tool for general scientific communication.

Given the nature of the Internet, there is no way to determine its precise size. However, there is evidence that the number of users is growing exponentially. According to an article in *Information Week*, there will be one billion users world-wide by the end of the 1990s (*Information Week* 1995, p.30).

Until the early 1990s, the major factor restricting the use of the Net was the lack of a central point for finding out what information is available. This lack of an easy way of searching and retrieving documents discouraged all but the computer-literate from exploring the resources available. This began to change with the arrival of tools such as WAIS (Wide Area Information Server), Archie, and Gopher. While this software was a step in the right direction, there were still limitations, especially the fact that only textual information could be displayed.

The World Wide Web

The World Wide Web (WWW), the first flexible, easy-to-use information retrieval processor, opened the resources of the Net to a much wider group of users. The Web has two main advantages over earlier systems:

1. It is 'hypertextual' which means that documents may be linked to other sources of information. Each link contains the name of the document being referenced, the address of the computer where it can be found and the method required to access it. These links are also known as Uniform Resource Locators (URLs). All of this is transparent to the user who simply clicks on a highlighted word to retrieve the document. The end result is a 'Web' of information.
2. It supports multimedia so that pictures, sound, and text can be displayed.

Two associated developments which helped to open up the Internet to a wider community were *Hyptertext Markup Language (HTML)* and a program called

Mosaic. Hypertext Markup Language is a format which standardizes the structure and layout of information in a document. Mosaic is a browser that makes it possible to access the Web using a graphical interface controlled with a mouse. Since Mosaic appeared in 1992, the choice of browsers has expanded; in the academic world Netscape has become the most popular browser.

Costs

At present Internet users pay only for access to the network, not for the amount of information transferred. For most academic users, the Internet is effectively 'free' since their access charges are paid by their employers in much the same way telephone charges are. Users can send as many messages, read as many files, and access as many databases as they like—anywhere in the world! Whether the Internet will continue to be free is uncertain. Some predict that interactive applications such as real-time, interactive video conferencing (which demand huge data rates) may lead to different grades of services.

The culture of the Net

Why do people make news, information, or personal profiles available on the Net? The Net has fostered a culture of open information exchange and has evolved a culture of sharing information and giving help. 'That commitment to information sharing survives today in people's willingness to post information on the Internet where anyone else can freely access it through browsers . . .' (Waldrop, 1994, p.880)

The question is whether this culture will survive as commercial organizations take an interest in the Net. Some predict that the nature of the Net will change and users will be required to pay for every character they send or receive.

Electronic learning resources: an overview

Although the Internet offers a whole range of new learning experiences and opportunities to medical students, it would be parochial to view the Net in isolation from other learning resources. In planning how to integrate Internet resources into the curriculum, educationalists need to think in terms of a continuum of learning resources. This studyscape consists of all the traditional resources (books, journals, patients, tutors), as well as old technologies (videos, slides, audio cassettes), and finally, electronic resources. This latter category includes:

♦ computer-assisted learning packages (CAL) e.g. tutorials, simulations
♦ computerized assessment packages, e.g. *QuestionMark*
♦ electronic textbooks, manuals, and atlases, e.g. *Textbook of Dermatology* on CD ROM; *Pathology TextStacks*
♦ standard software tools, e.g. wordprocessing, graphics, spreadsheets, databases, presentation packages, statistical packages
♦ bibliographic databases, e.g. Medline and CINAHL (Cumulative Index to Nursing and Allied Health Literature)

- Other databases, e.g. eBNF (Electronic British National Formulary); Toxline; Aidsline; the Cochrane Database
- image banks, e.g. The National Slide Bank of Medicine
- decision support systems, e.g. Iliad, DXplain, Quick Medical Reference (QMR)
- electronic patient records
- computer conferencing, telemedicine
- the Internet, e.g. e-mail, news groups, telnet file transfer protocols, the World Wide Web.

Educationalists who are new to this area and want further information should contact the CTI Centre for Medicine (CTICM) in Bristol, a nationally funded initiative to promote the use of computer-based learning resources in medical education (CTICM@bristol.ac.uk). The centre produces a regular newsletter and a resource directory. Staff in the Centre for Health Informatics and Multiprofessional Education (CHIME) are another source of advice (http:chime.ucl.ac.uk). You might also want to obtain a copy of the GHIFT database which contains information and resources to support education and training programmes in health informatics. This was funded by the Programme Board for the Education and Training of Clinicians in Information management and technology (IM&T). The GHIFT site is http://www.chime.ucl.ac.uk/GHIFT/. Finally, it is worth becoming acquainted with three other UK initiatives which have funded the production of courseware, templates, and other electronic resources: the Teaching and Learning Technology Project (TLTP) (http:www.tltp.ac.uk/tltp/); the Joint Information Systems Committee (JISC) which issues a catalogue of resources; and the Information Technology Teaching Initiative (ITTI) which also has a catalogue of products.

Some members of faculty may be inclined to dismiss these electronic resources on the grounds that they are untested and their benefits not proven. Tutors who are wrestling with the problems of designing and implementing a new curriculum, may feel that electronic resources do not come very high on their agenda. Staff who feel overwhelmed by the pace of change in medical education may perceive electronic resources more as a threat than as an exciting new opportunity. These technologies may be seen as diverting money from tried and tested means of delivering education, or as undermining the authority of tutors, or of taking students away from patients.

As more departments, tutors, and students gain experience in using electronic resources, some of these problems may resolve themselves. There are indications that only a minority of tutors are resistant to the introduction of new learning resources. Innovative medical schools are showing how computers can be used to support and enhance medical education. Schools such as Liverpool, Aberdeen, and Newcastle in the UK and The University of Washington (Seattle), Georgetown, and Harvard in the USA have started to explore ways of using electronic resources to support self-directed learning and problem-based learning.

Whatever your starting point with respect to technology-based learning, electronic resources pose a common set of challenges to curriculum developers and clinical tutors. There are eight issues which need to be addressed.

Table 4.1 Challenges posed by electronic learning resources

- ◆ Leadership of these developments
- ◆ Monitoring the quality of resources
- ◆ Infrastructure to access new resources
- ◆ Staff development
- ◆ Training and support for students
- ◆ Ethical and legal concerns
- ◆ Production of new learning resources
- ◆ Evaluating the learning outcomes

Leadership: organizational policy

The advent of new learning resources requires an institution-wide response. Instead of relying on individuals to informally assume the role of coordinating initiatives and developing an information strategy, deans of medical schools need to designate one individual to assume a leadership role. Those who are appointed to such positions need to work closely with curriculum committees, user groups, and service providers (librarians, computer services, etc.). They also need to maintain links with relevant groups outside the medical faculty and to keep abreast of trends in technology to ensure that there is a fit between the information needs of faculty and students (generated by the local curriculum) and the infrastructure in place for delivering information.

Quality of information

In a world of information explosion, the quality of the information is a matter of considerable concern. New learning materials need to be monitored both in relation to content and to ease of use. With the Internet, anyone is free to disseminate information.

> Because little of the medical information on the Internet is original research, most of the information is not peer reviewed in the manner traditionally used by medical journals. Publishers of medical journals own the copyright to articles they publish, and few of these journals make their articles publicly available over the Internet. In most cases the quality of the information on the Internet is determined solely by the institutions and individual persons who publish it. *Glowniak 1995, p.126*

Students will need help to develop the necessary critical appraisal skills to enable them to scan material rapidly and to distinguish between high quality information and less credible offerings.

Infrastructure

Electronic learning resources require an investment in infrastructure. To deliver these resources medical schools must provide computers, software, and networks. Computer labs and learning resource centres need to be staffed, and equipment needs to be maintained and renewed. If computer-based resources are to support the curriculum, students must be able to access resources wherever they happen to be studying: in the library, the laboratory, the ward, student residences, local family practices, out-patient clinics, or community health settings. Soon we will need to provide network access for students who come to medical school with their own machines.

Staff development

If tutors feel confident about using new learning resources, they will be motivated to seek ways to incorporate these resources into their modules. Although many basic medical scientists and clinicians are *au fait* with emerging technologies, it is a mistake to regard this group of experts as representative of the whole faculty. Medical educationalists need to survey staff expertise; such information should inform staff development programmes.

Workshops should not just focus on the technology and software design, but should also address the issue of how students could be expected to use these resources.

Support for students

Students need encouragement and incentives to use the electronic tools provided by medical schools. They may require help to develop both computer literacy and information handling skills (at least for the next several years). Because students vary enormously in terms of prior exposure to information technologies, there needs to be a variety of training materials and learning opportunities (ranging from structured tuition to self-help sheets). Unless students are provided with appropriate support, there is a danger that they may waste valuable time using these tools inefficiently. (This is particularly true of the Internet where the novice can easily get lost in cyberspace!) Negative experiences may lead students to avoid using these resources. Librarians have a key role to play in introducing students to electronic resources. As for incentives, module convenors and curriculum managers will need to consider the link between assessment methods and electronic learning resources.

Ethical and legal concerns

Electronic resources raise a variety of ethical and legal concerns. First, as electronic patient record systems (containing both administrative and clinical data) are introduced, medical schools, trusts, and professional bodies will need to agree an ethical framework to regulate the way in which electronic patient data is used in teaching hospitals. Patient consent needs to be obtained if their data is to be used for teaching purposes. (For a discussion of these issues see Murphy *et al.* 1993.)

Secondly, copyright, citation, and rules of conduct in the field of electronic communication need to be addressed. Copyright issues arise in the production of learning resources. Obtaining rights to use images and text in electronic publications will need to be carefully negotiated. (See Brennan *et al.*, 1996 for an analysis of what steps need to be taken.) Ways of citing electronic publications are starting to evolve; McKenzie (1996, pp.52–8) provides a very clear guide to matters relating to copyright and citation.

Networks enable medical schools and trusts to share information and allow students, administrators, and clinicians to connect to the Internet. In addition to the benefits, there are potential security problems. Personal and institutional data must be protected from access by unauthorized users. Although outside the remit of medical education, issues of safeguarding data, and protecting against viruses will arise in discussion with computer service departments.

Production of resources

Learning resources may be produced in-house, developed through academic consortia or purchased from commercial publishers. If readers are thinking about becoming involved in producing CD ROMs or other materials, they would be well advised to seek help from those who have experience of such projects. If you are unable to identify expertise in your medical school or university, the CTI in Bristol will be able to put you in contact with appropriate project groups.

Evaluation strategies

Medical education units play an important role in developing strategies for evaluating the impact of electronic resources on learning outcomes. This is a long-term exercise, as distinct from reviewing a particular package or tool. Such evaluations need to be linked to ongoing curriculum review, staff development, and academic audit.

Medical resources on the Internet: URL sites to explore

What makes the Internet of interest to the world of medical education is that it provides fast, free access to a large collection of technical, scientific, educational, and biomedical resources. This section seeks to provide an overview of these resources, and draws attention to some useful starting points for educationalists wanting to get an overview as to what is available. The library or computer service unit should be able to provide any help needed to access these resources. Full addresses of all the sites mentioned in this section are provided in the appendix to this chapter.

Uniform Resource Locators (URLs)

One term used in this discussions of Internet resources is URL, which stands for Uniform Resource Locator. All files on the Internet are classified by the method by which they are accessed and their location on a specific computer. This format is called the Uniform Resource Locator (URL) of the file. Web browsers use URLs to locate files. The **.html** extension to the filename (or possibly just **.htm** if the Web server is running Windows New Technology—NT) indicates an HTML document.

URLs must be typed exactly! If a URL does not work, check the spelling and the case. If a filename has changed, related information may be found by dropping the filename and ending the URL with the '/' symbol. If access is required to any of the sites listed in the appendix to this chapter, type in the complete URL.

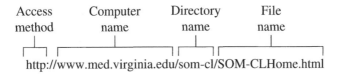

gopher://gopher.dfci.harvard.edu

Fig. 4.1 Components of a Uniform Resource Locator (URL). World Wide Web browsers use this format to locate documents. The leftmost set of characters identifies the mode of access. For the World Wide Web, the access method is the hypertext transport protocol (*http*). Other common access methods are telnet, FTP (file transfer protocol), and gopher. A colon and two forward slashes follow the access method. The next entries are 1) a computer name: 2) the directories that lead to the document, with entries separated by forward slashes; and 3) the name of the document or file. If the directory path and file name are omitted, as in the second example, the main menu or Web page at the site is displayed. Glowniak, 1995.

Finding resources

Methods of classifying or indexing documents on the Internet are still evolving. Because the Internet has no central controlling agency, there are no official registers of resources. However, several organizations have compiled indexes of Internet resources and have developed free search programs.

Internet catalogues and 'Virtual libraries' are good starting points for locating information to support the curriculum. Some Internet sites (for example medical schools) contain pointers to available medical resources (see Table 4.2).

Table 4.2 A selection of useful places for starting a search for material to support curricula

HyperDOC: National Institutes of Health's Online Information Services. This is the National Library of Medicine's gateway to Internet medical resources. **http://www.nih.gov/**

Martindale's Health Science Guide: a guide to Internet Resources on medicine and health care. (Also known as The 'Virtual' Medical Centre)
http://www-sci.lib.uci.edu/~martindale/Medical.html

Medical Matrix: A Guide to Internet Medical Resources. A database of clinical medicine resources on the internet, categorised by disease and specialty. Contains hypertext links. Sponsored by the Internet Working group of the American Medical Informatics Association.
http://www.medmatrix.org/Index/asp

Medical Resources. Good links to other sites. Bulletin Board for UK Libraries.
http://www.link.bubl.ac.uk/medicine

MedWeb Biomedical Resources (Emory University). A catalogue of resources on medicine and health care. **http://www.gen.emory.edu/MEDWEB/medweb.html**

OMNI (Organising Medical Networked Information Project). Project seeks to build a UK gateway to sources of biomedical information. Project brings together major UK organisations in the field of biomedical information. It aims to be a quality service, filtering, cataloguing and subject-indexing resources before they are added to the gateway. **http://www.omni.ac.uk/**

Physicians' Choice. A medical website which seeks to identify the most useful medical Web sites. Sites are reviewed by doctors. The reviews emphasize the quality and quantity of original content and its utility for the practising physician. **http://www.mdchoice.com/**

Virtual Library for Medicine: Oregon Health Sciences University host the medical section of CERN's World-Wide Web Virtual Library. **http://www.ohsu.edu/cliniweb/wwwvl/**

Yahoo (Stanford University) A general purpose search engine. Easy to use.
http://www.yahoo.com/Health/

Types of resources available for medical education

In searching the Internet, it is useful to have a conceptual map of the different types of resources available. Table 4.3 classifies Internet resources which are likely to be of interest to clinicians, students, and medical researchers. It is an amalgamation of a scheme devised by Robert Kiley, health sciences librarian at Frimley Park Hospital NHS Trust and one used by Bruce McKenzie (1996).

Table 4.3 Classification of Internet sites

Main types of sites	Examples of sites
Pointer sites: virtual libraries, catalogues, indexes	See list in Table 4.2
Academic sites (medical schools)	A list of world-wide medical schools on the WWW is available on: http://www.anat.dote.hu/~tore/medfak/
	Check the home page of your university or medical school
Agencies: key national and international health sites	Centre for Disease Control; National Institute of Health (USA); Medical Research Council (UK); UK Department of Health; National Library of Medicine; World Health Organisation
Clinical practice guidelines; protocols	Agency for Health Policy and Research (AHCPR) — seventeen clinical practice guidelines
Clinical specialties	Anaesthetics; general practice; neurology; oncology; public health
Databases	Genetics, immunology
Diseases	Cancer
Education: interactive teaching resources	From anaesthesiology to The virtual hospital and The visible human project
A list of URL addresses of useful sites is provided at the end of the chapter Electronic journals	*BMJ; JAMA; Journal of Epidemiology and Community Health*
Evidence-based medicine	Centre for Evidence Based Medicine (Oxford); Cochrane Centre; EBM Home Page (McMaster)
Image databases	Dermatology, haematology, The whole brain atlas
Patient education	Breast Cancer Information Clearing House; National Cancer Institute's patient information sheets
Primary health care	FAM-MED; UK primary care

Using bookmarks

As readers explore these various sites to locate material which may be relevant to their curriculum, they will want to be able to mark any they find interesting. Bookmarks (or hotlists) are a way of storing the URLs of WWW pages which might like be visited again. When a page is saved as a bookmark, it is added to a pull-down list where it can be selected the next time a visit is made to that site. This saves having to manually file the address and later retype it. Some Web browsers (e.g.Netscape) allow saving bookmarks as an HTML document, thereby making it possible to share your favourite sites with colleagues or students.

Other resources: E-mail, newsgroups, and discussion groups

Although the World Wide Web has gained the lion's share of attention, educationalists and tutors should also direct students towards the other communication tools available through the Net. Soon all medical students will have e-mail accounts and should be given guidance as to how best to use this facility. Faculty should point out ways in which e-mail can be used to support group work, making it easy for members of a tutorial or seminar group to share resources and to communicate with one another. Thought should also be given to how individual tutors might use e-mail to communicate with their groups (Duffy *et al.* 1995).

Students should also be made aware of the various electronic discussion groups and how they operate. They will need instruction in using file-transfer protocols (FTP) if they are to retrieve stored files in the public domain.

Two other potentially useful resources for medical students are newsgroups and mailing lists. Both are an extension of electronic mail and offer a means of communicating with others about medical and health-related subjects. Postings (i.e. earlier mailings) may be archived and there are often collections of FAQs (frequently asked questions) both of which can be searched. The difference between the two forums is that messages to newsgroups are *not* delivered to the user's mailbox, while messages in mailing lists are.

Newsgroups

A User's Network facility (USENET) is dedicated exclusively to discussion groups. New messages created at one site, are passed to other sites which choose to carry that particular newsgroup. The phrase *news*groups, as McKenzie points out, is something of a misnomer; the postings to most groups are not 'news' in the usual sense of the word. Of the thousands of groups which have been set up, more than one hundred have a health-related or medical focus. For medical educationalists, the most relevant groups are those which are designated as **sci.med.**—for example sci.med.radiology, sci.med.immunology and sci.med.pathology. Another newsgroup of interest to medical educationalists is **misc.education.medical**.

Newsgroups provide a way of answering a query when the information cannot be found either on the WWW or through conventional information sources. As anyone can read or post messages to these groups, the quality of information can be quite variable.

Some newsgroups are set up so that the titles of the postings (or 'articles') can be searched and only those of interest need to be downloaded and read. For a useful overview of these groups see Lincoln (1995) and for details on how to subscribe and search see McKenzie (1996).

Mailing lists

Mailing lists are a variant of personal e-mail. Each message sent to the list is automatically forwarded to all other participants. To join a list and receive messages, you e-mail a specially formatted request to the list. This process is referred to as 'subscribing' to the list. To contribute to a mailing list, you send an e-mail message with your comments to a special software program (often called a listserver) on the host computer. The listserver then automatically forwards the message to a list of e-mail addresses belonging to discussion group members (stored in the listserver software).

Glowniak (1995) suggests that mailing and lists provide some of the most varied and specific medical information on the Internet. Kleeberg and Masys (1995) have identified 300 medically related discussion group on the Net, and the number is growing rapidly (see Table 4.4).

Table 4.4 Discussion groups: medicine and health

Discussion groups of interest to medical students	
Addiction	Immunizations
Ageing	Medical students
AIDS	Nursing homes
Autism	Parkinson disease
Cancer	Schizophrenia
Clinical alerts	Stroke
Cystic fibrosis	Student health
Diabetes	Women's health
Emergency medicine	
Fitness	
Health management	
Health reform	

What is the value of these resources to students? Mailing lists and newsgroups can be used to '*eavesdrop*' in that they provide a chance to hear different views, listen in on debates, and find out what people in different medical schools and teaching hospitals think. Students can also be more active by putting questions to others, asking for help, and seeking other sources of information. Since new educational methods such as problem-based learning and evidence-based medicine stress the importance of learning how to formulate questions, a resource which allows students to ask questions and which provides very rich feedback is immensely valuable. Once students have mastered the basics of using the Internet and are primed on 'netiquette', the Internet offers unrivalled opportunities to engage in global tutorials.

So what must medical schools do to embed these resources in the curriculum? Table 4.5 describes ways of preparing students to use these resources.

Various internet sites provide details on how to find useful mailing lists. Tile.Net is a good place to start: http://tile.net/lists/. The Johns Hopkins Medical School Library site provides general information about Discussion Lists and Newsgroups: http://www.welch.jhu.edu/help/guides/wii/lists.html

Table 4.5 Encouraging students to use news groups and mailing lists

- ♦ Alert students to their existence
- ♦ Ensure students know how to join
- ♦ Introduce students to basic 'netiquette'
- ♦ Introduce students to archives and FAQs
- ♦ Initiate discussions on how to pose questions
- ♦ Warn students about information overload

How to harness the Internet to your curriculum objectives

The traditional approach to medical education has been to provide *all* the resources students required to carry out their studies on site. These resources have evolved from traditional libraries with books and journals, through to tapeslides and videos, to modern clinical skills laboratories equipped with mannequins, simulated patients, and communication suites, to computer labs with standard packages and courseware designed to support the curriculum, and, most recently, to learning resource centres. And, of course, hospital wards, with real patients, are a fundamental resource for clinical teaching.

Changes in the usage and range of learning resources provided to students are closely linked to rethinking about *what* should be taught (the content of the curriculum) and *how* it should be taught (teaching methods). In the UK, in the wake of the General Medical Council's review of medical education, and in the USA after the publication of '*Physicians for the twenty-first century*', all medical schools are seeking ways of reducing the amount of didactic teaching. Approaches to medical education such as problem-based learning, evidence-based medicine, and community-based medical education have implications for the types of learning resources required. The vision that has emerged requires a learning environment (or studyscape) where students find it easy to locate and use the resources that are appropriate to their learning needs and style. How does the Internet fit with this rethinking of medical education? What kind of learning resources can it provide? And what actions are needed to prepare students to use this resource?

Internet resources differ from more traditional resources in two important ways. First, they are not physically present on the campus. With the Internet we start to move towards a 'virtual' library or 'virtual' campus. Second, students need to become proficient in using electronic tools to access these resources and to find material relevant to their needs. In traditional educational programmes, students have been expected to develop two types of knowledge:

- Factual/theoretical knowledge—knowing *about* things
- Procedural knowledge—knowing *how* to do things (clinical skills)

The shift towards self-directed learning, and problem-based learning requires new knowledge and skills. Tomorrow's doctors must know *where* to access information and *how* to assess its validity and usefulness. The Internet makes similar demands: to make efficient use of the resources students must be able to analyse their information needs and to retrieve useful information from the vast amount available online.

How might students use the Internet?

To answer this question, we need to analyse the range of activities students routinely carry out and then see how the Internet can provide resources to support these activities. Table 4.6 identifies the main types of activities which students are asked to carry out.

Table 4.6 Examples of routine student activities

- Work as a group on a problem
- Engage in self-directed learning, e.g. research a topic such as the rise of tuberculosis
- Carry out a literature review
- Prepare a poster or leaflet for a community clinic or voluntary agency
- Write an essay
- Prepare a presentation for a group of health workers
- Design a research project
- Draft a research proposal
- Carry out a small piece of research
- Complete a grant application
- Design a questionnaire
- Critique and redesign a form used in general practice
- Design a clinical trial
- Specify the ethical and legal issues for a given domain (e.g. geriatric medicine)
- Design and carry out a clinical audit
- Take a patient's history
- Record patient information in case notes
- Make a case presentation
- Assess the relevance of evidence to patient management
- Develop a treatment plan
- Develop patient education material
- Prepare for an examination

The balance of these activities, of course, will vary from school to school and as schools experiment with variants of problem-based learning, activities will shift to meet the new course objectives. However, irrespective of local variations, the Internet is likely to prove a valuable resource for both tutors and students because it provides instant access to a wide range of case material for problem-based learning. (Tutors in problem-based curricula often note the difficulties of generating useful case material for teaching purposes.)

Problem-based learning places great demands on resources: working notes must be printed; images and reports need to be collected and stored; there must be coordinated distribution and retrieval of resources. Finally, all these resources must be revised and kept up-to-date. The Internet is cheap and multiple users can access the same resources simultaneously. It is possible for medical schools to set up pages which act as gateways to both local and global resources to support the curriculum. Here are some examples of such sites: Ben Gurian University of the Negev (http://medic.bgu.ac.il/med.edu/); Stanford University's MedWorld (http://www-med.stanford.edu/medworld/home/) and the University of California, Irvine (http://meded.com.uci.edu:80/)

Using the Internet as a learning tool

Despite the apparent differences in the nature of the tasks assigned to students, from the students' point of view the common requirement is to find relevant information. Using the Internet, medical students can access a wide range of information sources, and different types of information. Table 4.7 summarizes the various sources of information available on the Internet.

Table 4.7 Information sources and learning opportunities

Information sources on the Internet	Interactive learning opportunities
Electronic textbooks	Tutorials
Electronic journals	Interactive student lounge
Treatment protocols e.g. online database of the National	Case presentations; case studies; simulated patients
Cancer Institute's PDQ (Physician Data Query)	Medical images
Databases: bibliographic and other	Exams and quizzes
Patient education material	Discussion groups or newsgroups
Educational software programs	Virtual hospital
Study guides	Journal clubs
Teaching files	
Handbooks	

How Internet resources can supplement traditional resources

The Internet has some distinct advantages over traditional paper/library-based resources:

- It is cheap (or free).

- Under optimal conditions it is fast and convenient. There is no need to go to a special library, fill in request cards, or make photocopies—you can do it all from your computer.
- It provides access to up-to-date materials from government health departments, medical schools, research groups, and commercial organizations around the world.
- It allows students to make contact with other medical students and doctors around the world. They can listen in on or take part in global discussions.
- It enables students to obtain national clinical guidelines which can be compared with local practice.

Preparing students to trawl the Net

In courses which espouse the methods and concepts of problem-based learning, or evidence-based medicine, or which seek to engender self-directed learners, the ability to find and evaluate facts becomes much more significant than the ability to memorize facts. Helping students to know how to find and retrieve information become key learning objectives.

What must be done to prepare students to use the Internet in an efficient and effective manner? What skills are required to navigate this massive information base? To use the Internet, students will need to develop:

- an ability to assess their information needs in relation to the task in hand;
- an ability to formulate a problem so that they can search for information;
- an ability to identify and retrieve relevant information;
- critical appraisal skills;
- computer literacy.

What this analysis suggests is that medical schools must develop a coherent plan on how best to integrate Internet resources into the curriculum. When should students be permitted access? (During induction week? In their first tutorial? Later in the term?) What type of documentation should be produced? Should there be workshops? Who should be responsible for showing students these resources and providing guidance on how to use them effectively? (Librarians? subject tutors? small group facilitators?)

In the absence of a planned approach, it is likely that students will just be told to 'surf the Net'. This would be time-consuming and an abdication of academic responsibility. It would be far better to provide guidance, and set structured tasks with opportunities for discussion and feedback. Given their expertise in organizing information, in teaching search techniques and in evaluating sources, medical librarians should be part of any working groups which are developing materials and they should be viewed as part of the teaching team.

There are a set of standard questions which students need to be primed to ask: Is the source (or author) credible or reputable? Should I cross check the information against other information sources? What should I do if it contradicts what I've heard in lectures, or read in a course textbook or class handouts? Has the information been peer-reviewed in any way? Is there evidence, or citations to back up the claims? When was the information compiled and when was it last updated? Why is the information being provided?

A summary of the educational issues

If the 'Internet ward round' is to become a reality, medical schools will need to do more than simply provide networks and terminals. As mentioned earlier in this chapter, at the organizational level schools need to address a range of issues.

1. Staff development

The challenge is to ensure that all members of faculty become conversant with Internet resources. This goal is allied to the need to provide opportunities for staff to become computer literate. Training in the use of information tools needs to be seen as an ongoing activity rather than a one-off event so that tutors are able to keep up with advances in technology and feel that they are on a par with the student body. Staff development may be provided within the medical school or by central university. All newly appointed members of staff should be expected to attend training courses or workshops on the Internet which covers both the technology and how to navigate, as well as the educational issues. It is especially important that the needs of clinical tutors are met so that they are aware of what is available and know how to direct students to the relevant resources.

In designing courses for staff, it is important to have a clear idea of what they are seeking. Do they want a general overview? Are they looking for resources which could support a particular module? Are they wanting to set up pages with links to relevant sites? Do they want to become information providers?

2. An educational policy for integrating Internet resources into the curriculum

Internet resources will not have been purpose designed for your curriculum. Thought needs to be given as to how to embed and customize these resources to suit the local curriculum. Curriculum committees need to consider how Internet resources, along with locally produced electronic resources, are to be used to support the learning objectives of individual modules. Attention must be given to where these resources fit in with more traditional learning resources such as textbooks, journals, and locally produced reading lists. In the future, Internet resources will need to be considered when advising students what materials they should examine. The important message is that schools need a plan to integrate Internet resources into the curriculum.

3. Preparing students

In some respects the needs of students and tutors overlap. Both need training to enable them to make the best use of Internet resources. At the outset, the novice will probably find it useful to consult a 'A Master Resource' such as The Medical List or Medical Matrix (USA). OMNI (Organizing medical networked information project) is a UK initiative which seeks to build a UK gateway to sources of biomedical information. The next step will be to browse through some of the medical resources to get a feel for what is available. In the initial stages, you may want to direct students to those sites which have been designed for medical students.

New users may also find it profitable to engage in self-directed learning using one of the tutorial packages available on the Internet. One set of materials prepared in the UK is called TONIC (The Online Netskills Interactive Course). Information is available at the following URL: http://www.netskills.ac.uk/TONIC/ An American information scientist, Linda Goodwin, has prepared a list of online guides and tutorials. Pointers to this material may be found at the following site: http://www.duke.edu/~goodw010/wwwintro.html#Internet The BMJ provide a Guide to the Internet for Medical Practitioners, authored by Mark Pallen: http://www.tecc.co.uk/bmj/archive/7017ed2.htm

Having been introduced to some of the basic concepts and terminology, students should be shown how to set bookmarks. An important element of any introductory course should deal with critical appraisal techniques.

4. Ensuring that the key players work together

The Internet is about sharing resources. To develop an effective information strategy for the medical school, librarians, staff in computer departments, and in audiovisual units must work with medical education departments and clinical tutors. If we focus on the technology and neglect these organizational and educational issues, the 'Internet ward round' will not materialize.

> The process comes full circle back to academic medical institutions. The usefulness of the Internet hinges upon the policies these institutions create to aid the organization and dissemination of medical information, and in the means they use to make their constituents aware of the pitfalls and potentials of various technologies. Expertise in the provision and support of networks must be complemented by expertise in the maintenance and dissemination of biomedical knowledge bases. The central intellectual issue from before the introduction of network-based resources, remains unchanged: how does one properly classify, archive, and disseminate knowledge so that it may best serve the needs of others?
> *Frisse 1994, p.23*

Becoming an information provider

Although the Net was a by-product of scientific communication, the democratization of the Net in the wake of World Wide Web has resulted in a proliferation of information providers. Scientists continue to act as major information providers, but many more players are entering the field—from businesses to college students and individual hobbyists who want to share their enthusiasm with a wider audience. They do this by setting up a site on which they include their name and some basic information about themselves, often a picture or two, a list of 'cool links' to follow, and whatever other information they like.

Bruce McKenzie's book *Medicine and the Internet* (1996) provides suggestions for would-be information providers. Readers should have a look at the end section of

Chapter 15 (Becoming an information provider) and the section in Chapter 24 which gives advice on writing your own home page. The Yale C/AIM Web Style Guide, produced by the Yale Center for Advanced Instructional Media, is a widely acclaimed guide to how to design a high quality web site. The whole document can be downloaded. The site address is: (http://info.med.yale.edu/caim/manual/index.html)

Problems with the Internet

The general thesis of this chapter has been that the Internet offers a powerful set of learning resources to medical students. However, there are also potential problems regarding the Internet as a learning site or resource. Perhaps the single biggest complaint is that it is often hard to find things which are genuinely useful.

> The Internet in its present incarnation has been widely criticized by those wishing to use it for more than pure entertainment. Most criticism [dwells on] . . . the anarchic nature of the Internet, which has, ironically, permitted it to flourish. Specifically, it is difficult to locate what you want, and only a small proportion of content is actually usable. The Internet is rather vast, and in its vastness there is a lot of 'data' (as opposed to information)—but while the relative proportion might not be large, the absolute content of real information is significant. The trick is to know where to look before you go looking. *McKenzie 1996, p.81*

Table 4.8 presents a checklist of what are perceived to be the defects of the Net.

Most of these problems are not insurmountable and are being addressed. Efforts are under way to catalogue medical Internet resources and suggest directions for their development. Working groups are addressing the issue of quality control and standards. Ease of access is improving. More information and gateways are added each day and the underlying software is being improved. It is becoming easier to provide information. Methods for introducing order, such as special servers to compile and share indexes, are evolving. User interfaces are improving.

Looking ahead

Within the United Kingdom, all Higher Education Institutions are charged with developing an information strategy, setting out policies and approaches to the handling and use of information throughout the organization. Information strategy is seen as central to strategic planning overall. To work safely and cost effectively, it is important to ensure that all information is appropriately defined, fit for purpose and used and safeguarded responsibly.

The pace of technological change affecting academic institutions has challenged their ability to innovate in the field of educational computing. Attempts to deliver components of a curriculum and its assessment wholly through computer-based learning have had limited but increasing success. Much excellent work in the medical field dating back over twenty years has become outdated mainly through technological obsolescence. The hardware for which it was written no longer exists or the software tools are no longer available or supported. Gradually *de facto* standards established through commercial

Table 4.8 Problems associated with the Internet

- *Access problems.* The Internet is slow at certain times of the day when the 'traffic' is heavy. Slow response times are probably the biggest obstacle to using the Internet. There are often problems in downloading large files. URLs change and many resources are 'under construction'. The information on the Net is volatile and it can be frustrating to try to relocate information.
- *Lack of regulation and standards raises doubts about the quality of the information.* In a world where anyone is free to publish, how is the user to judge whether it is trustworthy? Much depends on the credibility of the source, the method by which the information was compiled, and the frequency of update. At present much of what is on offer lacks context. Agreed ways of inserting context into documents, making it clear where they come from, and how they relate to other documents on the Web, are required.
- *Navigation can be difficult.* Although there are catalogues and virtual libraries these need to be maintained. In the very fluid situation of the Internet, it is hard to keep these up-to-date.
- *The Internet incurs overheads.* Students and staff need training to learn how to readily access high quality material. Institutions must invest in terminals, networks, and technical staff.
- *Possible negative impact on other learning resources.* There is concern as to whether the Internet will lead to deterioration in the quality of other (traditional) information sources.
- *Financial costs.* Although at present the Net is 'free', there is the possibility that in the future charges will be introduced.
- *Information overload and problems of navigation* make it easy for the inexperienced user to waste a great deal of time 'surfing the Net'.
- *Impact on patient care.* One general worry voiced about electronic tools is whether information technology may lead to a reduction in the time students spend with patients and other human beings. Is there a danger that the Internet ward round may seduce students away from patients' bedside, away from discussions with fellow students, and away from interactions with live clinical tutors?

success or industry wide standards to which all manufacturers then work and produce products, have begun to take hold. In turn, this trend has begun to consolidate hardware and software platforms and open up broad markets for commercially viable innovation in educational computing products. Common software environments intercommunicating through industry-standard programming conventions provide opportunities for sharing and continuity of resources. These lessen the risk and increase the academic and economic advantages for institutions to become involved.

Even ten years ago, the concept of shared access to resources on the scale of the Internet, facilitated through common telecommunications standards, would have seemed quite improbable. Ten years before that, the desktop computer and local area network were not in evidence. Today, the capabilities of current technologies to deliver virtual reality environments over considerably higher capacity networks, to achieve considerably higher density of recording of information, thus encompassing large visual archives in portable media, are only beginning to find application. Already, the increasing numbers of people all over the world able to access the Internet strains the performance of the installed hardware to the point where remote access, particularly to the USA, is not fast enough for educational uses. There are ways to combat this by arranging to mirror frequently used resources on local hardware and by instituting what are called *caching* mechanisms so that any accessed page will be stored locally for a short period and can therefore be used when a further reference is made to the same location. Frequently used information is then gradually accumulated in the cache memory with a statistical algorithm governing the period of retention after its last local use.

The graphical user interface on the Internet is primitive by contemporary standards and will inevitably improve as hypertext mark-up language (HTML) gives way to more powerful languages such as JAVA, with capabilities for handling information using object-oriented programming techniques.

The power of processors and the capacity of storage devices has increased by three orders of magnitude per decade for the past four decades. This has mirrored several eras of semiconductor devices and now optical processing systems. The decades of seconds, millisecs, microsecs, nanosecs and towards picosecs have been matched with those of bytes, kilobytes, megabytes, gigabytes and toward terabytes. Computational power is still expanding through advances in parallel architecture of processors. The growing power has been applied to improving many aspects of user interface, now more intuitive and moving towards effective voice recognition systems. The growing capacity of optical communications and switching systems has been equally spectacular. Hence, on the key measures of standards, power, storage capacity, communications capacity, and usability, the computing domain has transformed itself through innovation many times over during the period and the technical frontiers have moved during this evolution. Cost has also been transformed; the huge sixties mainframe is now dwarfed by the capacity of the 90s desktop machine at a fraction of the cost. The poor fifties pundit who anticipated that the needs of the world for computing could be satisfied by a total of four large computers illustrates the risk of predicting the unpredictable.

The most adverse effect of this precipitate period of advance has been the long period of expensive distraction it has provided for many areas of education, which has struggled to find ways of embedding technology into their teaching and learning environments. The future potential has been at odds with the present reality at all times. Was the computer about to make the teacher obsolete? If not, how should institutions balance the roles of teachers and computers in delivering a curriculum: What machines should be bought? How should they be deployed and supported? What software should be developed and used? What should be taught about computing systems? How should activities be coordinated? Fortunately, the field of educational computing is now moving beyond technical innovation; content issues and quality issues are assuming their rightful place in driving forward strategies. We may expect the highest quality of learning resources and systems to emerge, many within a commercial framework but many as well in the public domain. Also funding realities within our institutions will mean that only those institutions which manage to balance teaching and research within a viable information strategy will be able to afford to continue as centres of excellence. The repetitive imparting of the same lecture courses, based on the same notes, to lecture theatres filled with bored students will be seen as second best to more innovative and valuable learning strategies, such as problem-based learning which can be delivered using substantial elements of information technology leavened by face-to-face tutor involvement, more and more absent in today's typical higher education institution.

References

Brennan, M., Williams, J., Huckaday, T., and Hammond, P. (1996). Whose image is it anyway? Ethical, legal and copyright issues in medical CAL. Computers in Medical Education Conference. CTI Centre for Medicine, Bristol.

Duffy, C., Arnold, S., and Henderson, F. (1995). Net-Sem – electrifying undergraduate seminars. In Darby, J. and Martin, J. (eds) *Using the Internet for Teaching*. Active Learning, No 2, CTISS Publications, University of Oxford.

Frisse, M.E., Kelly, E.M., and Metcalfe, E.S. (1994). An Internet primer: resources and responsibilities. *Academic Medicine*, **69**, 20–4.

Glowniak, J.V. (1995). Medical resources on the Internet. *Annals of Internal Medicine*, **123**, (2), 123–31.

Information Week (1995). Where's the Internet headed? July 17 1995, **536**, 30–36.

Kleeberg, P. and Masys (1995).

Lincoln, T.L. (1995). The importance of Internet newsgroups. *Journal of the American Medical Informatics Association*, **2**, 269–70.

McKenzie, B.C. (1996). *Medicine and the Internet: introducing online resources and terminology*. Oxford University Press, Oxford.

Murphy, J., Griffith, S., Duddle, J. and Machado, H. (1993) Educational Requirements of GEHR Architecture and Systems. EC AIM GEHR A2014, Deliverable No. 9, GEHR Consortium. URL: http://www.chime.ucl.ac.uk/Healthl/GEHR/EUCEN/gehr.htm

Waldrop, M.M. (1994) Culture shock on the networks. *Science*, **265**, 879–81.

Appendix A

Education sites on the Internet

Note: this does not purport to be a comprehensive list. The sites have been selected so as to include those that are well known and generally regarded as the best constructed.

List of world-wide medical schools on the WWW	http://anatomy-1.1.dote.hu/ ~ tore/medfak/
Anaesthesiology – WWW Study Guide, Year IV University of Queensland – Access via online Med Ed. AUS	http://gasbone.herston.uq.edu.au/
Anatomy, histology and pathology (LUMEN) Hyptertext medical education resources. Mixture of graphics and text. Medical Education Network, Loyola University, Chicago. USA	http://www.meddean.luc.edu/lumen/
Biochemistry – NetBiochem is intended to be a complete Medical Biochemistry centre which can be accessed over a computer network. USA	http://www-medlib.med.utah.edu/NetBiochem/NetWelco.htm
Bioethics resources compiled by MacLean Center for Clinical Medical Ethics in Chicago. USA	http://ccme-mac4.uchichago.edu/CCMEDdocs/EthLinks
BONES: The Biologically Oriented Navigator of Electronic Services. This page lists a variety of Internet resources of interest to health sciences educators. USA	http://bones.med.ohio-state.edu/bones/educator.html
Bristol Biomedical Image Archive. A collection of approximately 20,000 images for teaching medical, veterinary and dental science. UK	http://www.ets.bris.ac.uk/brisbio.htm

Cancer Teaching and Curriculum Enhancement in Undergraduate Medicine. University of Texas. USA	http://snapper.utmb.edu:800/ccenter/INDEX.HTML
Cardiology – The Virtual Heart – Describes all aspects of heart function and diseases; contains links to quick-time movies, to sound files and to many other cardiology pages on the Web. USA	http://sln.fi.edu/biosci/heart.html
Case Index by Patient History. University of Pittsburg – USA	http://path.upmc.edu:80/cases
Case Presentations – LARG*NET MEDICAL I-WAY A large array of case presentations categorised. Clicking on an anatomic or pathological group retrieves a case list. Cases include histories, images, clinical diagnoses and case comments. USA	http://johns.largnet.uwo.ca/
Case Studies (Clinical). Department of Defence. Includes Telemedicine, Radiology, Pathology, Obstetrics, Psychiatry, Emergency Medicine, Surgery and Internal Medicine. USA	http://www.matmo.army.mil/pages/casestudies/casestudies.html
CTICM – Bristol. Computers in Teaching Initiative, Centre for Medicine. A nationally funded centre to promote the use of computers in medical, dental and veterinary schools. UK	http://www.ets.bris.ac.uk/
Evidence Based Medicine. The Heatlh Information Research Unit (HIRU) site at McMaster is the best starting point for finding information relating to epidemiology, biostatistics, and evidence-based medicine. Canada.	http://hiru.mcmaster.ca/
GHIFT – Gateway to Health Informatics for Teaching. A database of information and resources to support education and training in IT and health informatics. UK	http://www.chime.ucl.ac.uk/GHIFT/
Gynecologic Oncology Tutorials. Covers main gynaecologic concers; also breast cancer and pain management – University of Washington. USA	http://gynecology.obgyn.washington.edu/Tutorials/Tutorials.html.
Harvard Medical Gopher – Clinical, public health, medical education resources. USA	gopher://gopher.who.ch/
Intern On-Call Handbook. This site includes helpful hints for problems commonly faced by housestaff on inpatient medicine and surgery patients. Oregon Health Sciences University. USA	http://www.ohsu.edu/cliniweb/intern/intindx.html
The Interactive Mecical Student Lounge. Peer Support includes a "conversation bulletin board" for peer support and links to libraries. resources, resources and medical department.	http://www.geocities.com/Heartland/1756/lounge.html
The Interactive Patient – Marshal University School of Medicine – An interactive medical education tool that simulates an actual patient encounter. User asks history questions, performs a physical exam, orders tests and submits a diagnosis and treatment plan. Detailed feedback is provided. USA	http://medicus.marshal.edu/medicus.htm

Learning Resource Centre (University of Michigan Medical Centre) – Educational resources including a thoracic radiology tutorial and a medical software catalogue. USA	http://www.med.umich.edu/lrc/lrchomepage/lrchome.html
The Medical Education Page – designed by a medical student. USA	http://www.primenet.com/ ~ gwa/med.ed/
Medical Education Software Archive. All software posted to this site is either public-domain, or shareware. University of California, Irvine. USA	http://sun3.lib.uci.edu/ ~ sclancy/med-ed/index.htm
Medical Textbook – CHORUS. Documents are indexed by organ systems that describe diseases, radiological findings, differential-diagnosis lists and pertinent Neuroendocrine system (head and neck), Cardiovascular system, Respiratory system, Gastrointestinal system.	http://chorus.rad.mcw.edu/chorus.html
MedWeb (Birmingham) Focuses on CME, undergraduate and postgraduate education. The base also for a unique computer-mediated assessment facility delivering MCQ's, short-type clinical cases and OSCE's. UK	http://medweb.bham.ac.uk
Meningitis Epidemic Case Study – Liverpool School of Tropical Medicine. UK	ftp://ftp.liv.ac.uk/pub/epidemic/
The Multimedia Medical Reference Library. Classroom Section contains pointers to Internet resources to support the medical curriculum (biased toward basic medical sciences). USA http://www.med-library.com/	
Nuclear Medicine Teaching File. Diagnosed Cases presented by organ system, disease category or imaging method. Computed tomographic, magnet resonance, radiographic and nuclear medicine images are accompanied by explanatory text and references. Washington University Medical Centre (St Louis, Missouri). USA	http://gamma.wustl.edu
Nuclear Medicine Teaching cases. Cases, images and discussion. At the present time, free access is permitted to these teaching files. The copyright is retained by the Joint Program in Nuclear Medicine. Harvard University. USA	http://www.med.harvard.edu/JPNM/.index.html
Nuclear Medicine Teaching File. Radiology and anatomy teaching files organised by pathology, anatomy, organ system. University of Washington (Seattle) USA	http://www.rad.washington.edu/
NUMS MedBank. A Critiqued Listing of Medical Education Resources available on the WWW. Access from the Northwestern University Medical School site. Designed by a medical student. USA	http://www.wmitc.nwu.edu/
Online Mendelian Inheritance in Man (OMIM). Online version of Victor McKusick's text. USA	http://gdbwww.gdb.org/

Ophthamology – Grand Rounds, original articles, links to other resources. Harvard. USA

http://www.meei.harvard.edu/meei/DJOhome.html

Paediatrics – Neonatology on the Web – Reference material, teaching files, clinical guidelines – USA

http://www.csmc.edu/neonatology/

Pathology – WebPath, a resource for pathology. Image base and tutorials. Online mini-tutoirals/discussions of various clinical pathology cover topics such as pap smears, amyloidosis, tuberculosis, and clinical chemistry. Internet Pathology Laboratory at the University of Utah in Salt Lake City. USA

http://www-medlib.med.utah.edu/WebPath/webpath.html

Pathology – The Uniformed Services University of the Health Sciences (surgical pathology) – Exam papers and quizzies. USA

http://wwwpath.usuf2.usuhs.mil/surg_path/student.html

Physiology – University of Arizona; contains text, tables, graphic figures, photographs, animation, movie and sound files pertaining to physiology. USA

http://www.physiol.arizona.edu/CELL/Default.html

Primary Care – GP-UK – focus on healthcare computing clinical problems, research, drug reactions, audit and education. UK

http://www.ncl.ac.uk/ ~ nphcare/GPUK/gpukhome.html

Primary Care Teaching Modules (Stanford University) – Designed to educate medical students and residents in primary care specialties. Includes: Dizziness & Screening; sinusitis & URI. USA

http://www-med.stanford.edu/school/DGIM/Teaching/Modules-index.html

Primary Care Teaching Topics. University of Chicago Includes Health Promotion and Prevention, Gastrointestinal Topics, Renal and Urology Topics, Cardiovascular topics, Pulmonary Topics, Haematology and Oncology Topics. USA

http://uhs.bsd.uchicago.edu/uhs/topics/uhs-teaching.html

Respiratory Medicine – ElectricDiffuseLung – A multimedia textbook from the virtual hospital on diffuse lung disease. USA

http://www.vh.org/Providers/Textbooks/DiffuseLung/DiffuseLung.html

Southampton University Biomedical Gopher (Microbiology, medical statistics, biomedical software, European medical information) UK

gopher://medstats.Soton.Ac.Uk:70/

Surgery: Interactive Teaching Project – University College London and other collaborators. UK

http://www.ja.net/SuperJANET/SuperJANET/SJ-Applics-Menu.html

Surgery – Online Surgery Notes. Personal notes made for the American Board of Surgery In-Training Examination, plus notes on miscellaneous surgical topics. USA

http://dbmi6000.mc.vanderbilt.edu:8000/intro.html

Summit – Stanford University Medical Media and Information Technologies Group – site is devoted to exploring new applications of computers in medical education. USA

http://summit.stanford.edu/

Teaching and Learning Technology Programme (TLTP) – UK

http://www.icbl.hw.ac.uk/tltp

Tropical Medicine Resource (TMR) – Wellcome Trust – UK	http://www.chime.ucl.ac.uk/
Virtual Hospital – Project of the University of Iowa College of Medicine, Department of Radiology. Oriented toward patient care and physician education. Continuously updated medical multimedia database. Contains multimedia textbooks, teaching files, clinical guidelines etc. Also a bibliography of multimedia computer-based education. USA	http://indy.radiology.uiowa.edu/ VirtualHospital.html
Virtual Medical Centre. Contains pointers to thousands of Internet multimedia medical teaching files, manuals, multimedia medical cases, and continuing medical education courses. USA	http://www-sci.lib.uci.edu/ ~ martindale/ Medical.html
Visible Human Project. A complete, anatomically detailed 3-D representation of the male & female body. USA	http://www.nlm.nih.gov/ extramural_research.dir/visible_human.html
Virtual Anatomy Project at Colorado State University (CSU) is working on generating a 3D geometric database of the human body. A future goal of the project is to develop a virtual human anatomy lab for undergraduate anatomy instruction. USA	http://www.vis.colostate.edu/library/gva/ gva.html
WebRounds. An interactive, on-line journal for medical students. It is a collection of case studies, experiences, career tips, special features, and useful links to medical web sites that will both entertain and educate. The site contains articles from medical school professors, practitioners, medical students, medical residents, researchers and authors. USA	http://www.wwilkins.com/rounds/
WebDoctor (CME). Contains a variety of resources on Anatomy, Cardiology, Emergency Medicine, Family Medicine, Geriatrics, Patient Simulations, Preventive Medicine, Paediatrics and Radiology. USA	http://www.gretmar.com/webdoctor/cme.html

5 Assessment

5   Assessment

David Newble

The importance of assessment

It is impossible to overestimate the importance of assessment. Involvement of teachers in developing assessment procedures is almost certainly the most critical educational task they will undertake. The methods they select and the content they include will have profound effects not only on what students learn but also on how students learn. Yet, in many institutions, assessment practices misdirect student learning activities in ways that may seriously undermine the aims of the curriculum. In addition, the organization and preparation of undergraduate examinations are often left to junior members of staff who have neither the experience, training, resources, nor the authority to produce tests of high quality. In the process of curriculum or course review, assessment is frequently something which is little more than an afterthought, following detailed consideration of the aims, objectives, teaching methods, and timetabling.

Nevertheless, it is hard to believe that academic staff are unaware of the profound influence of assessments (particularly examinations) on the attitude and behaviour of their students. Has there ever been a committed teacher who has not been frustrated by students asking whether the material being taught is going to be examined and, when the answer is 'no', finding a considerable lessening of their enthusiasm and commitment for what may be creative and stimulating activities? Yet, despite our growing understanding of the importance of assessment, and the development of better tools, there is little evidence of significant reform. Prominent British educator Graham Gibbs (1991) identified eight myths about assessment, the last being that assessment in higher education is improving. His view is that assessment is actually getting rapidly worse as a consequence of pressures on resources. This has reduced the moderating effect of a range of informal assessment procedures which are dependent on personal teacher–student contact, leaving only the formal allocation of marks which is 'stupid, destructive, and misleading' (Gibbs 1991, p. 4).

If this gloomy analysis is true, or even partially true, we, as responsible teachers, must undertake to do something about it. This will only happen with a better understanding of the purposes, principles, and methods of assessment coupled to a recognition that this is one of the major issues for medical education in the future.

Purposes of assessment

In the world of medical practice, tests are used for a variety of purposes including making diagnoses, guiding patient management, screening, and self-monitoring. The purpose determines the approach and methods chosen. Similarly, the purposes of measurement in the field of education are many and varied. A failure to clarify the purpose will lead inevitably to inappropriate and ineffective procedures. While this may appear to be stating the obvious, experience has shown that the purposes of tests are often not clear and that medical teachers may even have conflicting views on the purpose of the same assessment procedure. Some possible purposes are:

Measuring academic achievement

This is probably the most common and most readily understood purpose. Such tests are administered to allow the teacher or the institution to measure the achievement of the student. Most often this information is used for grading or ranking. Such assessments are often critical to the students' progress or graduation. They are referred to as 'summative' assessments and usually administered at the end of a course of study.

Setting standards

One of the most frequently identified purposes for the assessment of medical students is the need to satisfy registration bodies, employing institutions and the community that graduates are competent to practice. The intention is to certify the achievement of a minimal standard of performance. Ideally, such a standard should be an absolute one ('criterion-referenced') rather than a comparative one which is determined by performance relative to other students ('norm-referenced')

Diagnosing student problems

An important, but under-used, purpose of assessment is that of providing students with information on their progress within a course. The aim is to allow students to identify their strengths and weaknesses and to help them predict their likely success in the summative assessment. This then allows time and opportunity for remedial action. Such assessments are known as 'formative'. They may be administered by the teacher during the course, in which case the results should not count towards any end-of-course mark. They may also be developed as self-assessment tests which the students can use at their convenience. An important component to all such assessments is the provision of feedback (see Chapter 3). This may range from simply supplying the answers for a multiple-choice self-assessment test to providing individual counselling for students who find they are not progressing satisfactorily.

Encouraging good approaches to learning

The content and format of examinations have a profound effect on the way students approach their study and learning (Newble and Entwistle 1986). As discussed in Chapter

3, assessments form a major component of the 'hidden curriculum' or the perceived curriculum. For example an over-reliance on testing factual recall using multiple-choice tests will be likely to encourage a superficial, rote-learning approach to study. If a deeper approach to learning is a desired outcome of a course, then the assessment procedure must include and give appropriate weight to methods which require the student to understand and apply their knowledge and skills.

Demonstrating course and teacher effectiveness

An assessment may be administered to a group of students as a means of providing feedback to the teacher or institution on the effectiveness of a course. Such an approach is commonly used after the introduction of a new component of a course in order to judge its efficacy in achieving its intended outcomes in terms of the students learning. In the area of staff appraisal, or when there is need to provide evidence for promotion committees on teaching excellence, individual academics may wish to use such data to quantify their accomplishments.

Predicting future performance

In the world of business, aptitude tests are used extensively in an attempt to predict future job performance. In medicine, test results are often used for this purpose: school examinations for selection into the medical course; final examination results for choosing interns and residents. Generally speaking, such tests are not specifically designed as aptitude tests and, thus, it is not surprising that their predictive powers are often poor.

Designing an assessment procedure

If predictable outcomes on student learning and behaviour are to be achieved, extraordinary care must be taken in the design phase of curriculum and course planning. As a fundamental first step it is essential that the aims are clear. This will be evident if they can be written in the form of brief statements, with which everyone agrees, that describe the things the students should know or be able to do at the end of the course ('outcomes objectives'). It is usually adequate to specify these in fairly broad terms. For example: 'At the completion of this course the student will be able to *apply* the principles of . . .; be able to *perform* a . . .; be able to *communicate effectively* with . . .'

Having done this it becomes, in principle, a relatively simple matter to match these to an appropriate method of assessment. However, it will soon become obvious that one method of assessment is unlikely to be able to measure all objectives. For instance, in the example above, it would be impossible to measure validly three such objectives by a written test. 'Perform' and 'communicate' imply the need for observation of actual performance in a real or simulated setting. The important principle is that the definition of what is to be tested should determine the content and the methods of assessment.

A simple example of how this was applied to a short course on teaching basic clinical skills is shown in Table 5.1 (Newble 1982). A more complex example can be found in a recent book which outlines a procedure for developing a comprehensive assessment of clinical competence (Newble *et al.* 1994).

Table 5.1 Activities designed to help students meet the objectives of the course

Objectives	Teaching activities	Assessment
Take a comprehensive history	Tutor sessions with videotape recordings; ward practice	Tutor's opinion based on videotape recordings at end of course
Perform a complete physical examination	Viewing demonstration videotape; tutor sessions; ward practice; ward rounds with registrars	Tutor opinion; observation of screening examination by independent examiner at end of course
Write-up history and examination and construct a problem list	Problem-oriented case write-ups on ward patients; tutor sessions	Case write-ups
Decisions on diagnosis, investigations and management	Whole-group problem-solving sessions; case write-ups	Whole group sessions; case write-ups
Ability to relate to patients	Tutor sessions with review of videotape recordings	Tutor's opinion
Improve knowledge of medicine and surgery	Self-instruction; preparation of cases for presentation to the whole group; computerized self-assessment programmes; tape-slide tutorials	Whole-group tutor's opinion; self-assessment

What happens when things go wrong—a case study

In order to illustrate how a mismatch in assessment methods to curriculum aims can undermine the best of intentions, I will describe a salutary experience at my own institution (Newble and Jaeger 1983). In 1971, the medical school introduced a major curriculum revision. This included the completion of the formal teaching of clinical and paraclinical sciences by the end of the fifth year and the restructuring of the final (sixth) year into a series of full-time internships, with students having direct responsibilities for patient care.

An integral part of the changes in final year was the introduction of ward-based assessments, completed by the head of the unit in consultation with ward staff, at the end of each internship. This form of assessment replaced the traditional clinical viva previously administered to all students as part of the final examinations. The largely multiple-choice based knowledge tests in the major clinical disciplines were retained with the heaviest weight being allocated to medicine and surgery. Multidisciplinary clinical vivas were retained to help make pass–fail decisions on those students who performed unsatisfactorily on the ward assessments or in the final written examinations.

We believed that the Faculty's goals for the curriculum change were clearly evident. The removal of didactic teaching in favour of internships and the introduction of ward-based assessments demonstrated a commitment to improving the teaching and assessment of clinical competence in a real-world practice setting. However, it became evident within two years that something was seriously amiss. As the year progressed students were seen less frequently on the wards; tutorials and lectures were being requested; and increasingly more time was being devoted to learning from books. In other words despite strong support from staff and students for the curriculum reform, something was undermining its effective implementation.

The reason was easily detected from surveys and discussions with the students. They had soon discovered that the chance of obtaining an unsatisfactory ward rating was remote—in one early year only 3 out of 480 assessments were graded as unsatisfactory. The students' study strategy clearly was to avoid obtaining a pass–fail viva. The way to do this was to pass the written examination from whence almost all vivas emanated.

What was to be the subsequent strategy of the Faculty? There was no dissatisfaction with the final year objectives or the teaching programme. Ward ratings were seen as important for providing feedback and an incentive for attendance. The only option seemed to be to reintroduce a clinical examination for all students as part of the final examination in an effort to restore balance in the students' minds between the theoretical and the clinical/practical components of the course. There was an unwillingness to reintroduce the traditional viva as doubts about its reliability had been raised previously. This led to the development of a new test of clinical competence of which an objective structured clinical examination (OSCE) formed a major component. This is not the place to discuss the new procedure, but it is described in detail in the literature (Newble 1988; Newble and Swanson 1988). Suffice to say, the strategy was successful with students perceiving the need to devote more of their attention to ward-based activities in order to do well on the test of clinical competence.

This example underlines the importance of matching aims to assessment methods. Even apparently rational and well-meaning alterations to assessment procedures can produce unexpected changes in student behaviour. While the effects may not always be as important and as dramatic as in this case, it will generally pay to be sensitive to the effects that altering examinations have in the students' minds, remembering that the changes in behaviour may take several years to become fully manifest.

Using examinations constructively—a second case study

The previous case study illustrated how the aims of a whole course can be compromised by a mismatch with the assessment procedures. The power of the examinations to effect student learning can, of course, be used constructively to give the students not only broad directives but also quite specific messages. Often, we provide such directives through devices such as subject or disciplinary weightings or by requiring minimum pass marks on subcomponents of a multidisciplinary examination. Less frequently do we take equal care with the detailed content specifications of examinations, yet students are acutely aware of imbalances in content. The 'spotting' of possible questions from an analysis of past examination papers or from discussions with previous years students is a well-recognized phenomenon.

This inevitable aspect of student activity can be used to advantage if some components of the course have a higher priority than others. Another case study from our own experience illustrates this point (Jolly et al. 1993). Data was analysed from the OSCE stations in the test of clinical competence referred to in the previous section. Mean class performance was reviewed on stations which were administered more than once over a 12-year period. Re-using stations produced an average increment in scores of about 5–7% per repeat administration. The most marked effect was for a cardio-pulmonary resuscitation (CPR) station which was repeated five times. Class scores rose from an initial 45% to a plateau of around 80%. While most repeated stations in this examination were not selected specifically for the purpose of directing student learning, the CPR station was chosen for this purpose. This approach has a largely unexploited potential to specifically direct student learning in desirable directions.

Choosing the appropriate assessment methods

Clinicians are expected to have a knowledge of the tests and procedures available for aiding diagnosis and management. They are also expected to be able to select from amongst these in a way which is rationally based on an understanding of their value and quality. It would seem reasonable that medical teachers charged with the responsibility for selecting assessment procedures should have a similar level of knowledge about available educational tests. Yet, all too often this is not the case. Test methods are frequently employed in an arbitrary fashion without adequate attention to the purpose of the assessment and without due consideration of their strengths and weaknesses. End-of-course assessment procedures may not come under critical scrutiny during curriculum reviews and may remain unchanged and un-challenged for many years. They may even be the responsibility of totally separate bodies to those charged with developing and implementing the curriculum and individual courses. As a consequence a mismatch between aims and assessment becomes almost inevitable with the consequences discussed previously.

The first step must be to acquire a working familiarity with the test methods likely to be of value—what Ronald Harden (1986) has called 'the examiners' toolkit'. This is not the place for a detailed discussion of the attributes of individual methods but such information is readily available in standard texts on educational measurement and in books written with the medical teacher in mind (Neufeld and Norman 1985; Newble and Cannon 1994).

An example of an area in which choice of methods has received a considerable amount of attention in the last few years has been the assessment of clinical competence. Critical reviews of the strengths and weaknesses of current and potential methods are to be found in the books by Neufeld and Norman (1985) and Newble et al. (1994) and in a recent article by Van der Vleuten (1996). An illustration of an attempt to evaluate a range of methods used to assess aspects of competence can be found in the proceedings of the First Cambridge Conference on Clinical Assessment (Norman et al. 1985) in which participants reached a consensus based on available evidence and experience. For example (see Table 5.2) global ratings were recommended only for use in assessing personal qualities yet in practice are frequently used to assess other attributes. Multiple-choice tests were recommended for testing knowledge, and to a limited extent for reasoning and management, but may often be the single form of written test used in major examinations of competence. On the other hand, standardized (simulated) patients were recommended for assessing a broad range of attributes, particularly data gathering and physical examination skills, yet are seen infrequently in medical school examinations in most parts of the world.

Table 5.2 Recommendations on the use of evaluation methods to assess domains of competence
+ = of some use + + = of most use

Competence/Skill	Method								
	Global ratings	MCQ	MEQ	PMP	'Cambridge case/key features	Standardized patient	Patient rating	Direct observation	Mechanical simulation
Knowledge		++	++	+		+		+	
Interview/ interpersonal						++	++	++	
Data gathering, history		+	+	+++	+++		++		
Physical exam (technical)						+++		+	+
Reasoning/ diagnosis		+	+	+	++	+		+	
Lab utilization/ management		+	+	+	++				
Personal qualities	++								

(Reprinted with permission from Cambridge University School of Clinical Medicine)

In another article, which emanated from a later Cambridge Conference, a set of principles was defined for the selection of test methods to be used in the assessment of clinical competence (Newble *et al.* 1993). The first was that test methods should strive for a representation of reality (fidelity) that is appropriate to the clinical tasks being assessed; the second was that those clinical tasks should dictate the method by which they are to be tested; and the third was that there must be a recognition of the practical constraints on selecting the optimal examination methods. While these principles are related to the assessment of clinical competence they are equally applicable to any test situation. The underlying message is that the content, process, and personal attributes expected of the student should all be represented in the assessment procedure, not just those that are convenient to test.

Rarely will it be possible to implement fully such an 'ideal' assessment procedure and compromises will be necessary. However, the balance has often been too far on the side of expediency with inadequate attention being given to the ultimate quality of the test procedures and of the results on which decisions are taken.

The attributes of a good test

The judgement of whether a test used in clinical practice is good requires information on its specificity, sensitivity and cost-benefit ratio. The judgement of whether an educational test is good requires information on its levels of validity, reliability, and practicability. Validity requires establishing that the test measures what it is supposed to measure and reliability requires that it produces results which are consistent or reproducible.

Validity

Content validity is the first and major priority. It is determined by empirically establishing what is to be tested and ensuring that an adequate sample of this content is represented in the assessment procedure. In many medical schools, the process used to determine what actually gets into examinations is not clearly defined and any sampling procedure is likely to be rather crude, such as asking for a certain number of questions per topic or discipline.

To bring a more orderly and scientific approach to achieving high levels of content validity, the use of a blueprint has been strongly advocated to guide the selection of test content (Newble *et al.* 1993). Such blueprints are structured 'grids' which define the areas to be tested. Dimensions may reflect disciplines, organ systems, patient problems, intellectual processes (recall, interpretation, problem-solving), patient age, a range of clinical skills, prevalence, and so on. Agreement of faculty must be sought as to the appropriate balance of the chosen dimensions.

It must be remembered that there is no statistic which can be calculated to indicate whether content validity has been achieved. It is something which must be argued from the procedures used and evidence that the actual content of the test has matched the predetermined specifications.

There are other forms of validity, such as a criterion-related and construct validity, which it may be necessary to establish. The most important of these is criterion-related validity. For instance, for an aptitude test it is essential to know if the test is able to predict future performance (predictive validity). It may also be of interest to correlate students results on one test (e.g. a new test) with those on a previously validated 'gold standard' test (concurrent validity). These types of validity can be statistically expressed in the form of a correlation coefficient. Many tests in undergraduate and postgraduate medical education are used ostensibly as aptitude tests (e.g. intern selection; competence to be a specialist) yet few organizations could produce such validity data.

Reliability

Reliability is a statistical concept. It is reflected in statistical information on the consistency and generalisability of the test scores. Factors which influence reliability include the length of the test, the spread of scores, the level of difficulty and the objectivity of the marking. Generally speaking, reliability will improve when there are more items in the test; where the spread of marks is broad and even; where the level of difficulty is moderately high; and when errors due to inconsistent marking are minimized.

Various coefficients of reliability can be calculated. Classically, these consist of a variety of coefficients (e.g. test-retest; equivalent test forms; internal consistency using split-half or Kuder–Richardson methods; rater-reliability). Reliability coefficients of internal consistency, for example, are a standard part of the computer analysis of MCQ tests. Most examination co-ordinators would appreciate that a value of less than 0.8 for a coefficient is an indication for concern and a value of less than 0.7 is an indication for improving the quality of the test. Examiners are also aware of the potential for inconsistency when subjective marking is employed, for instance in essay tests or clinical examinations. High levels of marker reliability in such situations is very hard to achieve, even with tactics which may include examiner training, the preparation of model answers, the use of double-marking in essay tests, and the use of structured rating forms and multiple examiners in clinical examinations. As a general rule, reliability can be more effectively improved by increasing the number of items in the test than by tactics directed at correcting inconsistent marking. This strategy has been one of the reasons for using short-answer questions in preference to essays and multiple-station structured clinical examinations instead of the traditional clinical viva.

Reliability statistics based on generalizability theory are providing valuable insights into which factors contributing to error are most critical (Brennan 1983). This new approach to analysis is not well known in medical circles despite the fact that extremely interesting and valuable studies have appeared in the last few years in the medical education literature. Traditional approaches to reliability estimates, as described in the previous paragraph, are appropriate for multiple-choice and very short answer tests where objective marking is possible. In such tests the only significant source of variance in the students marks is the real differences in their performance on the test items. In clinical and viva voce examinations there are additional sources of measurement error which may confound, to varying degrees, the students 'true' scores. It is in such situations that the generalizability theory based approach is particularly appropriate.

The test of clinical competence developed at the University of Adelaide, and mentioned previously, was subjected to such a generalizability analysis with revealing results (Newble and Swanson 1988). Data was accumulated over four years on the written and OSCE components of this test. It might have been assumed prior to this analysis that the main source of error in the OSCE component would be the inter-rater agreement at the stations. Indeed the inter-rater reliability (correlations between pairs of examiners) was varied and in some instances unsatisfactory (average 0.7; range 0.38–0.91).

However, any problem in this area paled into insignificance when compared to the average inter-station correlations of less than 0.1. This problem undermined the reliability of the test to such an extent that a 90 minute OSCE circuit of 15 five-minute stations would have a reliability coefficient no higher than 0.5–0.6. The only way of achieving a level of reliability (0.8) suitable for fair decision making on individual student performances would have been to extend the test to four hours (40 stations).

This type of result has now been found for a wide range of tests used in medical education, including oral examinations (Swanson 1987), written and computer-based patient management problems (Swanson et al. 1987), and standardized patient-based examinations (van der Vleuten and Swanson 1990). However the low levels of inter-station or inter-item correlation do not reflect just the poor quality of the tests. They simply reflect the fact that the performance of a candidate on one case or situation is not a good predictor of performance on another case or situation. This phenomenon is now referred to as 'content (or case) specificity'. The implications are that there must be a broad sampling of clinical situations and skills for tests of competence and that these must be longer than those used in the past.

Another useful reliability statistic is the standard error of measurement (SEM) which provides an estimate of the amount of variation in the test score (Streiner and Norman 1993 p.88). It can be calculated from the knowledge of a reliability coefficient and the standard deviation of the test. It can provide a confidence band for candidates' scores within which the 'true' score is located. Such information may be extremely valuable when important decisions are being taken about whether a student should pass or fail. As one author puts it, the SEM 'makes it possible to interpret and use test results more intelligently' (Gronlund 1990).

Future developments in assessment

There seems little doubt that pressure from within and without medical schools and other medical examining bodies will see an increasing emphasis on improving the quality of assessment procedures. This may arise from a desire to direct students learning more appropriately or from a need to satisfy external review.

A concern to match assessment methods to defined outcome objectives will inevitably lead to more complex, multi-format examination and assessment procedures. It will be discovered that many apparently 'tried and true' approaches will be found wanting. For example conventional multiple-choice type examinations will not be adequate to test important higher-level thinking and decision making skills essential in medical practice. It is very difficult to use conventional MCQs to measure more than the recall of a body of factual knowledge, with results additionally fudged by technical limitations such as cueing. In addition, the much revered traditional clinical viva may finally have to be laid to rest or be combined with other approaches to clinically-based assessment (e.g. an OSCE) to achieve acceptable levels of reliability.

Those responsible for assessment will need to seek the advice of educationalists and test developers. In some areas they will receive objective advice which is based on well-conducted research. This will be particularly so in some areas of knowledge-based assessment and in the area of the assessment of clinical competence. Relatively new approaches like the OSCE and the use of standardized patients have been shown to be valuable additions to the examiner's toolkit, if used appropriately. There are also a range of new written test formats (e.g. long menu MCQs) which are less well established but have their attractions.

In other areas, the answers will be less precise. Two areas of major concern are those of assessing clinical problem-solving ability and on-the-job performance-based assessment. The former takes us to the cutting edge of test development. New understanding of the psychology of problem-solving is directing development. Unfortunately present methods purporting to measure clinical problem-solving, such as patient management problems, have been shown to have serious limitations.

Examinations will never be the complete answer to clinical assessment. If we are to have a truly valid assessment of competence the student must be observed in the real situation. This has to be an essential component of any procedure which aims to evaluate attitudinal, ethical, and interpersonal aspects of behaviour and performance. Unfortunately this brings with it major problems of reliability due to error variables relating to context, sampling, and rating.

Arguments will continue about whether the approach to clinical assessment should be a process one or one based on evaluating patient outcomes. There is no simple answer to this quandary but in general a process approach (i.e. looking at the components of competence) will be more appropriate in the undergraduate sphere while an outcome approach provides an attractive alternative possibility in the postgraduate sphere (e.g. audits of the outcome of patient care).

These are other practical aspects of assessment that will receive more attention. The need for longer and more complex assessment procedures will raise the issue of efficiency and cost-effectiveness. Such strategies are already emerging and include the use of sequential testing in OSCE type examinations and the 'key features' approach in tests of problem solving (see Page *et al.* 1995). Issues relating to scoring and standard setting will become a growing problem as more complex and multiformat procedures are introduced and also because of the increasingly litigious climate in which examinations are conducted.

References

Brennan, R.L. (1983). *Elements of generalizability theory*. American College Testing Program, Iowa City.

Gibbs, G. (1991). Eight myths about assessment. *The New Academic* **1**, 103.

Gronlund, N.E. (1990). *Measurement and evaluation in teaching* (6th Edn). Macmillan, New York.

Harden, R.M. (1986). Assessment of clinical competence examiners' tool-kit. In *Newer developments in assessing clinical competence*, (ed. I.R. Hart, R.M. Harden, and H.J. Walton), pp. 11–21. Heal Publications, Montreal.

Jolly, B.C., Newble, D.I., and Chinner, T. (1993). The learning effect of re-using stations in an objective structured clinical examination. *Teaching and Learning in Medicine*, **5**, 66–71.

Neufeld, V.R. and Norman, G.R. (1985). *Assessing clinical competence*. Springer, New York.

Newble, D.I. (1982). The way we teach basic clinical skills. *Medical Teacher*, **4**, 12–15.

Newble, D.I. (1988). Eight years experience with structured clinical examination. *Medical Teacher*, **22**, 200–4.

Newble, D.I. and Cannon, R. (1994). *A handbook for medical teachers* (3rd Edn). Kluwer Academic Publishers, Dordrecht, The Netherlands.

Newble, D.I. and Entwistle, N.J. (1986). Learning styles and approaches: implications for medical education. *Medical Education*, **20**, 162–175.

Newble, D.I. and Jaeger, K. (1983). The effect of assessments and examinations on the learning of medical students. *Medical Education*, **17**, 165–71.

Newble, D.I. and Swanson, D.B. (1988). Psychometric characteristics of the objective structured clinical examination. *Medical Education*, **22**, 325–34.

Newble, D.I., Dauphinee, D., Dawson-Saunders, B., Macdonald, M., Mullholland, H., Page, G., Swanson, D., Thomson, A., and van der Vleuten, C. (1993). Guidelines for the development of effective procedures for the assessment of clinical competence. In *The certification and recertification of doctors: issues in the assessment of Clinical Competence*, (ed. D.I. Newble, B.J. Jolly and R.E. Wakeford), pp. 69–91. Cambridge University Press, Cambridge.

Newble, D.I., Jolly, B.C., and Wakeford, R.E. (eds.) (1994). *The certification and recertification of doctors: issues in the assessment of clinical competence*. Cambridge University Press, Cambridge.

Norman, G., Bordage, G., Curry, L., Dauphinee, D., Jolly, B., Newble, D., Rothman, A., Stalenheof, B., Stillman, P., Swanson, D., and Tonesk, X. (1985). A review of recent innovations in assessment. In *Directions in clinical assessment* (ed. R.E. Wakeford), pp. 9–27. Cambridge University Schools of Clinical Medicine, Cambridge.

Page, G., Bordage, G., and Allen, J. (1995). Developing key-feature problems and examinations to assess clinical decision making skills. *Academic Medicine*, **70**, 194–201.

Streiner, D.L. and Norman, G.R. (1993). *Health measurement scales*. Oxford University Press.

Swanson, D. (1987). A measurement framework for performance-based tests. In *Further developments in assessing clinical competence*. (ed. I. Hart and R.M. Harden), pp.13–36. Montreal: Can-Heal Publications.

Swanson, D., Norcini, J., and Grosso, L. (1987). Assessment of clinical competence: written and computer-based simulations. *Assessment and Evaluation in Higher Education*, **12**, 220–46.

van der Vleuten, C. and Swanson, D. (1990). Assessment of clinical skills with standardised patients: state of the art. *Teaching and Learning in Medicine*, **2**, 58–76.

van der Vleuten, C. (1996). The assessment of professional competence: development, research and practical implications. *Advances in Health Sciences Education*, **1**, 46–67.

6 The continuation of learning

6.1 The preregistration year in the UK

Thomas H.S. Dent and Jonathan H. Gillard

Introduction

The months before and after graduation are among the most demanding and the most exciting in the career of a doctor. The preparation for final examinations in a medical school which follows a traditional pattern of assessment requires mental stamina and concentration and culminates in a longer and more demanding set of examinations than the students are likely to have experienced hitherto. After this, the medical student becomes a doctor: the longed-for prize at the end of undergraduate training and an alarming prospect for which few feel properly prepared.

The preregistration year is therefore a transitional one, falling at a particularly critical time in the medical career. Its transitional nature is one of the reasons why the definition and execution of quality improvements should be relatively easy. It is more straightforward to define the objectives of a period of training during which the knowledge, skills, and attitudes to be acquired are less sophisticated than those sought later in postgraduate training. All involved in preregistration training accept that house officers are inexperienced doctors from whom relatively little medical expertise can be expected and whose need for training is obvious and pressing. The precedent for them to be more closely supervised by more senior medical and nursing staff is well established. However, despite recent improvements, the preregistration year currently fails to deliver high quality medical education and needs reform (McManus *et al.* 1977; Christie 1980; Dent *et al.* 1990*a*; Gillard *et al.* 1993*b*).

In the UK before the introduction of the preregistration year, medical graduates could begin independent, unsupervised medical practice without further training. This was seen as particularly unsatisfactory for those entering general practice and the need for a period of postgraduate preregistration training was first identified by the Goodenough report (HMSO 1944). Preregistration house officer posts were introduced in 1951, designed to provide newly qualified doctors with supervised training in the setting of routine clinical care before they began less supervised work.

Over the intervening fifty years, these primarily educational goals have fallen victim to the changing nature of medical practice. The increasing pace and complexity of in-patient care have meant that little of the house officer's time is now available for education. Calman (1992) suggested that the year had three main objectives: acquiring knowledge (of common medical conditions, emergencies, and rehabilitation), acquiring skills (diagnostic, clinical, and decision-making), and developing attitudes (of caring, learning, and ethics). These high educational goals have however been difficult to achieve because of service commitments.

The setting for preregistration training

The determination of what constitutes suitable general clinical training in the preregistration year in the UK is a statutory responsibility of the General Medical Council (GMC) under the Medical Act 1983. Without the completion of a year in posts which satisfy the GMCs specifications, a doctor cannot be fully registered and begin more specialized postgraduate training. This control of the content of training and of access to promotion provides the GMC with an authoritative and potentially highly effective platform from which to direct change in the preregistration year. The GMCs recommendations are put into effect by regional postgraduate deans, who are usually senior clinical consultants with a high local reputation. Their regular visits to hospitals provide an opportunity to persuade, cajole, and remonstrate with the consultants to whom house officers are attached. By an iterative process over several years, standards should gradually improve.

House officers are keen to take up what education is available. They come to their posts excited in anticipation of practising medicine after the long period of undergraduate preparation. The prospect of having patients for whose care they have some responsibility and who will look to them as 'their doctor' during their in-patient stay is appealing and house officers are keen to complement the theoretical knowledge that they have acquired at medical school with practical skills and experience. House officers see this as the most rewarding aspect of their work and by demonstrating the connection between this and other aspects of training its relevance can be established. The establishment of this relationship between learning and experience accords with what is known to improve adult learning (Knowles 1990; see Chapter 3). The training needs to be conducted in time protected from encroachment by clinical work, implying an acceptance by superiors that it is at least as important. This is also a component of effective adult learning. Providing training mostly in small groups with other house officers reassures participants that their problems are not unique and allows them to raise problems more freely (Paice and Smyth-Pigott 1992). There are currently few, but increasing, competing priorities for junior house officers. They do not have to sit examinations, but their role in out-patient and pre-admission clinics is burgeoning and the necessity to travel between hospitals in the same Trust increasing. Nevertheless a training programme centred on the medical care of general medical and surgical in-patients, constructed from controlled and adequately supervised exposure to clinical work and relevant formal training in protected time would have great appeal to house officers. It is sometimes argued that house officers do not want more formal educational sessions after spending so many years in medical school, but the formal element of training is important to them: only 52% say there are enough educational meetings at their hospital (Gillard et al. 1993b). When house officers were asked about the formal educational meetings available to them, 83% were satisfied with the quality of the meetings but 47% were frequently or almost invariably unable to attend them because of clinical commitments.

However, other important elements of an effective context for adult training are absent from the preregistration year. There is little feedback from consultants on house officers' progress (Gillard *et al*. 1993*b*), it is seldom self-directed and active and the providers of formal training in this as in other phases of medical training do not regularly involve the learners in evaluation of what is provided (Grant *et al*. 1992).

In the rest of this chapter, we set out some of the reasons why preregistration training is defective and ways that the problem can be addressed.

Confused responsibilities

The potential for improving preregistration posts is marred by confused and overlapping responsibilities for quality assurance; the confusion is itself a product of the transitional nature of this phase of training. The GMC is statutorily responsible for setting the objectives and standards in undergraduate medical education and qualifying examinations, and itself periodically inspects medical schools and their examinations. It also makes recommendations about suitable settings and content for preregistration training (GMC 1992, 1997) but delegates responsibility for enforcing these to universities. Postgraduate deans are responsible to regional offices of the NHS Executive for funding the posts and directing and co-ordinating all postgraduate and continuing medical education in NHS regions (the populations of which, since the regional mergers, range from three to ten million), including the implementation of the GMC's recommendations. The final responsibility for assessing that a house officer has reached the standard required for full registration is in turn delegated to the consultant supervising the post, who has little to gain and much to lose by indicating that the trainee in question was not enabled to achieve that standard under his/her supervision. The standard required for full registration is not clearly defined, with the main qualification being the completion of the requisite period in a recognized post. Because different universities and postgraduate deans have different views of what constitutes suitable training, and in particular whether specialties such as paediatrics, ophthalmology, and neurosurgery are appropriate for the preregistration year, house officers graduated from one university may become fully registered after completing posts which would not have been acceptable under another university's jurisdiction. The postgraduate deans have sought a consensus among themselves on which specialties are suitable (Biggs JSG, personal communication). Finally, on 1 April 1996, deans became directly accountable to the Department of Health; the impact of this on the development of education at regional and local level is currently unclear.

In summary, the posts are regulated according to national recommendations interpreted differently in the areas overseen by different universities, enforced by deans with an accountability to the Department of Health but with the final judgement of attainment being made by a consultant accountable to neither. The GMC is able to exert influence over the small number of undergraduate courses leading to medical degrees but the span of control involved in dealing with thousands of posts in British district hospitals is well beyond its capacity. Universities internally determine the curriculum and examination system by which they will satisfy the GMC, but do not have that degree of control outside their walls in the hospitals where preregistration training occurs.

The widespread emergence of NHS Trusts under less central control has had considerable impact on the training of preregistration house officers. In order to improve efficiency, trusts are reducing the length of in-patient stays and making changes in procedures undertaken, and this is reducing house officers' educational experience. This will be compounded by the little access which house officers have to the increasing numbers of patients seen as out-patients and day cases. While more medical students are taking advantage of the shift from secondary and tertiary to primary care (see Chapter 4.1), this trend is not yet widespread for house officers and is a further threat to their education. The effective delivery of education is inseparable from the effective delivery of patient care and both are going through a period of rapid change and are under political and financial pressure at present. The drive to improve preregistration training is one among many that the NHS is trying to carry forward, and may yet fall victim to 'initiative fatigue'. The implementation of improvements in specialist medical training is and will remain the main priority of postgraduate deans.

In this setting of rapid and unpredictable change, it is difficult for standards to be maintained and improved in a co-ordinated and effective manner; instead, progress is piecemeal and slow, and without formal surveys it is impossible to know against what standard different posts and house officers are being assessed and to what extent the standards are achieved.

Hours of work

British doctors in training have worked excessive hours for many years, and house officers have been among the worst affected. In 1988/9, 75% of house officers in the Thames regions were on duty for 83 or more hours per week. Since then, an impressive programme of improvement driven by determined managers and supported by doctors has achieved large reductions in hours of duty, so that only 30% of Thames house officers were working 83 or more hours per week by 1992/3 (Gillard et al. 1993a). Reducing hours while maintaining training quality, continuity of patient care and doctors' income is proving difficult, but fatigued doctors can neither learn nor treat patients adequately and therefore the reduction in hours should be seen as a precondition to effective training and medical practice, not a competitor.

Casemix

The GMC recommends that the preregistration year should provide training in and experience of general medical and surgical patients. However, there is no definition of what constitutes an appropriate mix of patients and in particular the maximum acceptable proportion of patients from subspecialities such as orthopaedics or oncology. Particularly at large teaching Trusts, many patients have uncommon or complicated conditions which make them less suitable for preregistration training purposes than those in district hospitals.

Teaching hospital house officers have fewer patients under their care and are more likely to report that the patients are too few in number to enable them to acquire clinical experience at an adequate rate (Dent et al. 1990b). Teaching hospitals are inimical in other ways: house officers there admit fewer patients per week, the burden of inappropriate tasks is greater and, at least in 1988/9, the hours of work were longer. The belief that these posts are a prestigious start to a doctor's career operates as a perverse incentive, attracting graduates to posts they do not expect to enjoy or learn from simply because they are sought after and to have succeeded in securing one is a marker of ability.

There are also differences between the numbers of patients seen by house officers in different parts of England. Large and significant differences are found between eight English regions in the numbers of emergency (two-fold) and routine (1.8-fold) admissions which house officers were responsible for in an average week (Dent *et al.* 1995). The Thames regions offered significantly less clinical experience than those elsewhere. House officers in some regions have 30% more in-patients under their care than those elsewhere, with significant differences between Thames (mean 18.8) and non-Thames (22.4). Thames house officers are more likely to report having so few patients that they are not gaining sufficient clinical experience. This may exacerbate the deficiencies in London medical students' clinical experience recently identified by McManus and colleagues (McManus *et al.* 1993).

Skill mix

House officers work closer to the boundary between the roles and competencies of different professional groups than any other type of doctor and this, coupled with their lack of power in the working environment, has made them particularly vulnerable to the imposition of inappropriate tasks. These include injecting intravenous drugs, filing results in clinical notes, and finding beds for emergency admissions: these are usually more suitable for a nurse, ward clerk, or bed manager. House officers can also find themselves facing inappropriately delegated medical assignments for which they have inadequate training such as communicating bad news or controlling severe pain (Jolly and Macdonald 1989). These tasks use time that should be assigned for training or providing medical input into patient care, are not cost-effectively performed, and can lead to errors with fatal results. They also have a highly corrosive effect on house officers' morale and are ranked by them as the most important problem they face at work (Gillard *et al.* 1993*b*). In North America, by contrast, interns (the equivalent of house officers) are less likely to perform so many inappropriate tasks because of a greater cost-consciousness and unwillingness to use expensive staff for work that could be done by others.

House officers are young, short-term employees of organizations under constant change and financial pressure, working long hours in an unfamiliar and demanding role, dependent on a reference for their promotion and without local acceptance that the principal purpose of their appointment is to receive training, not to provide patient care. It is therefore not surprising that their professional time is open to encroachment from other groups who are unaware of the house officer's primary educational objectives and often themselves short-staffed and performing inappropriate work. House officers are uniquely vulnerable to systematic abuse and have suffered correspondingly high levels of psychiatric ill-health for decades (Firth-Cozens 1987; Small 1981). The educational potential of the year is marred by these unresolved conflicts.

Budget-holding postgraduate deans

A major obstacle to change in the preregistration year has hitherto been the powerlessness of postgraduate deans. Trusts and their consultants are often reluctant to implement deans' suggestions; if house officer training is persistently neglected, the only available sanction is withdrawal of university recognition, which obliges the hospital to fill the post with an overseas-trained or fully registered doctor, at some inconvenience and additional expense. However, this sanction is rarely used, as a high threshold has to be reached before a public declaration of a post's unsuitability can be made. Although appointing a senior consultant, often from the teaching hospital, as postgraduate dean may mean that professional and personal relationships could be used to advance educational causes, it may militate against a capacity for robust discussion and confrontation when circumstances demand it.

Postgraduate deans hold all of the salary of doctors in training (NHSME 1992) and remit this to Trusts employing the doctors in approved training posts. As a result, the hospitals in which doctors are training enjoy the fruits of the doctors' service contribution at a subsidized price. In return, the dean requires the hospital and its consultant staff to provide suitable training, and making use of the contemporary market paradigm of the NHS, draws up educational contracts to specify what has been agreed. If the hospital does not deliver this, the subsidy can be wholly or partially withdrawn. A large hospital spends several million pounds a year on junior doctors' salaries, and being obliged to raise this income through contracts with health care purchasers when its competitors are receiving it as educational subsidy will be an unwelcome prospect. Postgraduate medical education has thus adapted to the prevailing NHS culture and acquired a powerful method of credibly and flexibly influencing local decisions.

Consumerism

The teaching and training of doctors are now fashionable topics. In the last five years, the increasing subscriptions to medical education journals, the appearance of a series of articles on the subject in general medical journals, increased membership of medical education organizations and attendance at their meetings, and initiatives from the Chief Medical Officer and Department of Health, such as the Undergraduate Medical Curriculum Initiative Support Scheme, indicate that medical education is seen as an important mechanism to improve the quality of patient care. The consequent determination to ensure that training is provided to a high standard must now be converted into action, and consumers of medical education have a legitimacy here that they must exploit. Hitherto, they have had too passive a role and allowed programmes such as 'Achieving a Balance' (Department of Health 1987), and 'New Deal' ('NHS Management Executive' 1991) to be presented as concerned largely with improving doctors' career prospects or chances of a full night's sleep, rather than methods of enabling the profession to deliver safer and more effective care to patients. Similarly, there is a risk that medical education initiatives will appear to hinder the performance of clinical work by taking doctors in training away from the bedside. On the contrary, the gain from one recent educational initiative (allocating ward tasks to the appropriate professional group rather than according to tradition) is clinical as well as educational: when nurses rather than doctors gave intravenous antibiotics, the timing of doses and the recording of drug administration improved (Denton *et al.* 1991).

The status of doctors' training as a salient but fashionable topic brings with it the risk that attention will soon shift elsewhere and present initiatives will languish. Equally, if the regional postgraduate deans in particular cannot show beneficial results in terms of outcomes from their investment in education, ideally including impacts on patient care, then the activity may not be considered to represent adequate value for money and the attention of NHS policy-makers and the resources they command will be directed elsewhere. Two steps are needed to prevent this: first the structures by which medical education is directed must become more firmly enmeshed in the apparatus of the NHS so that the provision of education is seen as an everyday part of the service rather than something marginal which can be increased or decreased at will. Second, regional deans must acclimatize promptly to a very different managerial and professional task. They are now trying to achieve difficult objectives in an environment changing as fast as any other in the NHS. The resources available have increased proportionately, but this has brought the deans into closer proximity to those who see medical education as a call on limited resources which has to prove its effectiveness in competition with direct patient care.

Changes in London's hospitals

Change can be facilitated by overwhelming external forces which oblige all parties to accept its inevitability and allow the drawbacks of the old system to be dealt with *en bloc* when incremental improvement was proving very slow. The teaching hospitals in Inner London train almost a third of British medical students, many of whom have at least one of their preregistration posts at their Alma Mater. House officer training in London teaching hospitals is more defective than that elsewhere in the Thames regions of south-east England (Dent *et al.* 1990*b*). Despite the widespread impression that there were too many house officers in Inner London, supported by the evidence of differences in clinical experience referred to above, the decline in the number of in-patients at Inner London hospitals as they underwent temporary and permanent bed closures, merged and closed altogether has not been fully reflected in the transfer of house officer posts to district hospitals elsewhere.

The Tomlinson report (1992) recommended a reduction in the numbers of beds and hospitals in Inner London. However, the King's Fund, an independent advisory organization, originally a champion of rationalization in London, has now called for a review of London's health care and educational problems. Outside the Thames regions, a higher proportion of house officers report having so many patients that there was no time to learn from their job (Dent *et al.* 1995). The educational quality of the existing posts as well as those transferred would be improved by this change.

New initiatives

Two recent developments improve the prospects for preregistration training. The Calman report (Department of Health 1993) was concerned only with postgraduate medical training after the preregistration year, but the spirit of its recommendations is likely to lead to changes elsewhere. The development of defined curricula, the specification of criteria for completion of training (in place of the assumption that if a pre-determined period has elapsed since a trainee took up a post then *ipso facto* they are trained) and the increased emphasis on delivering training more intensively so that it can be completed by the trainee's early rather than late thirties: all these objectives are applicable to the preregistration year and their acceptance for one phase of training can be used to bring about change in another.

The second initiative results from the GMC's attempts to deal with the overload in undergraduate medical education by opening a debate on what are the essential knowledge, skills, and attitudes which all doctors need at graduation and whether undergraduates could be allowed to select areas to explore in greater depth. This is already the case in the preregistration year: the GMC specifies the key educational requirements before a post can be approved for preregistration training, but allows the local consultants and the post-graduate dean to develop other aspects of the post (such as exposure to subspecialties, the provision of formal educational sessions, and the balance between academic and service work) and of course allows applicants to select posts according to their interests. The 'core plus options' approach could be applied more extensively, however. Preregistration training in general practice is congruent with the GMCs existing recommendations and can offer experience of great breadth and value (Harris *et al.* 1985), but only two British medical schools provide it. If the notion of starting the design of training with the definition of minimum educational objectives and a complementary range of subjects suitable for deeper study was to spread, then the preregistration year could be seen as a phase of training in which undergraduate core learning was built upon, previous special interests developed and new ones taken up. This is only a restatement and development of existing practice, but it depends on the preregistration year being seen, like undergraduate training, as driven by externally determined educational objectives, the achievement of which is not assumed to have occurred with the passage of time but is checked by measurement of outcome. At present, the necessary exposure to service overwhelms the educational content and the house officer's objectives are seen to have been fulfilled, both by the consultant and the house officer, if the service tasks are completed satisfactorily.

Another scheme which might provide a model for improved training is the LATS (London Academic Training Scheme) programme run within the London Implementation Zone Educational Initiative (LIZEI). This scheme is a year long attachment for young post-trainee general practitioners to academic departments of General Practice in London. Its aim is to educate rapidly a cohort of GPs in research, teaching, and advances such as evidence-based medicine (EBM) and clinical techniques. The view is that such training at an early stage will galvanize subsequent clinical practice and the quality of patient care. With a modification of such a scheme perhaps house officers could spend 3–6 months of a post attached to a clinical unit with a view to increased reflection and study of particular aspects of the practice of medicine, or of techniques such as audit, EBM, and so on.

Towards better preregistration training

The original aim of the preregistration year, to provide supervised postgraduate clinical experience before independent practice began, has been overtaken by the development of further postgraduate training for all specialties, including general practice, and the acceptance that medical education continues until retirement. If the preregistration year is merely the start of this process, does it differ in any way from the rest of postgraduate training, does it offer anything unique or should we let specialized training begin directly after graduation? Conversely, can the educational objectives be attained in a year or should we extend it to two years (Richards 1992). This idea is unpopular with house officers (Gillard *et al.* 1993*b*) and universities, but it is indicative of the extent of the problem that it has appeared from a distinguished source and received some support.

The novice graduate needs to begin to practise medicine in as controlled and supervised an environment as possible. The increasingly complex, cost-contained and specialized context of modern medicine makes this even more desirable. The preregistration year cannot therefore be supplanted by a less educationally oriented introduction to clinical work. Nor are the aims and objectives set out by the GMC unsatisfactory. What is lacking is a robust mechanism to ensure that they are achieved. Educational or learning contracts (see Chapter 3) may well provide the mechanism that universities require, but if they do not, the GMC should actively look for another.

House officers would derive more benefit from their preregistration training if they were more empowered. They have some influence over the post they are allocated (Gillard and Dent 1988), but little reliable information on what the post will be like. Job descriptions for house officers are notoriously inaccurate and should be supplemented by reports of house officers who have completed the post. All house officers now receive an induction course in their first week of service. Their predecessors, who from 1 August each year become Senior House Officers, are retained in post for a few days to enable service cover to be given while induction takes place (Gillard *et al.* 1993*a*). This practice is effective, simple and relatively cheap. Previously, not to pay house officers for attending these courses (the practice of many Trusts) implied that the organization did not value their time and gave a demoralizing but often accurate indication of what lay ahead.

House officers usually move to a different hospital for their second six-month post, and their lowly and marginal role in the hospital is exacerbated by the brevity of their presence. If both posts were in the same hospital, they would develop greater knowledge of the organization and would therefore be more effective, would have greater stability in their personal lives and might represent a more worthwhile avenue of investment for the hospital (Dowling and Barrett 1992). Educationally inadequate posts would be less likely to be tolerated if their effects were not counteracted by a second training location.

The use of incentives rather than punishments is a more effective way to make change happen (Donabedian 1989). Consultants are willing to increase their involvement in house officer training, but lack skills and time and do not see the preregistration year as an educational process (Wilson 1993). The King's Fund (Towle 1991) and the Standing Committee on Postgraduate Medical Education (SCOPME 1992) have also identified the lack of training for senior doctors in how to train as major deficiencies in the British system, though steps to recruit staff to provide this training are under way (Biggs *et al.* 1994). Postgraduate deans should consider giving clearer guidance on what they and house officers expect, and providing the training consultants need in order to deliver training more effectively. The consultants' as well as the house officers' time needs to be protected for training. More imaginative ways of increasing consultants' commitment to preregistration training should be sought: universities could provide special recognition or honorary titles to consultants who excelled, a consultant's achievement in this area could be considered in allocating merit awards (a scheme under which consultants select colleagues for substantial pay increments based on excellence in research, clinical care or, rarely, teaching) or other forms of performance related pay and high quality training could be publicised via 'Good Job Guides' so that more attractive applicants sought the post.

The monitoring of posts' quality is at present very haphazard. Because house officers apply to the GMC for full registration at the end of the preregistration year, the GMC is in a position to request completion of a postal questionnaire at that time or even make it a condition of registration. Postgraduate deans could also undertake this on a regional basis.

In 1997, the GMC issued *The New Doctor*, its revised recommendations for the preregistration (GMC, 1997) year. The new recommendations are a repsonse to the failure of the previous set to bring about change. It reveals some sense of urgency, and broadens the educational scope of the pre-registration year by including themes such as critical appraisal and teamwork. A welcome feature is its recognition of the need to reduce confusion over responsibility. The duties of postgraduate deans and supervising consultants are specified and it indicates that consultants will need training to fulfil those duties. The GMC clearly expects postgraduate deans to deal with defective posts, stating that 'universities should exercise control over [preregistration house officers'] clinical duties, hours of work, . . . night duty commitment and personal study time'. It is also suggested that more structured appraisal of preregistration house officers will be introduced in future.

It is revealing that the GMC's response to the non-implementation of its last set of recommendations is to issue more and exhort everyone to try harder. The obstacle to progress is not a lack of standards, and publication of new requirements is unlikely to have much impact. The GMC is hampered by its need to work through deans, universities, Trusts and training consultants to raise standards. It has access to neither incentives nor sanctions. *The New Doctor*'s effectiveness depends on it galvanizing other parties to try hard to succeed. Initial signs are encouraging, with the Association for the Study of Medical Education proposing a national assessment for house officers, structured appraisal by training consultants at specified intervals, and formal training in their training role for consultants by August 1999 (see also Jolly, 1997).

Preregistration training has languished despite efforts to overcome its defects. The present ascendancy of medical education, the increasing influence of postgraduate deans, and the latest GMC recommendations have set the stage for another attempt. What made a difference in other areas of persistent inertia, e.g. hours of work, was determined intervention from the Department of Health; perhaps there is no other force which can overcome the resistance to improving the educational quality of postgraduate medical training in the UK.

References

Biggs, J.S.G., Agger, S.K., Dent, T.H.S., Allery, L.A., and Coles, C. (1994). Training for medical teachers: a UK Survey 1993. *Medical Education*, **28**, 99–106.

Calman, K.C. (1992). The preregistration year. In Downie, R.S. and Charlton, B. (Eds.). *The making of a doctor: medical education in theory and practice* pp.00–00. Oxford University Press.

Christie, R.A.S. (1980). The preregistration house appointment: a survey in Manchester. *Medical Education*, **14**, 210–3.

Dent, T.H.S., Gillard, J.H., Aarons, E.J., Crimlisk, H.L., and Smyth-Pigott, P.J. (1990*a*). Pre-registration house officers in the four Thames regions: I. survey of education and workload. *British Medical Journal*, **300**, 713–6.

Dent, T.H.S., Gillard, J.H., Aarons, E.J., Crimlisk, H., and Smyth-Pigott, P.J. (1990*b*) Pre-registration house officers in the four Thames regions: II. comparison of education and workload in teaching and non-teaching hospitals. *British Medical Journal*, **300**, 716–18.

Dent, T.H.S., Gillard, J.H., Aarons, E.J., and Smyth-Pigott, P.J. (1995). Variation in clinical experience of British house officers: the effect of London. *Health Trends*, **27**, 22–6.

Denton, M., Morgan, M.S., and White, R.R. (1991). Quality of prescribing of intravenous antibiotics in a district general hospital. *British Medical Journal*, **302**, 327–8.

Department of Health and Social Security United Kingdom Health Departments, Joint Consultants Committee, Chairmen of Regional Health Authorities. (1987) *Hospital medical staffing: achieving a balance: plan for action*. London.

Department of Health (1993). *Hospital doctors: training for the future*. DoH, London.

Donabedian, A. (1989). Institutional and professional responsibilities in quality assurance. *Quality Assurance in Health Care* **1**, 3–11.

Dowling, S. and Barrett, S. (1992). *Doctors in the making: the experience of the preregistration year*. School for Advanced Urban Studies, Bristol.

Firth-Cozens, J. (1987). Emotional distress in junior house officers. *British Medical Journal*, **295**, 533–6.

General Medical Council (1992). *Recommendations on general clinical training*. GMC, London.

General Medical Council (1997). The New Doctor: recommendations on general clinical training. GMC, London.

Gillard, J.H. and Dent, T.H.S. (1988). The allocation of house officer posts: a UK survey. *Medical Education*, **22**, 342–4.

Gillard, J.H., Dent, T.H.S., Aarons, E.J., Crimlisk, H.L., Smyth-Pigott, P.J., and Nicholls, M.W.N. (1993*a*) Preregistration house officers in the Thames regions: changes in quality of training after four years. *British Medical Journal*, **307**, 1176–9.

Gillard, J.H., Dent, T.H.S., Aarons, E.J., Smyth-Pigott, P.J., and Nicholls, M.W.N. (1993*b*). Preregistration house officers in eight English regions: a survey of quality of training. *British Medical Journal*, **307**, 1180–4.

Grant, J., Chambers, E., Hodgson, B., Kirkwood, A., Morgan, A. (1992). *Formal opportunities in postgraduate education for hospital doctors in training*. SCOPME, London.

Harris, C.M., Dudley, H.A.F., Jarman, B., Kidner, P.H. (1985). Preregistration rotation including general practice at St Mary's Hospital Medical School. *British Medical Journal* **290**, 1811–13.

HMSO (1944). Report of the interdepartmental committee on medical schools. (Goodenough Report) HMSO, London.

Jolly, B.C. (1997) Assessment and Appraisal, Medical Education, **31** (Suppl 1.) pp.20–24.

Jolly, B.C. and Macdonald, M.M. (1989). Education for practice: the role of practical experience in undergraduate and general clinical training. *Medical Education* **23**, 189–95.

Knowles, M. (1990). *The adult learner: a neglected species*. Gulf Publishing Company, Houston.

McManus, I.C., Lockwood, D.N.J., and Cruickshank, J.K. (1977). The preregistration year: chaos by consensus. *Lancet* **i**, 413–6.

McManus, I.C., Richards, P., Winder, B.C., Sproston, K.A., and Vincent, C.A. (1993). The changing clinical experience of British medical students. *Lancet* **341**, 941–4.

National Health Service Management Executive. (1992). *Funding of hospital medical and dental training grade posts* (EL (92)63). NHSME, London.

NHS Management Executive. (1991). *Junior doctors: the new deal*. Department of Health, London.

Paice, E. and Smyth-Pigott, P. (1992). Improving the preregistration period. *British Journal of Hospital Medicine*, **48**, 215–17.

Richards, P. (1992). Educational improvement of the preregistration period of general clinical training. *British Medical Journal* **304**, 625–7.

Small, G.W. (1981). House officer stress syndrome. *Psychosomatics*, **22**, 860–9.

Standing Committee on Postgraduate Medical Education. (1992). *Teaching hospital doctors and dentists to teach: its role in creating a better learning environment*. SCOPME, London.

Tomlinson, B. (1992). Report of the inquiry into London's health service, medical education and research. HMSO, London.

Towle, A. (1991). *Critical thinking: the future of undergraduate medical education*. King's Fund, London.

Wilson, D.H. (1993). Education and training of preregistration house officers: the consultants' viewpoint. *British Medical Journal* **306**, 194–6.

6.2 Service-based learning in hospital medicine: integrating patient care and training in the early postgraduate years

Janet Grant

Background

Postgraduate medical education is based in clinical practice. That is a given that everyone accepts. Our own research work (Grant and Marsden 1988, 1992; Grant *et al.* 1989) has provided the evidence and it has been replicated many times by other workers.

However, the advent in British hospital medicine of partial shift systems can deter the regular presence, as a group, of junior doctors in either service or teaching contexts. It also can mean that doctors no longer get the opportunity to follow a patient through from admission to diagnosis and treatment. They can have a partial view of a patient's current history and its resolution. Added to this, patients themselves are staying in hospital for shorter periods, as increased throughput per bed becomes a management criterion. Clinical experience thus decreases with decreasing times in in-patient stay. A shortened overall period of training does not add any comfort to the observer of this picture.

As the clinical experience of doctors in training threatens to become less satisfactory, the conditions of the seniors who teach them offers no compensation. Senior doctors are busier than ever with increasing demands on their time from the service and from the need to become involved in the management of their departments. Added educational responsibilities will not fall on their deaf ears or on unwilling hearts, but simply on most senior doctors who have no contractual time for education (although they have a contractual obligation) and who are already overcommitted elsewhere.

And there are new educational responsibilities. There are demands for evidence of the training that junior doctors receive. The medical Royal Colleges have the professional responsibility to ensure that a proper training is specified and delivered. These agencies lay down the content and processes of postgraduate training. The Department of Health also specifies standards and recording systems for postgraduate training.

What is missing from this picture, is often any support for the senior doctors to teach, or for the junior doctors to learn. There is increasing clarity of standards but, at this stage, perhaps less to help their practical delivery.

It is to practical development and support that the profession must now turn. Acceptable and workable solutions will only be developed if this context of SHO training is recognized and educational systems are designed that will fit into that context and not strain it further. This means that we should recognize the conditions of teachers and learners, and the strengths as well as the weaknesses of postgraduate training as it has developed, so that we are realistic about what can and cannot be altered.

Learning from practice

Service-based learning is a UK system of senior house officer (SHO) training that has been developed in paediatrics, accident and emergency, and anaesthesia which takes this context into account and builds on what is still, despite its faults and problems, an appropriate model of professional training because it is founded on professional clinical practice.

The strength of the traditional integration of service and training is not to be underestimated. Although it is well recognized that the apprenticeship aspects of postgraduate training leave something to be desired, it would be as well to recognize that most professions, in the end, move away from isolated academic learning and towards taking up the skilled and responsible practice of that profession in a controlled and guided manner, in the context of practice. This, however imperfectly, is what postgraduate medical training does. But it can be problematical.

One of the many challenges for the recently qualified and registered doctor is that of finding a new way of learning. The young doctor who is in a training grade has to cope with the inherent contradiction of his or her position: of being obliged to demonstrate competence to care for patients while also recognizing and articulating a need to learn and to be trained. This contradiction is frequently skated over, often not recognized and rarely addressed or analysed. Yet it is at the root of many of the issues and problems of the early postgraduate years.

None the less, there is no dispute about the power of such practice-based, 'situated learning' (Lave and Wenger 1991) in developing professional skills and the high-level problem-solving thinking which characterizes the master of the craft. Situated learning describes the process whereby the trainee begins working with limited, peripheral participation and limited responsibility; gradually, over years, moving towards central participation and full overall responsibility. The training programme therefore should be planned around those experiences which provide the proper context for learning to take place. Situated learning describes postgraduate medical education and indicates to us the ways in which that education can be supported and developed to build on its strengths.

Traditional approaches to early postgraduate training

Until recent times there have been two major approaches to early postgraduate training. The first involves opportunistic 'teaching' by seniors as part of the general melange of the service experience. Thus seniors, who are also suffering from the competing pressures of their roles as clinicians cum teachers cum managers, have grasped the educational opportunities of the ward round, and have added to it small 'tutorials' or mini-lectures about the clinical problems that are being reviewed. Sometimes, junior doctors judge this, rightly or wrongly, to be less educational than their seniors would hope. The seniors are giving teaching, but the juniors do not feel that they experience learning (Grant and Marsden 1988).

The fundamental reason for this is found in the doctor–learner contradiction. On a ward round, the trainee is doing his or her best to show complete competence, to demonstrate that the patient has been properly clerked, that the right tests have been ordered, that the right thoughts about the patient's condition have been considered. The trainee carefully edits every utterance to avoid the glaring error, the embarrassing *faux pas*, the revelation of anything less than competence and confidence. The trainee does everything possible to demonstrate that he or she has few outstanding learning needs. On top of that, the ward round will have given rise to more clinical work and time is pressing. An impromptu lecture from the consultant can often be just another barrier to getting the service work done. These are not the characteristics of a climate for learning.

The second approach to early postgraduate training is to opt for dedicated time for formal learning of one sort or another. Following on from the half-day release scheme for trainees in general practice, there has been a consistent call from hospital-based educationalists for 'protected time' away from the service for training during the early postgraduate years. The time called for is usually a half day per week, although experience and pragmatism have seen this target shrink visibly in many quarters.

Protecting educational time from the service is more easily said than done. This is even true of the general practice vocational training scheme trainees. One study (Bouchier Hayes *et al.* 1992; Styles *et al.* 1994) revealed that only 37% of VTS (general practice) trainees working on hospital attachments attended more than 75% of the available study half-days, while 14% attended less than a quarter of the half-days on offer and 10% of VTS trainees attended none. The two main reasons for non-attendance were pressure of work (67%) and inability to find cover (45%).

Protecting the trainee from patient care perhaps does not make great educational sense, anyway. It is in clinical work that the trainee learns to become an effective clinician. It is not protection from the service that is required: it is support for teacher and learner to make that service of patient care even more pointedly educational.

Recognizing reality, building on strengths: the development and evaluation of service-based learning

The reality of service pressures, lack of time for training, lack of money and resources, and lack of staff who are dedicated to teaching must first be accepted if pragmatic, practicable, and achievable solutions to the problems of early postgraduate training are to be found. Crying for a moon made up of dedicated half-days for training, or hoping that a mini-lecture on a ward round will suffice can only lead to further tears.

Instead, we can begin from where we are, and build on current conditions, not asking anyone to change their ways entirely, but encouraging everyone to alter just a little, in ways that they feel comfortable with. We can accept that the service will predominate, because a choice between a lecture or seminar and a patient is no real choice at all. We can also take to heart the central tenet and strength of postgraduate training in medicine: that learning from providing patient care is the best learning of all. And we can find ways of making that work to high standards of assured educational excellence.

With this approach in mind, we undertook over a period of six years a carefully planned series of projects which have culminated in a supportive approach to SHO training: service-based learning in paediatrics, accident and emergency and anaesthetics. The example described here involved training senior house officers in anaesthetics. However, there is no reason why service-based learning should not be used in any specialty or at any stage of postgraduate training.

The aims of the project were to:

- describe and evaluate the actual training conditions of SHOs;
- identify the recognized and unrecognized opportunities for training that SHO posts have;
- identify the necessary characteristics of good practice in SHO training;
- design a new system of SHO training that could be integrated into the current conditions of any SHO post;
- test the feasibility of the new system in theory;
- recruit pilot sites to develop the system in practice and tailor it to their needs and conditions;
- test the system in practice.

The original design for service-based learning was achieved by the stages shown in Fig. 6.1.

Service-based learning materials for subsequent specialties, such as anaesthetics, have taken advantage of this original research so are developed through the stages shown in Fig. 6.2.

The detailed derivation of service-based learning is described elsewhere (Grant and Marsden 1988, 1992). Overall, it was developed through rigorous research in the field, consultation and planning in collaboration with clinical departments, and repeated testing in practice of each element of the materials. Recent steps taken by the medical Royal Colleges and postgraduate deans to define syllabus and process aspects of training has meant that, by negotiation, these can also be incorporated into these materials.

Such an approach to educational development is generally referred to as 'action research' (McNiff 1993). Although this might seem over-cautious, it is designed to ensure that the project always remained and remains grounded in the experience and conditions of its target audience. It also ensures that the problems which are identified really are the problems that are experienced by teachers and learners and that the solutions which are offered are the solutions that the target audiences can identify as their own. The importance of these factors in managing changes in medical education is central (Gale and Grant 1990, see Chapter 8) and will be disregarded at the educational developer's peril.

Evaluations (Grant and Marsden 1992; Grant et al. 1994) show that the outcome of the process has been a set of learning materials which is:

- flexible enough to fit in with the prevailing conditions in clinical departments;
- robust enough to use the same documentation and to display the same positive educational characteristics across different departments
- amenable to use in a wide variety of ways (Stanton, 1997)

Service-based learning has also been shown to be associated with an enhanced educational climate, better agreement between seniors and juniors on the educational quality of the department and higher scores on flexibility of diagnostic thinking (Stanton 1996).

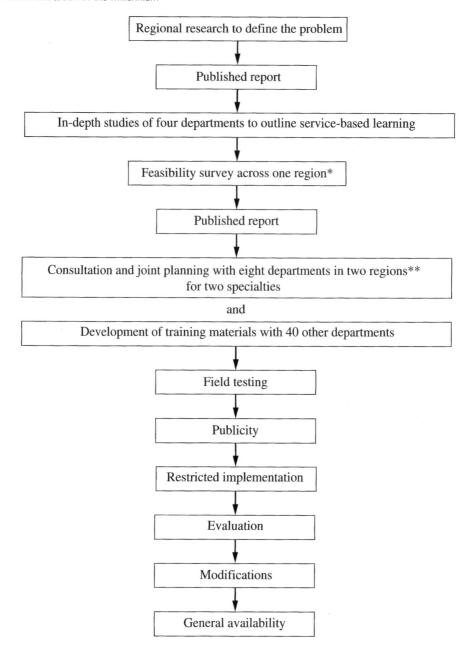

Fig. 6.1 Stages of development for the original educational design of service-based learning

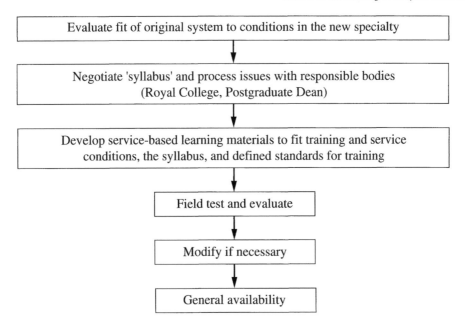

Fig. 6.2 Stages of development of service-based learning for subsequent specialties

The materials are also:

♦ educationally sound
♦ based on integrating service and training
♦ responsive to the needs of the syllabus for each specialty
♦ tailored to the individual learning needs of each doctor in training.

Service-based learning: the materials

Service-based learning is elegantly simple. It systematizes all the valued forms of learning which SHOs currently undertake and supports them to ensure their educational effectiveness. It makes clear what education and training are offered by a clinical department. It also ensures basic features such as syllabus coverage and feedback on performance. The elements of service-based learning are represented in Fig. 6.3. The five types of educational activity they support are outlined below.

Practice-based learning

Our research and development work showed that SHOs like to learn by following up for themselves the problems they have encountered and things they know they need to learn more about as a result of their clinical practice. However, they sometimes do not know how to set about learning more, or they simply do not find the occasion on which to decide how to follow up the necessary new learning.

The SHO's Educational record encourages a greater conscious focus on discussing and reflecting on clinical experience.

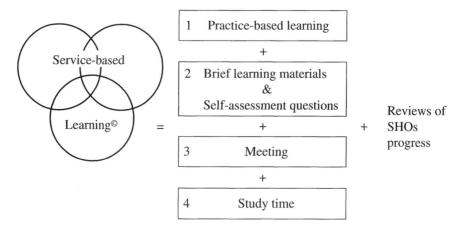

Fig. 6.3 The elements of service-based learning

The topics covered by practice-based learning are noted against the syllabus, and a note of the learning plan can also be made against that same syllabus list. Fig. 6.4 shows a page from the SHOs educational record where such events can be recorded against the college syllabus.

Brief learning and self-assessment

SHOs often want to be able to read about a condition, a procedure or a treatment during the working day, as part of their service work. Yet most reported that they did not have appropriate resources that were problem-focused and brief to read. Accordingly, the service-based learning materials include volumes of specially written brief learning materials (BLMs) which cover the syllabus and the practice of the specialty for an SHO in a practice- or problem-related way. Each specialty might have as many as 400 BLMs. Fig. 6.5 presents part of a BLM to indicate the style of these.

The BLMs are grouped into topics and each topic has an associated set of self-assessment questions and model answers. This supplies the SHOs' need to judge their own progress.

BLMs are read as part of the daily work of patient care, for private study, in preparation for meetings and in many other ways. Seniors often choose to base seminars on the BLMs or on the self-assessments. BLMs can allow the trainee to fashion a personal course. They also can extend the trainee's learning to beyond the experience offered by the department. SHOs can record when they have completed the self-assessments, as shown in Fig. 6.6.

Meetings

Most departments offer educational meetings. These may be in lecture format, or in a range of other interactive and participative formats as well. Our evaluations have shown that SHOs appreciate a variety of approaches.

Meetings attended are also noted down against the relevant syllabus item so that syllabus coverage can be monitored.

College syllabus, related BLMs, learning plans, meetings, & study time

Syllabus topics	Learning method which covered the syllabus topic			
	Related BLMs	Practice-based learning (Note the plan against the related syllabus topic)	Related meeting attended (tick)	Related study time taken (tick)
FOR YOUR FIRST SIX MONTHS 1. Care of the patient				
1.1 Resuscitation				
1.1.1 Basic life support	43.1.A	✓		
1.1.2 Advanced life support	43.1.B,C,D,E,G			
1.2 Intravascular access				
1.2.1 Peripheral venous	9.2	✓		
1.2.2 Central venous	9.3			
1.2.3 Arterial	9.4	✓		
1.3 Pre-operative care	7			
1.3.1 General assessment	7.1		✓	
1.3.2 Premedication	8.1		✓	
1.3.3 Consent	10.1		✓	
1.3.4 Airway assessment	9.5		✓	
1.3.5 Preparation of patient	7.1		✓	
1.3.6 DVT prophylaxis				
1.4 Operative care	10	✓		✓
1.4.1 Positioning of patient	10.5			✓
1.4.2 Protection		✓		✓
1.4.3 Electrical safety	4.2			✓
1.5 Common problems				
1.5.1 Hypotension	11.2, 38.6, 40.2			
1.5.2 Hypoxia/hypercapnia	1.2.G, 40.2			

Fig. 6.4 SHOs record of education

Group 11: Recovery and Postoperative Care
Item 2: Oxygen Therapy in Recovery

The recovery nurse will give your patient oxygen. Have you ever asked why?

Q
Think of three reasons for giving oxygen to postoperative patients. Think about your answers and compare them with the list below.

A
Reasons for giving O_2 in recovery.
• Respiratory depression from opiates
• As a safety margin against respiratory obstruction
• To counter diffusion hypoxia
• Because normal V/Q relationships are disturbed by general anaesthesia
• Intra-op blood loss will have disturbed O_2 carrying capacity

OK. So let's agree that patients need O_2 post-op, but
• how much?
• for how long?
• how are we going to give it?

HOW MUCH?

For most reasonably fit patients undergoing routine surgery we are only dealing with the first four reasons given above. So we are only aiming for about 30% O_2. The actual amount doesn't matter provided it's more than room air.

Practice Point
If you are in doubt or worried about a patient give 100% O_2 via a rebreathing bag and face mask. There should be one in every recovery room. Then think your way through the problem or call for help.

Q
Who needs more O_2?

Practice Point
As an SHO, if your patient needs more than 30% O_2 for any more than a few minutes you need senior help and your patient will probably need an HDU or ITU post-op.

A
Cases involving:
Large blood loss
Long anaesthesia
Intercurrent disease

Q
Does anyone need less than 30%?

A
Yes. Those patients with COAD who are on hypoxic drive. But these days it is rare for COAD to that bad.

Practice Point
You should not anaesthetise anyone in this group when you are alone.

Note: most patients with COAD are not relying on hypoxic drive to make them breathe.

Q
Now would be a good time to wrack your brains and write down the normal respiratory drive.
What make you breathe?
Where are the chemoreceptors?
Where is the respiratory centre?
What effect will hypoxia have on this?
Draw a graph of minute volume against $PaCO_2$.

A
No chance!
If you can't remember, look it up properly in a respiratory physiology textbook, such as *West's Respiratory Physiology*.

Patients with COAD who are on hypoxic drive will need accurate concentrations of oxygen, usually 24% maximum. See below for how to give accurate concentrations.

HOW LONG?

This may seem a blinding glimpse of the obvious but you only know how long it is needed if you measure the effect of withdrawing the oxygen.
• Use a pulse oximeter on all your patients in recovery.
• Give O_2 for an arbitrary time (say, for 10 minutes or until awake).
• Withdraw the added O_2.
• Continue to measure SaO_2 – see if it drops.
• If it does drop, give the O_2 for longer.

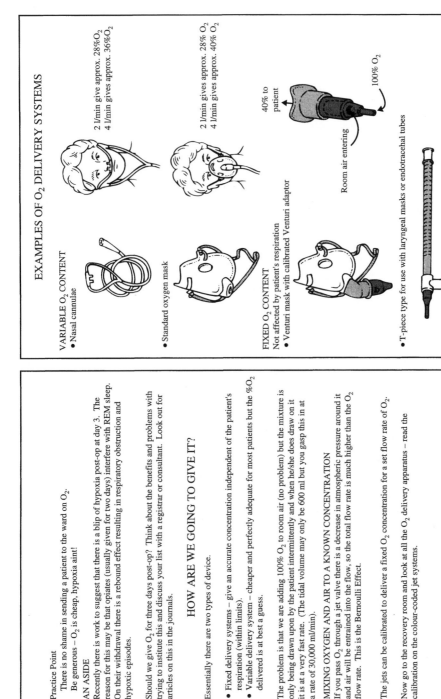

EXAMPLES OF O$_2$ DELIVERY SYSTEMS

VARIABLE O$_2$ CONTENT
• Nasal cannulae

2 l/min give approx. 28%O$_2$
4 l/min gives approx. 36%O$_2$

• Standard oxygen mask

2 l/min gives approx. 28% O$_2$
4 l/min gives approx. 40% O$_2$

FIXED O$_2$ CONTENT
Not affected by patient's respiration
• Venturi mask with calibrated Venturi adaptor

40% to patient

Room air entering

100% O$_2$

• T-piece type for use with laryngeal masks or endotracheal tubes

Practice Point
There is no shame in sending a patient to the ward on O$_2$.
Be generous – O$_2$ is cheap, hypoxia aint!

AN ASIDE
Recently there is work to suggest that there is a blip of hypoxia post-op at day 3. The reason for this may be that opiates (usually given for two days) interfere with REM sleep. On their withdrawal there is a rebound effect resulting in respiratory obstruction and hypoxic episodes.

Should we give O$_2$ for three days post-op? Think about the benefits and problems with trying to institute this and discuss your list with a registrar or consultant. Look out for articles on this in the journals.

HOW ARE WE GOING TO GIVE IT?

Essentially there are two types of device.

• Fixed delivery systems – give an accurate concentration independent of the patient's respiration (within limits).
• Variable delivery system – cheaper and perfectly adequate for most patients but the %O$_2$ delivered is at best a guess.

The problem is that we are adding 100% O$_2$ to room air (no problem) but the mixture is only being drawn upon by the patient intermittently and when he/she does draw on it it is at a very fast rate. (The tidal volume may only be 600 ml but you gasp this in at a rate of 30,000 ml/min).

MIXING OXYGEN AND AIR TO A KNOWN CONCENTRATION
If you pass O$_2$ through a jet valve there is a decrease in atmospheric pressure around it and air will be entrained into the flow, so the total flow rate is much higher than the O$_2$ flow rate. This is the Bernoulli Effect.

The jets can be calibrated to deliver a fixed O$_2$ concentration for a set flow rate of O$_2$.

Now go to the recovery room and look at all the O$_2$ delivery apparatus – read the calibration on the colour-coded jet systems.

Fig. 6.5 Example of brief learning material style

LIST OF BRIEF LEARNING MATERIALS AND SELF-ASSESSMENT QUESTIONS COMPLETED

There is no need to record which BLMs you have read, but you should indicate which Self-Assessment Questions you have completed, by ticking the appropriate box.	SAQ Completed *Tick*
GROUP 1 PHYSIOLOGY	
ITEM 1 Cardiovascular a) Basic Cardiac Physiology - Circulation b) Basic Cardiac Physiology - The Heart c) Control of blood pressure and peripheral vascular resistance d) Special circulations: cardiac, respiratory, cerebral, renal e) Normal values: volume, rate, pressure, output f) Cardiovascular response to anaesthesia	
ITEM 2 Respiratory a) Gas exchange; ventilation perfusion b) Oxygen carriage and dissociation curves c) Ventilation d) Mechanics of ventilation e) Artificial ventilation f) Normal values g) Respiratory response to anaesthesia h) Blood gases	
ITEM 3 Nervous System a) Nerve conduction b) Spinal cord; brain stem; midbrain; cortex c) Autonomic nervous system d) Pain e) Motor system f) Cerebrospinal fluid; control of intracranial pressure f) Nausea and vomiting	
ITEM 4 Renal a) Fluid and electrolyte balance, compartments, normal values b) Renal function c) Body Water Regulation ITEM 5 Haematology a) Sickle Cell Anaemia and Thallasaemia b) Clotting, coagulation and DIC ITEM 6 Endocrine a) Pituitary; thyroid; parathyroid; adrenal ITEM 7 Gastrointestinal a) Acid secretion, emptying b) Pancreas and Kidney	

Fig. 6.6 Example of brief learning material listing and record of self assessments completed

Study time

Educational time away from the department is negotiated at the beginning of an appointment, and the topics noted against the syllabus. In many departments where study leave is not negotiated at the beginning of an appointment, it is never taken at all. It is expected that where the first three strands of service-based learning activity are working well, there will be less need for educational time away from the department.

Reviewing progress

Service-based learning incorporates many Deans' and Colleges' requirement (and many trainees' unmet wishes) for the trainee and senior to meet once or twice every six months to review progress and give feedback on performance in a planned way. These occasions also allow a review of the education and training offered by the department. The meetings are guided by reference to the trainee's educational record and self-assessments.

Materials

The materials for service-based learning are elegantly simple. They consist of:

◆ The SHOs *Educational record and self-assessment questions*. This is a booklet, which is kept by the SHO. Figures 6.3, 6.4 and 6.6 are taken from such a booklet.
◆ Brief learning materials (BLMs): each department, or separate working location within a department, has a set of BLMs, usually bound in three volumes each of about 130 BLMs. These are used at the work location, although SHOs do sometimes purchase or acquire their own copies for home study.
◆ Model answers: each department keeps one set of *Model answers* to the self-assessment questions. The SHOs refer to these themselves.

In addition, the materials include a set of *Guidelines for consultants*, offering advice about using service-based learning materials, and a set of overhead transparencies for use by the consultant when introducing new trainees to them.

Conclusions

Service-based learning is a structured and flexible, individually tailored approach to early postgraduate training which overcomes many of the major problems and builds on all the great strengths of training experienced at that stage:

◆ It supports individual trainees to learn systematically and effectively as part of their service commitment.
◆ It focuses on the clinical experience, and intensifies that training. This will become increasingly important as the training period decreases.
◆ It offers practical support to both trainee and teacher in terms of learning resources, documentation and does not demand reorganization or increased funding or staffing.

- It encompasses the standards set by bodies responsible for education and training.
- It provides evidence of training offered and received.
- It encourages dialogue and feedback between senior and trainee.
- It builds on the strengths of postgraduate learning which is situated in clinical practice.
- It is flexible enough to fit in with a large range of departmental conditions.
- It does not make unrealistic demands of teacher or learner during times of great intensity of clinical work.

Service-based learning has the strength of building on current valued training methods, of ensuring that the training opportunities of each department are fully exploited and of demonstrating in a public, recorded manner that training does occur as part of the service experience of the trainee.

References

Bouchier Hayes, T.A.I., Golombok, S., Grant, J., Rust, J., and Styles, W.McN. (1992) *The Hospital component of training for general practice*. Report to the Nuffield Provincial Hospitals Trust.

Gale, R. and Grant, J. (1990). *Guidelines for change in postgraduate and continuing medical education*. Joint Centre for Education in Medicine, London.

Grant, J. and Marsden, P. (1988). *Senior house officer training in south-east Thames*. 2 volumes Joint Centre for Education in Medicine, London.

Grant, J., Marsden, P., and King, R.C. (1989). Senior house officers and their training. *British Medical Journal*, **299**, 1263–8. 2 parts.

Grant, J. and Marsden, P. (1992). *Training senior house officers by service-based learning*. Joint Centre for Education in Medicine, London.

Grant, J., Marsden, P., Perez-Avila, C., Stanton, F., and Waring, C. (1994). *Service-based learning in practice: an evaluation report of the first six months*. Joint Centre for Education in Medicine, London.

Lave, J. and Wenger, E. (1991). *Situated learning: legitimate peripheral participation*. Cambridge University Press, Cambridge.

McNiff, J. (1993). *Action research. principles and practice*. Croom Helm, London.

Stanton, F. (1996). *An evaluation of service-based learning in accident and emergency*. Joint Centre for Education in Medicine, London.

Stanton, F. (1997). *Approaches to the use of service-based learning in anaesthesia*. Joint Centre for Education in Medicine, London. Unpublished report.

Styles, W.McN., Grant, J., Golombok, S., and Rust, J. (1994). Vocational training for general practice: attendance rates at release courses. *Education for General Practice*, **5**, 66–70.

7 Perspectives on the quality of medical education

7.1 Historical and theoretical background

Brian Jolly

> My method, hitherto unknown here, and possibly anywhere else, is to lead my students by
> the hand to the practice of medicine, taking them every day to see patients in the public
> hospital, that they may hear the patients' symptoms and see their physical findings. Then
> I question the students as to what they have noted in the patients and about their thoughts
> and perceptions regarding the causes of the illnesses and the principles of treatment.
> *Sylvius 1679, p. 907*

Introduction

Clinical exposure is an important part of medical training. The intention of this chapter
will be to illuminate some of the characteristics and products of learning, by medical
students, in the clinical setting. The studies referred to here were carried out in the
context of courses in the UK, Canada, and Australia. Most were completed during a
period in which the primary location of clinical teaching was the ward, the lecture
theatre, or the out-patient clinic, all usually in a large teaching hospital. As pointed out
in Chapters 1 and 4, the movement of clinical education into the community has been
slow to materialize and confined to a small number of (mostly new) schools. Nevertheless 'hospital' based educational research has covered a wide variety of learning
environments and includes the structure and function of clinical attachments, ward
based teaching (including bedside teaching), the learning of technical skills, academic
work in a clinical context, and the use of out-patients. The activities undertaken by
students in such settings will probably overlap and duplicate considerably primary care
and social, community and laboratory based medical disciplines, because many of the
activities used by these disciplines (e.g. bedside teaching at home and walk-in clinics) are
similar to those discussed here. The challenge for medical education is to search for ways
to enhance the quality of clinical education first by comparing students' experience to
what modern educational theory and practice can offer and second in adapting common
practices in clinical education to new circumstances.

Some groundwork has been laid in Chapter 2, Here we will discuss two questions; why
is clinical education important; where did it come from? These issues are discussed under
the canopy of the historical development of clinical education. Then the major goals of
clinical education as perceived by modern educators are addressed, the common
practices of clinical teaching are described, and finally a focused review of research

on clinical teaching and learning is presented. Later in the chapter we will stress the importance of strengthening the quality of the educational environment by close monitoring and by staff development.

The historical development of clinical education

Why clinical education?

The answers to such a question might seem obvious. But the history of clinical education has been littered with unchallenged assumptions. Some activities that are now taken for granted were, only a few centuries ago, unheard of or proscribed. It is difficult to envisage medical education without a clinical (patient-based) component. Yet for four hundred years prior to the seventeenth century much, if not all, of the preparation for practice as a physician was carried out by reading not by clinical contact (O'Malley 1970). This almost total reliance on the printed word was eventually challenged only by the development of empiricism in Europe. The pressing need to verify theoretical assertions in terms of patient outcome created both clinical work and clinical education. The balance between practical and theoretical work had, in fact, swung backwards and forwards since mediaeval times. The equilibrium was dependent either on the interests and personalities of those in positions of power or on other significant events. For example, in the late sixteenth century the rapid availability and expansion of knowledge in books consolidated medicine as an academic, not a clinical, discipline. The emphasis has changed at different times in different places. The development of Italian, Austrian, and Dutch clinical 'schools' from 1600–1850, and the reorganization of American medical education initiated in 1908, can be seen as manifestations of the superiority of practical or of theoretical orientations respectively, both of which are engaged in a perennial tension. These forces pivoted around two central questions: what should the primary focus for medical education be – the needs of the patient or the demands for scientific rigour; and where should learning activity take place, the clinic, or the library?

In many ways this has been a debate about what constitutes *quality* in medical education: the outcome hinging on the extent to which each side has predominated in the argument. At the beginning of the twentieth century the quality of doctors was seen to have been jeopardized by their lack of scientific rigour. In the effort to build this in, much was sacrificed. Now the agenda, and the focus, have shifted back towards the needs of the community and the patient, and we need again to appraise what educational activities are beneficial and/or feasible within the developing health care systems.

The following sections look at these issues in a little more detail, starting with a historical perspective. They challenge the notion that medical education has been developing progressively. Rather, its educational purpose and content has often been defined either by scientists or by physicians. Often the same developments have taken place in different countries at different times. Within this framework significant historical events and the work of educationally influential personalities, like Flexner (1910) and Osler (1906) should be seen as convenient, but unique, conceptual landmarks rather than as points on a medical educational (pedagogical) continuum that absorbs, and benefits from, all influences.

Where did clinical education come from?

Clinical education was conceived, born and nurtured in the hospital setting in the seventeenth and eighteenth centuries. 'The hospital is the only proper College in which to rear a true disciple of Aesculapius' John Abernethy: cited in Osler 1906. Hence the emergence of the bedside teaching method and the evolution of the characteristics typical of clinical training as we know it today were influenced by two important features. The first was the notion of the physician's personal responsibility for the patient. This was the stimulus for the systems of apprenticeship and patronage in clinical education that dominated Europe for several hundred years. The second was the fact that for much of the seventeenth and eighteenth centuries, external observation was the only method of identifying patients' signs and symptoms and of formulating diagnoses. Observation was a skill that had to be learnt, and there were few means of objective verification of the results. Hence the prowess of physicians to see, hear, and feel the essence of the disease process reached near mythical proportions. However it is also important to grasp that this expertise was not universally seen as academic wisdom.

The model both for the clinical component and, to a certain extent, for its linkage with a university education, was developed in Padua by Giovanni Battista da Monte (d,1551).

> . . . it is Da Monte who usually receives the credit for developing such clinical instruction to the point where it was remarked upon by non-Italian students as an unusual and commendable novelty of the Paduan curriculum.
> *O'Malley 1970, p. 95–6).*

The nature of this model was that students

> accompanied their teachers to the bedside in order to observe the patient's countenance; then talk with him about his symptoms: thereafter note his pulse and observe everything necessary to gain a knowledge of the particular illness.
> *O'Malley 1970, p.96.*

and its purpose, succinctly, was to

> put the students in a position to combine theory and practice so that they might thereby become experienced physicians.
> *Kink 1854.*

We have seen in Chapter 2 how the theoretical development of medical education must be linked to practical experience. However, historically, the hospital as a location for clinical experience was often divorced, both physically and intellectually, from the university, the traditional seat of culture and learning. This separation had a direct effect, from time to time, on all early attempts to educate doctors, whether in Paris, Padua, or Vienna (Coury 1970, p.146).

Likewise, at the Universities of Oxford and Cambridge in the early sixteenth century there was no requirement or facility for a clinical component to medical education – the decreed course being entirely lecture- and book-based (O'Malley 1970). However, despite this lack of local clinical opportunity, only Oxbridge scholars were eligible for election to the College of Physicians. Hence, to gain any clinical experience in the eighteenth century such candidates had to travel to London, which had hospitals but no university, to see and investigate patients. Nearly one hundred years later, this separation of academic and practical aspects of medicine was enshrined by the General Medical Council (GMC) in the UK as the statutory model for the whole country. This divorce between theory and practice was then extended throughout the western world by colonial development and academic proliferation (Poynter 1970).

In western countries, current models of medical education are descended from these European beginnings, with additions and adumbrations derived from North America and it is worth discussing briefly how this development occurred.

Nineteenth century European medical education had been itself a hybrid of two influential genres. First, *the seventeenth-century apprenticeship system*, where one practitioner would undertake the personal supervision of a few (exclusively male) trainees over the course of several years, typically in a hospital setting. Second, *the collegiate system* of undergraduate training, developed at the Universities of Vienna, Padua, and Leiden, and subsequently successfully exported to their European neighbours during the eighteenth century. In this model traditional scholarship preceded and was then interspersed with clinical attachments. Hence medical schools at Edinburgh, and St Bartholomew's, (which had educational facilities modelled precisely on those at Padua), developed four-year courses in which attention was paid first to basic scientific endeavour and then to clinical expertise. Also at that time the clinical examination of a hospital patient was introduced into the assessment system for the award of the MB. This appeared first in Cambridge in 1842 (Poynter 1970) and rapidly spread to all medical schools. By 1861 such courses became the standard that the General Medical Council, founded in the UK in 1858, adopted as suitable for national accreditation. The period of training was extended to five years in 1892, and six in 1920. Commonly, the last year of this training was as a graduate house-officer.

It is informative to consider briefly how the house-officer year emerged as an educational experience both because it is a universal part of clinical training, and because of its influence on earlier parts of training (GMC 1993). The house-year was partly a product of the Viennese medical school system of *famuli* (servants to professor), in which senior students had, as part of their educational contract, to 'take turns in nursing those who were put under their charge day and night' (Lesky 1970, p.221). It is also related to the Napoleonic institution of *internes and externes*; divisions of junior doctors whose job it was to assist their seniors with an array of menial but essential tasks. In 1788 entry to these internships in Paris (that, like their current counterparts in the UK, all became vacant on the same day) was decreed to be by competition through written and oral examinations (Lesky 1970).

Hence the groundwork for the typical traditional curriculum seen today was laid as far back as the early seventeenth century: a two or three year basic science course, followed by clinical attachments and then a major examination to enable admittance to an even more intensive clinical responsibility after which the student became fully qualified. It is against this background that the modern clinical curriculum of the last ninety years needs to be viewed.

Trends in the Twentieth Century

In North America a review by Abraham Flexner (1910) at the end of the last century effectively decided the course of medical education for the next. His review resulted in a comprehensive increase in the emphasis on scientific, single discipline-oriented, predominantly laboratory-based studies in the medical curriculum—an idea that had its foundations, after 1850, in the most developed of the German schools. Subsequently, Johns Hopkins became the flagship of the post-Flexnerian fleet of North American medical schools. The important features of Hopkins were:

> Recruitment of faculty based upon a nationwide search for outstanding men. . . . To require for admission graduation from . . . an approved four year scientific school. . . . A logical sequence of training in basic science for two years, with emphasis on laboratory work (and) . . . medical school and hospital were interlocked and interacting from the start.
> *Welch 1916; cited in Field 1970*

The 'interlocking' of medical school and hospital was, however, not enough to secure the academic integration of clinical and basic disciplines. Even though it had originated in Europe this renewed alliance with science was re-interpreted by European schools as a further validation of one highly desirable characteristic of the profession—scientific rigour. Johns Hopkins became the school to which most UK colleges aspired. Its scientific research reputation soared. Together with dramatic expansion in student numbers, these factors effectively put an end to the one-to-one apprenticeship model that had begun to decline in the middle of the nineteenth century and resulted, on both sides of the Atlantic, in a very similar pattern of education. The outcome was a number of relatively homogeneous courses possessing the following deep rooted characteristics (Tosteson 1990; see also Chapter 1);

- a clear separation between basic and clinical sciences
- the teacher (both clinical and basic scientist) framed in the role of expert
- piecemeal clinical exposure in different clinical units.

Moreover, in Europe as well as espousing the above characteristics, many countries continue to develop large-cohort lecture-based courses with high failure rates and little or no organized clinical contact. In essence these features constitute the basic blueprint for medical education, although important changes of emphasis have taken place. Currently, in most schools clinical education is preceded by a two, three or four year preclinical phase in which basic and human sciences, and possibly pathology, are taught. There follows a three- (UK and Australia) or a two-year (the Netherlands, Canada, and USA) undergraduate period of clinical attachments to, or rotations around, clinical departments. This is usually followed by an intensive one-year attachment (as house officer or intern) in a hospital. In most countries the house officer attachment comprises six months of medicine and six months of surgery. Family medicine internships were introduced but were few in number (e.g. see Eary *et al.* 1978), although they are now quite common in this field. The house officer (intern) year is universally intended as a continuation of training, although the amount of formal education that is involved has been seriously questioned in the UK by independent researchers, and professional and government bodies. (Grant and Marsden 1989; SCOPME 1992 GMC, 1997.).

However the most recent major challenge to the Flexnerian model, one that is developing considerably (ACME-TRI 1993), has come from the Association of American Medical Colleges report on Physicians for the twenty-first century (AAMC 1984, see also Chapter 1). This report unequivocally restored patients, and their families, (see Chapter 2) as the primary focus of medical education. In it, the role, value of, and appropriate structure for clinical education was carefully described and general principles identified. In brief these include:

1. Medical faculties (as opposed to individual specialists) should specify the clinical knowledge, skills, values, and attitudes that students should develop.
2. Faculties should describe the clinical settings appropriate for clinical clerkships.
3. Teachers should have adequate preparation and the necessary time to guide and supervise students in clinical clerkships.
4. Clinical performance should be assessed.
5. Basic science and clinical education should be integrated to enhance the learning of key scientific principles and to promote their application to clinical problem solving (AAMC 1984, pp.14–19).

It is the last of these issues that will become the most challenging for the future development of clinical education. Even though far from achievement, it is the first time that such a notion has been put so forcefully, certainly by a national institution, since the age of enlightenment. Such principles have also increased interest in problem-based learning (PBL) as one of the primary methods of integrating basic science with clinical expertise in an appropriate manner. However most research on clinical education has been carried out primarily in traditional settings, in Canada, the UK, and Australia. Hence it is useful at this point to outline the major differences and similarities between these national educational programmes.

International similarities and differences

Without doubt, the changes introduced by Flexner in America were overdue, but they effectively stagnated the further development of courses for sixty years. Paradoxically, when schools in Europe began to look west for new ideas, they saw their own curricula and philosophy mirrored in the waters of Boston, New York, and Baltimore. American revolution in medical education hence consolidated European orthodoxy. The effect of this was to ratify the separation between the clinical and the academic environments. Any student who wished to lay hands on a patient had first to complete a 'scientific' education. As a result colleges of medicine, almost exclusively, now take students who have previously specialized in science. In the UK, and in most other European courses, intake is direct from secondary school. Until very recently the predominant difference between North American, and UK and Australasian models of medical education, has been the former's reliance on a graduate intake and the use of a four-year medical programme. However, three schools in Australia have recently gone over to a graduate entry, four-year clinical, largely problem-based programme.

The other principal difference between North American and UK/Australasian courses is the extent to which clinical skills are summatively assessed. In North America national examinations, until very recently, did not feature a clinical component. In the UK all schools include up to three separate evaluations (medicine, surgery, and obstetrics and gynaecology) of clinical skill in their final examinations, which directly license them to practise as junior doctors.

Nevertheless the clinical environment for North American, and particularly Canadian, students is very similar to that of their UK counterparts. Canadian students usually have a four-year course prior to internship, only the first two years of which are predominantly basic science. For example at the University of Toronto, the last two years are spent in teaching hospitals. The first of these 'clerkship' years was undertaken entirely in one large general hospital rotating round various clinical attachments, whereas the second year was spent following specialties in a variety of locations. In traditional schools in the UK and Australia, for example University College and Adelaide, students were usually attached to more than one hospital in every clinical year. In most other respects the clinical rotations are very similar.

The goals of clinical education

It might be thought from the preceding discussion, that charting the relationship between educational outcomes and clinical activity would be a simple matter. However, this is far from the truth. There is as little consensus on which outcomes should be measured (see Chapter 1) as on what the most appropriate learning methods should be.

In educational terms it is useful first to define goals or objectives, then to choose methods appropriate for achieving those goals and finally to assess the outcomes, comparing these with the original specifications Stenhouse 1975; Davies 1976; Newble and Cannon 1991). In most non-medical educational settings attempts to inculcate a variety of complex skills and behaviours would entail considerable attention to the specification of the proposed end product. In the case of the doctor, the clinical component of medicine, at its essence, involves:

> . . . identifying, recording and analysing symptoms presented in individual cases as a basis for diagnosis and treatment. Relentlessly inductive, clinical medicine requires accuracy in observation and testing to determine deviations from established norms. *MrGrew 1985.*

The fulfilment of this task (and more) is the goal of clinical education. However, surprisingly, less than 25% of the published studies of clinical education address these goals. Until very recently, most of the educational literature dealt with the educational process chiefly in terms of characteristics and activities of the teacher (e.g. see Irby 1978; Mattern *et al.* 1983) rather than with the objectives, length, structure, or function of the period of clinical attachment. In these studies of clinical teachers the worth, and hence the purpose, of the clinical experience is frequently assumed to be self-evident. In an early study, Reichsman *et al.* (1964, p.150) formulated the principal objectives of clinical teaching as:

a) to help students learn methods of observation and other clinical skills;

b) . . . acquire a body of information c) . . . develop capacity for clinical reasoning d) to effect modifications in students attitudes and behaviour.

Recently in a questionnaire and observational study of out-patient (OP) teaching at St Bartholomew's, Towle (1992) asked 51 senior clinicians to identify the objectives and the value of such sessions. The group identified twenty different objectives, and majority consensus (by 31 staff) was reached on only one area—the physical examination and the detection of physical signs. The other objectives identified included history taking (21), patient management (18), developing appropriate attitudes to patients (12), communication with patients (10), and presentation skills (4). The value of clinical work was seen in even more equivocal terms, the most common, but still with only nine physicians agreeing, being 'seeing how doctors and clinics work in the real world' (p.6). There was much more precise agreement, from 37 respondents, about the problems associated with such teaching, namely staffing, workload, and time availability (see Chapter 7.2).

Furthermore, criticisms of clinical education have rarely been levelled at its aims, but frequently at the process or outcomes (see Lowry 1992a, b). Part of the problem has been in defining precise outcomes in a professional environment in which graduation is merely a halfway house to independent practice. 'Is there an end product?' asks Lowry in one of her articles (Lowry 1992b).

Two coexisting, but antithetical, views of the end product are current in the UK, and these can be seen as further examples of the perennial polarity between the academic and the practical. In 1980 the GMC first attempted to define the principle objective of basic medical education as; 'the knowledge, skills and attitudes which will provide a firm basis for future vocational training' (GMC 1980 p.3). However in a recent set of guidelines, (GMC 1993) a 'complementary' goal has been added; to produce a graduate who can function as a preregistration house officer (intern). The former is aimed very much at creating a self-directed learner capable of further development, but the latter attempts to ensure competence in a wide range of clinical skills focused on the job of the house officer. Neither takes sufficient account of the movement of health care into non-tertiary hospital locations.

What does educational activity in clinical settings usually consist of?

McLeod and Harden (1985) summarize the components thought to contribute to a clinical education. These comprise:

♦ Bedside small group tutorials, in which students discuss a patient, sometimes at the bedside, with a more senior practising physician.
♦ Ward rounds, in which students tour with consultants (attendings/senior physicians) and their staff in order to discuss appropriate management of cases on the ward.
♦ independent patient contact in which students 'clerk' (interview, examine, and summarize in writing) a patient. This can be done in a variety of settings including the ward, out-patients, the patient's home, in general practice, etc.
♦ Classroom discussion, based either on patients or on an academic topic.

Other activities, not specifically mentioned by McLeod, would include attendance at operations, special procedures (e.g. radiography), post-mortems, and clinical case conferences, at both medical and paramedical level (psychiatric reviews, physiotherapy, etc.). All of these events, of course, can be (and are) supplemented on many occasions by an array of educational techniques such as lectures, reading, laboratory classes, and so on.

The activities undertaken by students in the studies reported later reflect this diversity. In their attachments of between four and ten weeks to general medical and surgical units, ward work, attending lectures and teaching rounds, clerking patients and writing patients' notes feature prominently. Other specialty attachments might be to the accident and emergency, renal, or endocrinology departments, and so on. Nevertheless such specialties increasingly provide more general medical or surgical experience.

In addition the assessment of clinical competence is now an essential component of the educational process. As we have seen this was not always the case (see p.174). Additionally modern developments have also made this a field in its own right (Newble et al. 1994a). The most significant progress has been the recognition that the mode and weight of assessment greatly modify the educational activities of students (Jolly *et al.* 1993, Newble and Jaeger, 1983), and the introduction of the Objective Structured Clinical Examination (OSCE; Harden and Gleeson 1979) in the late 1970s. This procedure, that challenged and in some cases replaced examination of one patient as the primary means of clinical assessment, allowed reliable and valid assessment and increased the scope of clinical examinations to encompass a wider range of clinical tasks.

Research on educational outcomes and processes in the hospital setting

There are probably several reasons for the lack of rigour in the definition of the purpose of clinical education. First, the historical development of medical education, as we have seen, was linked to a system of patronage and apprenticeship. Second, in the university this was reflected as 'person culture' (Handy 1976; Arluke 1980), where academic units derived their *raison d'être* from the intellectual and personal characteristics of one or two key personnel. This culture permeated both the practice of medicine and the organization of medical schools and can be seen in the operation of the ward round, the hierarchy of medical departments, the centrality of the professorial staff and so on all developed from the apprenticeship model. Some of the inherent control rules of this model—roundsmanship—have been identified by Arluke. Essentially they act to move the focus of educational activity away from the patient and more towards the academic and game-like aspects of professional interaction (Arluke 1980). There is also the historical legacy of the existence of clinical teaching pre-dating ratification by Universities. In addition until the mid-1970s there was virtually no educational research on or external scrutiny of medical courses at the consumers' level.

It is therefore not surprising that the respective educational model, especially in the UK, for the content of clinical education in traditional settings, is constructed more like a recipe for minestrone soup than a carefully planned educational experience. Courses were organized by departments through various specialty studies. Although there are usually introductory courses, and a short period of general medicine and surgery, these are followed by many topics, specialties and environments, all dissected into barely digestible units fed to the students in a fairly random order. The exact recipe in each school depends very much on the individual chef. For example, in 1973 the GMC commissioned a national study of the curricula in UK medical schools. All schools returned a comprehensive questionnaire on the construction and delivery of their courses. There was substantial variation between schools in the length of clinical attachments and the amount of patient-based clinical experience offered. As the GMC (1977 p.57) pointed out, 'There is enormous variation, even when only the major specialties are under consideration, and due to circumstances often rather than policy'. For instance, the length of attachments for 'general surgery' in the first clinical year in two schools picked at random was 7 weeks and 20 weeks. Furthermore, within any medical school students are frequently attached to different clinical units within the same subject area. Hence two students nominally attached to 'medicine' might nevertheless have completely different educational experiences. Such haphazard experience is widely reported (Kowlowitz *et al.* 1990; Jolly and Rees 1984; Hunskaar and Seim 1983). The problem with clinical education as currently construed is that the apprenticeship system has left a legacy of an ideology but not the means to implement it.

Consequently it is often difficult to know what is the precise educational diet for students even within one medical school. In Toronto this led to the instigation of a database, first in the preclinical school (Project Oracle), to track the students' encounters with content and process throughout their undergraduate education. Students kept logs of what had been covered and by what type of teaching. This was later expanded to the clinical course (Chin *et al.* 1988). Data on topic, hands on/patient based experience, literature available or referred to, and other indicators of clinical teaching were collected by two students from each of a first year clinical rotation and fed into a computer database.

The principal studies of the function of clinical education have come from sociological perspectives (Becker *et al.* 1961; Armstrong 1977; Atkinson 1977). In these the assumption is made that the purpose of clinical education is to turn ageing adolescents into young doctors, and that this is accomplished as much by a socialization process, concerned with mores, beliefs, and attitudes, as by educational development. Such studies are concerned with documenting the formation of and constraints on the socialization process. As Atkinson (1977, p.97) says: 'Although it takes place within the social and physical context of hospital life, the reality of bedside teaching is a carefully managed version of medical work.' Whether Atkinson is right or not about learning being a 'carefully managed version of medical work', his, and other sociologists' perspective on the purpose of clinical education is that it is a rite of passage designed to teach students how to cope with 'being' a doctor. This view has also been adopted by some educationists (Fleming 1986).

The clinical work of a hospital unit is supposed to serve as an organizational framework for discrete educational experiences. However, while the predominant tradition of clinical education throughout the world stems from bedside teaching, the amount of teaching actually taking place at the bedside, or in the presence of the patient, is highly variable, and as patient availability decreases so do opportunities for learning (McManus *et al.* 1992). Four studies designed to monitor educational activity in hospital settings (Chesser and Brett 1989; Payson and Barchas 1965; Reichsman *et al.* 1964; Mattern *et al.* 1983) found evidence that the time devoted to clinical activity was erratic or even non-existent, ranging from 0–25% of students' time on the ward. For example unpublished data from another cohort in the Chesser and Brett study, indicate that on a typical week of clinical attachments some students were receiving about twelve hours of bedside teaching, while others were receiving none. Mattern found that of six attending physician teams studied, only three visited the bedside for educational purposes. Teaching rounds continue to be a focus for education, but their organization still leaves little time for bedside teaching and development of clinical skills. Miller *et al.* (1992) recently found that within teaching rounds 63% of the time was spent in the conference room, 26% in hallways, and only 11% at the bedside.

There is a growing literature on the programme evaluation of clinical teaching and its methodology and on the detailed analysis of 'expert' teachers' activities. Reviews have attempted to identify a number of features that seem to contribute to student satisfaction and good teaching. Some of these have purportedly been validated in terms of resultant student abilities. For example Anderson *et al.* (1991) showed that results on an objective structured clinical examination (OSCE) in neurology reflected differences in students' ratings of their teachers on attachments to four hospitals for their immediately preceding neurology rotations, and Higgin and Harasym (1993) that students returning from some obstetric and gynaecological attachments did not do so well on a focused OSCE. More recently research has demonstrated location to be a potent variable in learning diagnostic skill, even overriding the effects of centralized curriculum design (Bordage *et al.* 1989; Wolfhagen 1993). Jolly (1994; *et al.* 1996), however, found that not only was student experience highly individualized, even within one attachment, the quality of the individual's learning environment was not particularly indicative of outcome on an OSCE only a few weeks later.

Nevertheless most early research on clinical settings concentrated almost entirely on the characteristics of the teacher (Irby 1978; Weinholtz *et al.* 1986). Later work has highlighted the need to look at the whole clinical environment (Chesser and Brett 1989; Towle 1992) and at student input (Stritter *et al.* 1975; Bennard and Stritter 1989). Chesser and Brett, using ratings of clinical attachments at The London Hospital, identified six major factors in student satisfaction with clinical teaching: feedback to students; clinical exposure; staff–student relationships; organization and delivery of teaching; involvement with the business of the 'firm' (a small group of doctors working with one or two consultants) and the degree of acuteness of medicine. The most important of these factors was feedback to students which accounted for 23% of the variance in student satisfaction in their study. They also showed that, although feedback and acuteness is important for all attachments, organization of teaching was relatively more influential on medical firms, while degree of clinical experience was more significant on surgical attachments. The necessity of feedback has been supported by numerous studies. Further research (Wolf and Turner 1989) also highlighted the perceived value of showing personal interest in students, reviewing histories and supervising physical examinations. This study also showed, as have others (Matttern *et al.* 1983; Bennard and Stritter 1989), that staff consistently overestimate how frequently they undertake certain teaching activities, especially those that they value highly.

Recently the role and practices of the 'good clinical teacher' have been extensively reinvestigated by Irby (1994*a*, *b*). Irby's earlier work studied the existence of common factors in the perceptions of good teaching: structure, feedback, and opportunities for student activity, for example. This recent research has taken a much more focused and detailed look at the rationale of individual clinicians and at how they organize and discharge their educational responsibilities. Furthermore, in these studies and in an outstanding comprehensive review of teaching in the out-patient setting, a number of useful guidelines for teaching are revealed (Irby 1995):

- Provide continuity by having longer attachments or create specific opportunities for patient follow-up (much like an educational version of clinical 'real-life').
- Engage students in continuous self-directed and collaborative learning (Jolly and Ho-Ping-Kong 1991 and see below).
- Devise faculty development initiatives to help teachers to: target instruction better, use time more appropriately, teach to learners' needs, be highly selective in what they teach, observe and give feedback to students, and create a supportive environment for learning.

There has been a great deal of interest lately in the need for self-directed or problem-based learning (Tosteson 1990; Barrows and Tamblyn 1980). It is often believed that the clinical environment carries the capability for such learning. However, 'teaching' ward rounds often have little opportunity for students to contribute; Foley *et al.* (1979) found that student contribution to teaching and business rounds was even less than that in lectures. Student input was significant only in patient management conferences and morning reports. Moreover, the content of such teaching as exists was frequently unconnected with patient care, clinical skills, doctor–patient communication, or management. Such observational studies of ward rounds 'in action' found that discussion often focused on minutiae, or on esoteric or scientific aspects of the case not amenable to bedside investigation. In one early study characteristics commonly attributed to ward-round teaching—patient examination and doctor–patient communication, occupied a small percentage of the round (Payson and Barchas 1965). Perhaps this is not surprising given that most studies have been conducted in high profile, university affiliated teaching hospitals (the Payson study took place at Yale). Research has consistently suggested that work-related, patient-based experience is more frequent and prolonged in district, community, or other non-teaching / non-affiliated hospitals, although most researchers do not directly suggest why this should be the case (Payson and Barchas 1965; Wakeford 1983; Lockwood *et al.* 1986; McManus *et al.* 1992; Brett and Chesser 1992). A number of factors could contribute; there may be fewer students per patient, more staff time per student, or generally more patients. However, the rules operating in major teaching hospitals may also inhibit real problem-focused activity (Arluke 1980).

As we have seen early research on clinical education typically concentrated on the aspirations, goals, and actions of senior clinical teachers, or on the perceptions of staff and students of these (see also Weinholtz *et al.* 1986). However, at least one factor-analytic study (Stritter *et al.* 1975) had found that one of the characteristics critical to 'good' clinical teaching was the ability of the clinician to 'provide a personal environment in which the student is an active participant' (p.878). This included the provision of opportunities to practice both technical and problem solving skills. However, in a complex clinical environment, such provision is not always straightforward. For example we have already seen how Atkinson (1977) and Armstrong (1977) have both pointed out that the problem solving process for the student, becomes distorted by the milieu of the ward round, and often leads to behaviour quite different to that associated with solving *de novo* clinical problems. Hence professional activity towards which students are progressing cannot always be packaged in an educationally acceptable framework (Fleming, 1986).

There have been recent attempts to counteract these problems. In Toronto, in 1988 (Jolly and Ho-Ping-Kong 1991) a course change had taken place that directly reflected work-related ideals and activities, and afforded the opportunity of studying a situation in which students' contribution to clinical education was both valued and encouraged. This was the student 'Grand rounds' programme. Professional 'Grand rounds' (GRs) are interdisciplinary patient-based fora for medical staff commonly held once a week in major teaching hospitals. In GRs staff present and discuss particularly interesting, important, or problematic cases. They are sometimes open to students, depending on the institution. These 'rounds' are not typically ward-based, mostly being held in large discussion rooms or lecture theatres, but nevertheless form one of the landmarks of the working week in a busy teaching hospital in most UK, North American, and Australasian countries. Typically (GRs have been observed by the author in the UK, Australia, and Canada) between twenty and forty senior physicians attend the medical grand round. GRs had been instituted just for students in the University of Toronto affiliated teaching hospitals. These student grand rounds evolved precisely from a rationale attempting to relate students' activities more to the work of the hospital and in providing them with more meaningful clinical exposure (University of Toronto 1982–86). Work related experience at an undergraduate level had not often been studied in clinical education. We attempted to unravel the aims and outcomes of these grand rounds through qualitative and participant observation strategies. In particular the study also attempted, by comparison with some British work on ward-based patient presentations (Fleming 1986) to analyse the boundary between the socialization and the educational functions of professional work-related activity.

With increased interest in problem-based or self-directed learning there has been concomitant attention given to creating a more problem based environment in clinical settings. Studies have shown increased diagnostic ability and slightly decreased or equivalent maintenance of factual knowledge in students from problem-based learning (PBL) curricula (Phelan *et al.* 1993; Schwartz *et al.* 1992); but the most salient and persistent outcome is that students consistently find PBL more enjoyable and motivating, although slightly more anxiety provoking, than traditional educational methods (Blosser and Jones 1991).

Most of this research highlights an important feature of clinical education, namely that assumptions about the amount of instructional activity taking place in clinical environments are not well founded. Although the concept of 'clinical experience' has been the driving force behind the later stages of medical training, it is difficult to find its equivalent in organized educational activity. Nevertheless it is true that students emerge from medical school, as house officers (interns) on the ward, with the knowledge, skills, and attitudes that enable them, however rudimentarily, to practise medicine. So there are obviously educational outcomes and presumably these derive from learning experiences. The gap between research on the quality and the reality of education may be because research has tended to concentrate on what the medical teacher does, rather than what happens to students and other aspects of the environment. From this chapter, one of the outstanding issues needing further research is what is actually happening to students and what is the connection between the measurable outcomes of clinical education and its content or process. This is as true of traditional courses as it is of innovative ones. If more can be understood about the constraints, inadequacies and successes of the students' experience, organized or otherwise, then a more appropriate rationale can be developed for clinical education.

Summary

In the preceding section several roles have been identified for educational research in the clinical setting, along with some initial findings about students' and teachers' views of clinical teaching. It has been shown that it is often difficult to know precisely what has been taught and sometimes why it has been taught in the first place. Some studies have attempted to analyse positive and negative features of clinical education, but until recently have ignored the students' contributions to their own education. Also researchers have generally overlooked the clinical environment, concentrating much more on teaching or learning activities. Moreover very few attempts (however see Murray *et al.*, 1997) have been made to link educational activity in the clinical setting with outcome.

The shortage of knowledge about clinical education is the context in which research presented in the remainder of this chapter and elsewhere in this book (Chapters 3 and 6) should be seen. Many curricula resemble the minestrone model (p.179). An end-of-course evaluation in one school (Jolly and Rees 1984) had shown that clinical teaching was perfunctory, and varied in quality and quantity. The students were sometimes humiliated on the wards, teaching was often cancelled, the curriculum stressed the retention of factual knowledge and the course had no discernible philosophy or goals. Previous examinations of the effects of undergraduate clinical education had mostly investigated students' perceptions. They had not taken advantage of the fact that their views might change once they qualified and started to work (see Chapter 6 and Jolly and Macdonald 1989). Furthermore at that time very little was agreed about precisely what skills and attributes house officers were expected to demonstrate on the job, and where they had learnt these. These deficiencies are beginning to be redressed, but slowly. In following sections of this chapter a clinical teacher gives views on the conflicting demands of clinical work and teaching, including attempting to define global objectives for the clinical course. Educational researcher Peter Bouhuis discusses the issues pertaining to the roles of teachers and learners in medical education and then Lewis Elton and Angela Towle discuss the framework of staff development which needs to take place to foster a more rational approach to clinical education.

References

AAMC (Association of American Medical Colleges) (1984). *Physicians for the twenty-first century*. Report of the panel on the General Professional Education of the Physician. (GPEP Report) AAMC:Washington.

ACME-TRI (1993). Educating medical students: achieving change in medical education—the road to implementation. *Academic Medicine*, **68**, (Supplement S1), 1–49.

Anderson, D.C., Harris, I.B., Allen, S., Satran, L., Bland, C.J., Davis-Feickert, J.A. *et al.* (1991).

Comparing students' feedback about clinical instruction with their performances. *Academic Medicine*, **66**, 29–34.

Arluke, A. (1980). Roundsmanship: inherent control on a medical teaching ward. *Social Science and Medicine*, **14A**, 297–302.

Armstrong D. (1977). The structure of medical education. *Medical Education*, **11**, 244–8.

Atkinson, P.A. (1977) The reproduction of medical knowledge. In (ed.) Health care and health care knowledge, R. Dingwall, C. Heath, M. Reid, and M. Stacey. pp. 83–106. Croom Helm, London.

Barrows, H.S. and Tamblyn, R. (1980). *Problem-based learning: an approach to medical education*. Springer Publishing Company, New York.

Becker, H.S., Geer, B. Hughes, E.C., and Strauss, A.L., (1961). *Boys in white: student culture in medical school*. University of Chicago Press, Chicago.

Bennard, B.C. and Stritter, F.T. (1989). Teaching medical students in ambulatory clinics: prescribed vs. actual practice. *Proceedings, Research in Medical Education*, 141–6. Association of American Medical Colleges, Washington.

Blosser, A. and Jones, B. (1991). Problem-based learning in a surgery clerkship. *Medical Teacher*, **13**, 289–93, 295–8 (Discussion).

Bordage, G., Morin, F., and Leclere, H. (1989). Comparison of the diagnostic performance of students of the old and new medical curriculum at the Laval University. *Union Medicale Du Canada*, **118**, (187–95).

Brett, M. and Chesser, A. (1992) *Auditing clinical teaching*. Address to the Association of for the Study of Medical Education, London Meeting, April 1992.

Chesser, A. and Brett, M. (1989). Clinical teaching in context: a factor analysis of student ratings. *Research in Medical Education*. Proceedings of the twenty-eighth annual conference, Association of American Medical Colleges, pp. 49–54.

Chin, V., Jolly, B.C., and Cohen, A. (1988). Use of a Database for curriculum monitoring—a clinical application. *Proceedings of the Conference on the Application of Computers to Medical Education*. University of Toronto, Canada, April 1988.

Coury, C. (1970). The teaching of medicine in France from the beginning of the 17th century. In O'Malley, C.D. (ed). *The history of medical education*. pp. 121–172. University of California Press, Los Angeles.

Davies, I.J.K. (1976). *Learning by objectives*. Kogan Page. London.

Eary, L.E, Kobernick, M, and Vanderwagen, W.C. (1978) Pilot experience of a family practice-based combined clerkship. *Journal of Family Practice*, **7**, 541–6.

Field, J. (1970). Medical education in the United States: late nineteenth and twentieth centuries. In (ed. C.D. O'Malley). *The history of medical education*, pp. 501–530. University of California Press, Los Angeles.

Fleming, W. (1986). Good professional reasons for poor educational practice: the interaction of medical and educational work in presenting cases during junior clinical clerkship. Proceeding of the *Society for Research in Higher Education*, Imperial College London. SHRE Publications, Guildford.

Flexner, A, (1910). *Medical education in the United States and Canada*. Carnegie Foundation, New York.

Foley, R. Smilansky, J. and Yonke, A. (1979) Teacher-student interaction in a medical clerkship. *Journal of Medical Education*, **54**, 622–6.

General Medical Council (1977) *Basic medical education in the British Isles*: the report of the GMC survey of basic medical education in the UK and the Republic of Ireland. (Vol. 1) Nuffield Provincial Hospitals Trust, London.

General Medical Council (1980) *Recommendations on basic medical education*. GMC Education Committee, London.

General Medical Council (1993) *Guidelines on undergraduate medical education* GMC Education Committee, London.

General Medical Council (1997). The New Doctor. London: GMC.

Grant, J. and Marsden, P. (1989). Senior house officers and their training. II Perceptions of service and training. *British Medical Journal*, **299**, 1265–8.

Handy, C. (1976). *Understanding organisations*. Penguin, Harmondsworth.

Harden, R.McG. and Gleeson, F. (1979). Assessment of clinical competence using an objective structured clinical examination (OSCE). *Medical Education*, **13**, 41–51.

Higgin, J.R. and Harasym, P.H. (1993). Using the OSCE to identify strengths and weaknesses in learning at three teaching hospitals. In *Approaches to the assessment of clinical competence*, (ed. I. Hart, R.McG. Harden, and H. Mullholland.) pp.00–00. Proceedings of the fifth Ottawa Conference on Medical Education 1992, Dundee.

Hunskaar, S. and Seim, S.H. (1983). Assessment of students' experiences in technical procedures in a medical clerkship. *Medical Education*, **17**, 300–4.

Irby, D.I. (1978). Clinical teacher effectiveness. *Journal of Medical Education*, **53**, 808–15.

Irby, D.I. (1994*a*). What clinical teachers in medicine need to know. *Academic Medicine*, **69**, 333–42.

Irby, D.I. (1994*b*). Three exemplary models of case-based teaching. *Academic Medicine*, **69**, 947–53.

Irby, D.I. (1995). Teaching and learning in ambulatory care settings: a thematic review of the literature. *Academic Medicine*, **70**, 898–931.

Jolly, B.C. (1985). Unpublished data from Room for Improvement.

Jolly, B.C., and Ho-Ping-Kong, H. (1991). Independent learning: an exploration of student grand rounds at the University of Toronto. *Medical Education*, **24**, 334–42.

Jolly, B.C. (1994). *Bedside manners: teaching and learning in the hospital setting*. Maastricht: University of Limburg Press.

Jolly, B.C., Newble, D.I. and Chinner, T. (1993). Learning effect of re-using stations in an objective structured clinical examination. *Teaching and Learning in Medicine*, **5**, 66–71.

Jolly, B.C. and Macdonald, M.M. (1986). More effective evaluation of clinical teaching. *Assessment and evaluation in Higher Education*, **12**, 175–190.

Jolly, B.C. and Rees, L.H. (1984). Room for improvement: an evaluation of the undergraduate curriculum at St Bartholomew's Hospital Medical College. Mimeo. SBHMC.

Jolly, B.C., Jones, A., Dacre, J.E., Elzubeir, M., Kopelman, P., Hitman, G. (1996). Relationship between students' clinical experiences in introductory clinical courses and their performance on an objective structured clinical examination (OSCE). *Academic Medicine*, **71**, 909–16.

Kink, R. (1854). *Geschichte der kaiserlichen Universitat zu Wien*. University of Vienna, Vienna.

Kowlowitz, V., Curtis, P., and Sloane, P.D. (1990). The procedural skills of medical students: expectations and experiences. *Academic Medicine*, **65**, 656–8.

Lesky, E. (1970). The development of bedside teaching at the Vienna medical school from scholastic times to special clinics. In *The history of medical education* (ed. O'Malley, C.D.) pp.217–234, University of California Press, Los Angeles.

Lockwood, D.N., Goldman, L.H., and McManus, I.C. (1986). Clinical experience of clerks and dressers: a three year study of Birmingham medical students. *Journal of the Royal Society of Medicine*, **71**, 38–42.

Lowry, S. (1992*a*). Whats wrong with medical education in Britain? *British Medical Journal*, **305**, 1277–80.

Lowry, S. (1992*b*). Curriculum design. *British Medical Journal*, **305**, 1409–11.

McManus, I.C., Sproston, K.A., Winder, B.C., and Richards, P. (1992). The experience of medical education: changing perceptions of final year students. *Proceedings of the Fifth Ottawa International Conference on Assessment of Clinical Competence*, Dundee.

Mattern, W.D., Weinholtz, D., and Friedman, C. (1983) The attending physician as teacher. *New England Journal of Medicine*, **308**, 1129–32.

McGrew, R. (1985). *Encyclopaedia of Medical History*. Macmillan, London.

McLeod, P.J. and Harden, R.M. (1985). Clinical teaching strategies for clinicians. *Medical Teacher*, **7**, 173–89.

Miller, M., Johnson, B., Greene, H.L., Baier, M. and Nowlin, S. (1992) An observational study of attending rounds. *Journal of General Internal Medicine*, **7**, 646–8.

Murray, E., Jolly, B.C. and Modell, M. (1997). Can students learn clinical method in general practice: a randomised cross-over trial. *British Medical Journal*, **31**, 913–16.

Newble, D.I. and Cannon, R. (1991). *A handbook for clinical teachers* (2nd edn). MTP Press, London.

Newble, D.I. and Jaeger, K. (1983). The effect of assessment and examinations on the learning of medical students. *Medical Education*, **17**, 165–171.

Newble, D.I., Jolly, B.C., and Wakeford, R.E. (ed.). (1994*a*). The certification and recertification of doctors: issues in the assessment of clinical competence. Cambridge University Press, Cambridge.

Newble, D.I., Dauphinee, D., Dawson-Saunders, B., Macdonald, M., Mulholland, H., Page, G. *et al.*, (1994*b*) Guidelines for the development of effective and efficient procedures for the assessment of clinical competence. In Newble, D.I., Jolly, B.C., and Wakeford, R.E. (ed.) *The certification and recertification of doctors: issues in the assessment of clinical competence*, pp. 69–91. Cambridge University Press, Cambridge.

O'Malley, C.D. (1970). Medical education during the renaissance. In *The history of medical education*, (ed. C.D. O'Malley), pp. 89–104. University of California Press, Los Angeles.

Osler, W. (1906). *Aequanimitas*. McGraw-Hill, New York.

Payson, H.E. and Barchas, J.D. (1965). A time study of medical teaching rounds. *New England Journal of Medicine*, **273**, 1468–71.

Phelan, S.T., Jackson, J.R. and Berner, E.S. (1993). Comparison of problem-based and traditional education student performance in the obstetrics and gynaecology clerkship. *Obstetrics and Gynaecology*, **82**, 159–61.

Poynter, F.N.L. (1970). Medical education in England since 1600. In *The history of medical education*, (ed. C.D. O'Malley), pp. 235–250. University of California Press, Los Angeles.

Reichsman, F., Browning, F.E., and Hinshaw, J.R. (1964). Observations of undergraduate clinical teaching in action. *Journal of Medical Education*, **39**, 147–163.

Schwartz, R.W., Donnelly, M.B., Nash, P.P., and Young, B. (1992). Developing students' cognitive skills in a problem-based surgery clerkship. *Academic Medicine*, **67**, 694–6.

SCOPME (1992). Teaching hospital doctors and dentists to teach: its role in creating a better learning environment. Standing Committee on Postgraduate Medical Education (SCOPME), London.

Stenhouse, L. (1975). *An introduction to curriculum research and development*. Heinmann, London.

Stritter, F.T., Hain, J.D., and Grimes, M.D. (1975). Clinical teaching re-examined. *Journal of Medical Education*, **50**, 876–82.

Sylvius, F. (1679). Epistola Apologetica. In *Opera medica*, p.907. Elsevie and Wolfgang, Amsterdam.

Tosteson, D.C. (1990). New pathways in general medical education. *New England Journal of Medicine*, **322**, 234–8.

Towle, A. (1992). Outpatient teaching at St Bartholomew's Hospital Medical College. Mimeo, SBHMC.

University of Toronto (1982-1986). Curriculum renewal documents. Mimeo, Faculty of Medicine, Deans Office.

Wakeford, R.E. (1983). Undergraduate students' experience in 'peripheral' and 'teaching' hospitals compared. *Annals Royal College of Surgeons of England*, **65**, 374–7.

Weinholtz, D. *et al.* (1986). Effective attending physician teaching. Research in Medical Education. *Proceedings of the twenty-fourth annual conference, Association of American Medical Colleges*, 151–6.

Wolf, F.M. and Turner, E.V. (1989). Congruence between student and instructor perceptions of clinical teaching in paediatrics. *Medical Education*. **23** (2), 161–7.

Wolfhagen, I. (1993). *Kwaliteit van klinish onderwijs* (quality of clinical education). University of Limburg, Maastricht.

7.2 Clinical work and teaching

Jane Dacre

Introduction

Most working doctors teach. In a 'teaching' hospital environment, there is an increased emphasis on this and, indeed, the Trust is paid a sum of money (service increment for teaching, SIFT) to allow teaching to continue. However, there are problems related to the career development of junior doctors. At the moment, progress through the medical ranks is based more on a doctor's research output than their teaching ability or experience. Promotions and appointments are biased towards candidates with a large number of publications on their curriculum vitae. There is no recognition of teaching other than in an informal way within each medical school (Dacre *et al.* 1996) The financial support given to an academic department by the local university is based on the number of papers produced, and the number of grants awarded to that department. This kind of assessment reduces the priority given to student teaching, Departments with a poor teaching record (at least as far as students are concerned) are often those that concentrate their efforts in research areas, and so generate a high income for the medical school. This difficulty has been appreciated by many medical colleges, but the system is still pervasive and biases academic departments against putting significant resources into their teaching programmes.

This section is based on experience wholly in a hospital setting. Undergraduate teaching in the general practice setting (see Chapter 4) is an area that is evolving and expanding—particularly since the GMC recommendations on undergraduate education (GMC 1993) are beginning to take effect. Nevertheless, the new guidelines on general clinical training (GMC 1996) also reinforce the need for all hospital based senior doctors or supervisors to be competent teachers. This step will bring the secondary care practitioners into line with their training counterparts in primary care whose efforts in this direction have long been recognized.

Who teaches?

Although all doctors are expected to teach, the majority of working doctors have no formal teaching qualifications, and have often had no instruction on how to teach. Some are naturally good at it, and do well intuitively, others tend to muddle through. As a junior doctor one's teaching experience historically began as a House Physician or

Surgeon. Students report that they learn a great deal by shadowing house staff. However, students may spend several hours hanging around, waiting for something to happen. House officers are usually very keen to show their new found knowledge, and work well with students, instructing them in history taking and practical procedures in a pseudo-apprenticeship arrangement (after all the junior doctors are not yet 'masters' of their craft). As the junior doctors progress through their career there is more of a formal emphasis placed on teaching. However, the amount of teaching done still depends very much on the interests of the doctor concerned. It is difficult for junior doctors to continue teaching during their senior house officer years as they have significant clinical responsibilities. They are also frequently studying for postgraduate examinations such as MRCP and FRCS. This may encourage their teaching as they are keen to impart their knowledge to others, but often the knowledge that they impart is very detailed and can be quite difficult for the students to understand.

By the time junior doctors reach registrar level, teaching is a significant part of their week and they will have a regular weekly commitment to the student for bedside teaching in addition to occasional small group sessions and lectures. This commitment increases at the senior registrar level and also at the consultant level where in addition to having regular teaching sessions and giving lectures, the teaching activities for the Firm are organized.

Teaching methods

Teaching methods used by doctors are very variable. This is because although they know their subject they have never been taught how to impart it and so they tend to rely on the methods that have worked when taught themselves. There is little consistency and usually no feedback, so poor teachers may not be aware of their deficiencies.

The most common form of teaching on the wards is 'bedside teaching' (see Chapter 7.1). The students will either have taken a history from or examined a patient and they will then present this to the teacher, who will make suggestions on how their presentation can be improved. In general, they may be observed examining the patient and be given feedback on their examination technique. Recently it has been noted that most medical students are not observed whilst taking their history and although doctors listen to the final version when students present the case, we are sometimes not aware of the steps they have taken to reach this stage. Examination technique however, is observed more often and is taught very well. The difficulty with this is that there are several slightly different (idiosyncratic) ways of performing an adequate examination and the students may become confused if such differences of technique are not made explicit.

The advantages of bedside teaching are that the students see the doctor as a role model and in this realistic setting they are assessing a real patient under real circumstances. There is no shortage of medical and ethical issues on every ward. Bedside teaching is ideal for small groups and it is also easy for relatively inexperienced teachers to use a problem-solving approach as this is the way they have assessed the patient themselves. Unfortunately, bedside teaching is usually limited to the patients available on the ward. On a specialist firm, or at a quiet time of year, the variety of clinical material may be limited. This causes difficulties in planning a comprehensive teaching programme; for example, during the course of the teaching attachment a patient with a large spleen, or another serious and important condition, may not be admitted.

Interruptions

Wards are very busy places and in addition to the doctors own interruptions caused by medical emergencies and bleeps, there are events related to the patient that are important for their wellbeing, such as lunch time and visiting. On a day when the firm is 'on call', it is often impossible to balance teaching commitments with professional ones and although the majority of clinical material comes into the hospital during this period it is very difficult to spend enough time teaching and advising students. Students may end up as passive observers and it may be up to them to participate in the care of that patient. This is no problem for some medical students but causes significant difficulties for the more diffident students, who will see less clinical material as a result. Also most hospital systems are not conducive to students' participation in many of their activities.

Changes in health care provision

Changes in health care provision in recent years have had an adverse effect on traditional medical student teaching. It is becoming more difficult to run the kind of traditional apprenticeship scheme alluded to above. Patients are staying in hospital for shorter periods, and there is an increase in day care. This reduces student access to patients on the ward. Although teaching still continues in the out-patient setting, it is difficult to allow enough time for teaching, in addition to keeping the waiting list to below six weeks, and the patient waiting time in clinic to below thirty minutes, as stipulated in the Patient's Charter.

On the wards, the increase in through-put of patients increases the workload of junior and senior doctors, by having an increasing number of patients to see and deal with. This decreases teaching opportunities as the patients are not around for long enough for the students to see them. Such difficulties have promoted the rapid expansion of skills centres and related simulated patient programmes (Dacre and Nicol 1996).

The welcome reduction in the hours worked by junior doctors to 72 hours per week has had a negative effect on teaching time. Junior doctors have to be very much more efficient in getting their work done during the time allocated and issues, such as teaching, that are not directly related to patient care tend to be forgotten and marginalized. During their reduced hours junior doctors are also expected to take an active part in clinical audit. The 'knock-on' effect of these changes is that consultants are playing an increasing role in the education and supervision of junior staff in both clinical and administrative matters, this leaves less *time* for undergraduates.

In summary, there are difficulties teaching medical students at the same time as participating in ordinary clinical work. The traditional teaching methods are under great strain due to the changes in clinical practice and health care provision. To improve this situation, support and recognition of good clinical teachers needs to be increased. With the current interest in medical student teaching across the country, and the new GMC guidelines for medical education, the system should improve.

References

Dacre, J.E., and Nicol, M. (1996). The development of a clinical skills centre. *Journal of the Royal College of Physicians of London*, **30**, 318–24.

Dacre, J.E., Griffith, S.M., and Jolly, B.C. (1996). Rheumatology and medical education in Great Britain. *British Journal of Rheumatology*, **35**, 269–74.

General Medical Council (1993). *Tomorrow's doctors: guidelines on undergraduate medical education.* GMC Education Committee, London.

General Medical Council (1996). *The new doctor: recommendations on General Clinical Training.* Draft document for consultation. GMC Education Committee, London.

7.3 The teacher and self-directed learners

Peter A.J. Bouhuijs

Introduction

Teaching in medicine has always been an important aspect of the physician's professional job. The Hippocratic Oath, which is still considered as a valid description of the tasks of physicians, stipulates that the physician will teach his professional knowledge and skills to future generations of physicians. In many languages physicians are called 'doctor' which means teacher. For a long time, medical education consisted of apprenticeships during which a junior learned the trade by working with a senior physician for some time. Although the teaching in medicine at medieval and renaissance universities also contained some formal teaching, students would usually stay with one or a few professors who would teach all relevant (and irrelevant) aspects of medicine. The Renaissance ideal of the learned man, who was supposed to be knowledgeable about most aspects of life dominated the teaching of medicine for a long time. The practical use of what was learned in universities was limited, and in many countries only limited funds were given to universities to pay for stipends and buildings. In the nineteenth century, the rapid evolution of the sciences caused major changes in university teaching. New disciplines emerged and it was no longer possible to teach everything that was known. Von Humboldt in Germany introduced the idea of a formal medical curriculum which would be based on sciences. This model was advocated later by Flexner in his reform of US medical education. Gradually this model was introduced in most countries around the world (Jolly 1994). Disciplinary teaching and specialization replaced a holistic model of expertise. It is clear that these changes affected the role of medical teachers deeply. Today, medical schools are composed of twenty or more departments, which are themselves sometimes divided in various sections, each of which covers a different aspect of medicine. The great teachers of the past have been replaced by experts in specialized areas of the medical sciences.

Major developments have also occurred in the way information is collected, reproduced, and transmitted to students. In the seventeenth century, anatomy at Dutch medical schools was taught during winter months since artificial cooling was not available. Book printing was very expensive, so students did not own books. Today imaging techniques, colour reproduction, cheap printing, computer simulations, videotaping, computer databases, and Internet facilities provide students with excellent opportunities to learn without requiring a teacher to transmit the available information. Students may no longer rely on a teacher's knowledge as the main source of information. The prevailing educational culture still considers the teacher as the person who determines what, when, and how learners will learn, and views direct teaching as the central role for teachers. However, a change is needed in view of new developments in medicine, health care, and educational technology.

What then is the role of the teacher under these new conditions? In this chapter we will develop the idea that the central role of teachers is the management of student learning. This not a new role, but historically, the role of the teacher as a central knowledge base for students has obscured it.

Management of learning

Creating an environment in which students can learn effectively and efficiently is the core managerial role of teachers. Management includes giving direction, providing learning opportunities, and evaluating outcomes of learning.

The main questions for teachers are: what should be learnt and how should it be learnt? The main difference now is that answers need to be formulated in a dynamic environment: the knowledge explosion and the changes in health care delivery require a redefinition of how we educate physicians to be capable of taking up their roles for the next twenty-five years. The knowledge and skills base of the graduate should not only enable them to function according to current standards, but also to provide means for further development. 'Learning to learn' is a crucial skill to keep up with the changes indicated before.

Shaping the learning environment therefore means two important things:

1. Providing students with relevant information and practice opportunities needed to develop a knowledge and skills base.
2. Designing the environment in such way that active learning is encouraged.

The first requirement implies that teachers are experts in their field, can make connections across disciplines, and have an overall view of the requirements of the profession. The second requirement implies that teachers have a good understanding of the conditions of learning. This includes general knowledge of how people learn, various modes of instruction, and knowledge of specific learning difficulties in their own field (Irby 1994).

In order to educate physicians who have a lifelong interest in learning, it is generally assumed that the way physicians are educated should reflect an interest in learning. Active learning, which means that the learner is learning by making deliberate connections between what he knows already and the content to be learned, exploring alternative solutions to a problem, and looking for meaning in the learning task, is considered an important ingredient of programs promoting learning to learn. Self-directed learning has a wider implication than active learning, since it also points to the responsibility of the learner in the learning process. Teachers find self-directed learning more threatening to their position than the idea of active learning since it has implications regarding their authority.

In the modern world professionals can only survive when they keep up with the developments in their field. That responsibility is handed over to them on the day they graduate, and it is therefore natural to prepare them for that part of professional life by increasingly making them responsible for their own learning. Active learning and self-directed learning are usually connected with problem-based learning. In this educational approach cases or actual patient problems are the starting point for the students' learning process. They analyse the problem and define learning objectives in small groups. After exploring the learning issues through self study, they report and discuss the results in the following group session. But active learning and self-directed learning can also be promoted in other curriculum strategies.

Managing learning seems to be contradictory to the concepts of active learning and self-directed learning. In reality they are not, since teachers play a major role in defining the learning environment in which students can develop their knowledge and skills, and they also represent the professional standard for students. In the following sections the various roles of teachers will be explored further.

Shaping the learning environment

Curricula are often constructed on the assumption, that learning occurs because a teacher is delivering content in a lecture. Promoting active learning and self-directed learning implies that teachers consider themselves as designers of learning situations. Based on their knowledge of the field teachers select and present topics, concepts, and problems in such a way that learners become actively involved. Selection is a key word here, since no teacher is able to present all available and relevant knowledge within the time frame of a curriculum. It is evident, that selection of content should be in line with professional standards.

In designing the learning environment several educational design parameters have to be taken into account as well:

1. *Complexity of the learning task*. Active learning requires the learner to explore and adapt their existing knowledge structure in view of new information. If there is little connection, meaningful learning will be more difficult. Obviously what is needed is a certain optimal complexity, since very easy learning tasks will not result in active exploration either.
2. *Learner involvement*. Intellectual curiosity is the motivating force which stimulates the learner to learn. Building upon existing interests of learners (i.e. using real life examples they can relate to) is a good way to promote learner involvement.
3. *Learner's logic*. Teachers are experts in their field. They have an overview of their field which makes it obvious for them to present topics in a certain order, usually according to a general disciplinary framework. Learners do not possess this overview and may need a different route of entry to the field. Cognitive research also suggests that learners in many fields have misconceptions which are obstructions to further learning. It is essential to take the learner's logic into account in developing a learning environment to promote active learning.
4. *Learner's needs*. The design of a learning environment to promote self-directed learning should enable learners to define and fulfil their learning needs. Within the boundaries of professional requirements to be met at graduation, learners should

increasingly have control over their way to reach those goals. In other words, the freedom to choose how and when to learn. Flexible learning environments are needed to achieve this requirement.

There is a wide variety of activities which promote active learning. Questioning students during a lecture to make them reflect critically on a topic is a modest way to do this. Small projects, field studies, or writing a paper on a specific topic are ways to involve students in an active way. Grand rounds, clinical conferences, and other forms of patient related activities offer opportunities for students to become self-directed learners provided the format of the sessions allows students to contribute. The Arabic philosopher and physician Avicenna (980–1037) provides an early example of how to do this. He is said to have had his students placed in concentric circles around a patient. The freshmen would start to try to find the explanation, then the more experienced would join in. At last, Avicenna himself would reach conclusions on the case. Allowing students to try to experiment is an important way of promoting their involvement and understanding.

New technological opportunities such as computer databases, expert systems, and simulations offer new means to make students more responsible for their own learning. Some of these new opportunities are excellent tools to stimulate or support self-directed learning. Computer access to libraries, databases, and research notes provide opportunities to search, to select, and to read information at home, at your own pace. Learning how to use those tools in an appropriate way will soon become part of the professional standard in any field of knowledge. More advanced tools, such as expert systems, allow learners to develop and test hypotheses, and shape their view on how to analyse professional problems.

Problem-based learning could be considered as an overall strategy to create a curriculum which promotes self-directed and active learning.

Problems, usually a written example are the starting point of the learning process. Students analyse these problems in small groups guided by a tutor. Students consider the issues in the particular case, discuss mechanisms involved in the problem, and finally develop a list of learning goals, which then try to fulfil for the next tutorial. Between the tutorial sessions (usually two tutorials a week) students use the learning goals to guide their own study. They may study from books, prepared hand-outs, videotapes, computer simulations, or lab work. At the next tutorial session they report back on their findings and check whether their understanding of the case is satisfactory. Since the learning goals of the students determine to a large extent their study activities between two sessions, the quality of examples is an important issue. Thus the central task of teachers is to develop series of cases that enable students to learn important aspects of the medical sciences. The design parameters mentioned before play a crucial role. For a more extensive discussion on case and course construction in PBL the reader is referred to Boud and Feletti (1991) and Bouhuijs *et al.* (1993).

The general rule in designing an effective learning environment is to pose the question, whether students can find and understand content by themselves without detailed teacher guidelines or presentations.

The teacher as a professional model

Being a teacher inevitably involves becoming a role model for students. From a learning point of view there are advantages and disadvantages. Expert behaviour in action is certainly an important motivating factor for learners and a rich source of learning opportunities. The downside is that imitating expert behaviour does not necessarily mean that learners have an insight into the underlying assumptions of a professional's behaviour. Cognitive research suggests that expert behaviour involves frequent short cuts in reasoning which are based on broad experience in the field. Donald Schön (1987) has pointed out that reflection on professional performance is needed to transmit the core of professional behaviour.

Teachers can be models in other ways as well. The teacher can be an example of how to learn as a professional: how do you keep up with new developments, which resources do you use, how do you fit learning into your daily routine work?

Coaching the learner

Although one might be tempted to conclude that teachers play a modest role as promotors of self-directed learning, at various points learners need guidance in their development. This is a central issue with problem-based learning in the debate around the role of the tutor. In PBL small groups of students analyse cases, define learning objectives, study independently, and report back in a tutorial group. These groups are guided by a tutor. Schmidt and Moust (1995) investigated the factors in tutor behaviour which have an effect on student learning. Three factors play a role here. The first one is the level of expertise in the area of study: the use of expertise has a positive influence on learning outcomes. Clearly providing learners with additional information and feedback plays a role here. The second factor is cognitive congruence, which could be described as using expert knowledge in relation to the needs of the learners (asking the right questions, asking for further explanations, pushing students to address certain issues). The third factor is general interest in the learner (social congruence). This could be described as a social factor which includes the teacher's concern for group climate, having understanding for the position of a student, and for concerns students may have. The three factors are not independent, but there is considerable variation possible between tutors. An excellent tutor scores highly on all these factors, but the total effect on learning outcomes is rather limited: learner characteristics and the learning task determine outcomes to a large extent. One could draw an interesting parallel here between the role of the tutor and the role of a sports coach. A good sports coach has a good understanding of the game, knows how to improve the skills of his players, and has a good eye for the team process and for the individual players.

The analogy also illuminates the nature of expertise in the field needed to be an effective tutor. Like a sports coach it is important to know what learners need to understand and to spot weaknesses in their reasoning. Knowing specific details seems to be less essential for a teacher. Like a sports coach he himself is not supposed to perform all the tricks that he wants to see in his players. Another interesting parallel between the tutor and a sports coach is the aim they have: developing knowledge and skills which may differ from their own, and which may even lie beyond their own level of expertise.

Coaching the learner is not restricted to problem-based learning. Clerkships are clear examples where teachers could promote self-directed and active learning by taking up a coaching role. Students frequently complain about the lack of guidance, support, and feedback provided during clerkships (Jolly 1994). This makes it harder for them to develop themselves into professionals in the real sense.

The teacher as an assessor

Assessment of learning outcomes is a necessary component in professional education to ensure that professional standards are met. In medicine, the expectations of society also influence the assessment process. Educational institutions generally take this responsibility seriously. The ideal of self-directed learning includes an ability to understand the limitations of the knowledge and skills a person possesses and implies voluntary self assessment as a way to check knowledge and skills. After graduation physicians are supposed to be able to judge for themselves what their limitations are, and self-directed learning is a way to prepare students for this part of professional life.

There is quite a difference between the ideal of self assessment and the responsibility as viewed by the medical schools (or independent exam boards). This is not only a philosophical issue, since it is well documented that learning processes are influenced by exams. Self-directed learning in its true sense generally results in a much greater variation in what students actually learn. A standard exam will mostly contain a limited number of questions on issues that the teacher considers important. If the things students learn are not sufficiently represented in the questions, students will be punished for not having studied those topics important to the teacher. In other words, they will be punished for studying according to their own interests. This sends a strong message to students that they cannot ignore: follow the teacher.

There are no easy answers here for this dilemma, but the key issue is to develop assessment strategies which cope with the natural variety in learning outcomes as a consequence of self-directed learning. A second issue is to develop assessment strategies which give students a greater responsibility for the assessment process.

There are several ways to use standardized tests in a self-directed learning environment (van der Vleuten et al. 1996). Adding test items on a broader range of topics will give students a chance to demonstrate which areas they covered; giving students an option to select a number of questions out of a wider range is a similar approach. New computer technology makes it possible to draw a selection of questions from a test item bank according to the characteristics of the learner.

Another approach is to develop test situations resembling the original learning task either using paper and pencil formats and computer simulations (Schuwirth et al. 1996) or objective structured clinical exams (OSCE).

Students can be more involved not only by giving them options to answer certain questions on a test, but also by introducing learner's reports, peer evaluation, and case reviews. These assessment methods require students to be assessors of their own work or of the work of fellow students, and give them a chance to develop their self assessment skills (Snadden et al. 1996).

Perspective

Self-directed learning is sometimes opposed by teachers who fear for their role as a teacher. The message of this chapter is that the role of the teacher is different, but not less important nor less demanding. Creative teachers will certainly enjoy the challenges of shaping a learning environment which motivates learners to develop themselves into independent professionals.

References

Boud, D. and Feletti, G. (1991). (ed.). *The challenge of problem-based learning*. Kogan Page, London

Bouhuijs, P.A.J., Schmidt, H.G., and Van Berkel, H.J.M. (ed.). (1993). *Problem-based learning as an educational strategy*. Network Publications, Maastricht.

Irby, D.M. (1994). What clinical teachers in medicine need to know. *Academic Medicine*, **69**, 333–42

Jolly, B. (1994). *Bedside manners: teaching and learning in the hospital setting*. Maastricht University Press, Maastricht.

Schmidt, H.G. and Moust, J.H.C. (1995). What makes a tutor effective? A structural-equations modelling approach to learning in problem-based curricula. *Academic Medicine*, **70**, 708–15.

Schön, D.A. (1987). *Educating the reflective practitioner*. Jossey-Bass Publishers, San Francisco.

Schuwirth, L.W.T., Van der Vleuten, C.P.M., Stoffers, H.E.J.H., and Peperkamp, A.G.W. (1996). Computerised long-menu questions as an alternative to open-ended questions in computerised assessment. *Medical Education*, **30**, 50–5.

Snadden, D., Thomas, M.L., Griffin, E.M., and Hudson, H. (1996). Portfolio-based learning and general practice vocational training. *Medical Education*, **30**, 148–52.

Van der Vleuten, C.P.M., Verwijnen, G.M., and Wijnen, W.H.F.W. (1996). Fifteen years of experience with progress testing in a problem-based curriculum. *Medical Teacher*, **18**, 2, 103–9.

7.4 Staff development and the quality of teaching

Lewis Elton

Most people would be very concerned, if they were operated on by untrained surgeons, if their cars were designed by untrained engineers, or their children taught by untrained teachers. In other words, we expect our bodies, our cars, and even our children to be in the hands of professionals, when they need attention. Yet when our children reach student age, it has been considered quite normal until recently that their professors should be untrained, and this may well still be the majority view within the profession of university teachers. Yet the very fact that such people are untrained calls into question the statement that they constitute a profession (Elton 1992; Warren Piper 1992). They are of course trained experts in *what* they teach, but they have normally had no training in *how* they teach. Furthermore, the *how*, of teaching is not confined to personal competencies as a teacher in the classroom; possibly even more important are the competencies of curriculum design, which greatly influence the *what* of teaching, and the attitudes which teachers bring to their varied teaching tasks. As there is now a concern both inside and outside universities, about the quality of teaching in universities, there ought to be a corresponding concern about the absence of training and development of university teachers. We shall address these two concerns in turn.

Quality: its control, assessment, and enhancement

Quality has two quite different meanings. There is the colloquial meaning, where quality is synonymous with excellence, and where a Rolls Royce is of higher quality than a Mini. The underlying philosophy is that of Plato, who postulated the existence of ideals, to which real things approximated. Within higher education, the concept of a gold standard of a British degree is essentially platonic. The other and more technical meaning of quality is often expressed as 'fitness for purpose', i.e. quality is a measure of the extent to which an entity achieves what it is designed to achieve for a specified purpose. With that definition, both a Rolls Royce and a Mini could be of high quality, in terms of the extent to which they can satisfy the very different purposes for which they are designed. In higher education, a degree course would be of high quality, if it achieved the educational objectives for which it had been designed. Since this second meaning of quality has the authority of Aristotle, we are clearly dealing here with a long standing argument. Since we shall in fact need the concepts represented by both meanings, we shall give the first the name 'standard' and the second the name 'quality'.

Unfortunately, giving names to concepts does not necessarily make it possible to use these concepts operationally. Thus when two universities, say the universities of Camford and of Bruddersford, have very different institutional missions, then their degree courses will be very different from each other, both in concept and in delivery. Yet, while the Higher Education Funding Councils accept this in principle, in practice they still expect both to provide education 'at degree level', whatever that may mean, and preferentially to use certain teaching and learning methods that are approved of by those who understand such things. In other words, even when quality relates to different purposes, it is still to be governed by certain absolute standards. It is all very confusing, but it actually helps in the understanding of the problems associated with quality to know that it is difficult to tackle them in a wholly logical fashion.

Quality control at its crudest is the control of the inputs and outputs of a production process through the quality specified for each and the rejection of those that fall below it. A good example is the way that most universities in the UK, have used A level grades and finals examinations as their main forms of quality control. More recently, certain process controls have been added in connection with the quality of teaching which students received. How effective such controls are in maintaining quality is now being judged, at some expense, through the quality audits of the Committee of Vice Chancellors and Principals (Academic Audit Unit 1991) and, at much greater expense, by the quality assessment of the Higher Education Funding Councils in England, Scotland, and Wales (see e.g. HEFCE 1992). None of these processes will by themselves lead to an enhancement of quality, which—in view of the current lack of professional training of university teachers—is most readily achieved through the provision of staff training and development. But for that the resources are much more meagre than for audit and assessment.

Broadly speaking there are three levels of quality enhancement; to improve what is bad, to improve what is good, and to do things differently but better. Each requires a different set of activities and strategies for success, as is indicated in Table 7.1. Each also requires a different approach to assessment and associated funding; the HEFCE idea that the same approaches can be used to identify and reward/punish at the two extremes of 'excellent' and 'unsatisfactory' is far too crude. On the other hand, there is one thing that they all require: the recognition of teaching, in its broadest sense, as being of equal importance as research as a university activity, accompanied by appropriate resourcing and by rewards for excellence (Elton and Partington 1993). Each also requires a different approach to staff development and training as is shown in Table 7.1, to which we now turn.

Staff development and training

Clearly, all concerned with teaching—and this includes not only academic teachers, but all who impinge on the overall learning experience of students, whether in direct support of teaching or in a more administrative capacity—must have a basic training to fit them for their tasks. This is now in general, although not always adequately, provided by initial training programmes, but the word 'initial' is unfortunate here, for a similar basic training is also needed by those who, while experienced, are untrained. More than sixty such courses are now formally accredited by the Staff and Educational Development

Table 7.1 Quality enhancement

Levels	Activities	Strategies
Improve what is bad	Advice and basic training Counselling Threats	Student evaluation Staff appraisal
Improve what is good	Curriculum development New teaching methods	Self-reflection and improvement Institutional support and rewards
Differently and better	New teaching and learning support Technical support Institutional change	Research and development in teaching and learning Serious training Self-instructional training materials Diploma courses

Association. New entrants are in general very willing to undergo such training, but for the rest the processes of student evaluation and staff appraisal are essential to ensure that those who need training most will undergo it. This will 'improve what is bad'. To 'improve what is good', it is generally not necessary to provide training courses. Good teachers have learned from reflecting on their teaching (Schön 1983). What they need in order to improve their teaching and their courses, as comes out very clearly from the experience of the Enterprise in Higher Education Initiative (EHE) (Wright 1992) is institutional support and opportunities for self-improvement. They also should perceive the possibility of being rewarded for teaching excellence. Finally, in a rapidly changing environment, it is not enough to improve what is good, because much that was good in an earlier environment, is good no longer. What is needed then is to do things 'differently and better' but in what way to do things differently may be far from clear. This is where research and development in teaching and learning becomes essential, combined with a serious training programme, with the possibility of it leading to postgraduate qualifications. One highly cost-effective way of providing such a training programme is through self-instructional training materials (Cryer 1992), supported by local mentoring.

While the above provides a structure for staff development and training, it says little about the ethos that should underlie it. Brown and Sommerlad (1992) characterize the ethos, by identifying three approaches to staff development, the fragmented, the formalized, and the focused (see Table 7.2). The first is still the most common in academia, while the third is the one favoured by progressive industry. While each accepts that training must cater for both individual and organizational needs, each is associated with a very different ethos: the fragmented approach sees training largely as remedial; the formalized approach recognizes the need of all staff for lifelong training and development; but only the focused approach links the needs of the staff and the organization for which they work into a unified and mutually supportive whole, thereby causing a 'learning organization'. Only the third approach enables organizations to adapt to change successfully.

Table 7.2 Approaches to staff development

Fragmented	Training is a cost, not an investment; not linked to institutional goals; perceived as a luxury; based in a training department; primarily knowledge based.
Formalized	Training is systemic (part of career development); linked to human resource needs; linked to appraisal and individual needs; focused on skills as well as on knowledge; carried out by trainers and line managers.
Focused	Training is a continuous learning process; essential for organizational survival; linked to organizational strategy and individual goals; on-the-job as well as through specialist courses; the line manager's responsibility; tolerant.

Institutional change

Quality enhancement at all three of the levels characterized in Table 7.1 necessitates substantial change, both of the institution and the individuals in it. This is most obvious at the third level, since it is associated with a changed external environment, but it is equally true at the lowest level, where individuals have to develop a radically different approach to their job, from the traditional one where teaching was a 'private activity between not always consenting adults' and governed by the teacher's academic freedom. At the middle level, it would appear at first sight that change is a minor consideration, since, as has been so clearly shown in the EHE initiative, the so called 'good' teachers do not need to change; all they appear to need is a chance to do what they want to do. Unfortunately, this is not entirely true and the enthusiasm of even the most dedicated wanes in the absence of institutional recognition and rewards (Elton 1991). The major change needed is then not in the primary area of the improvement of teaching, but in the secondary one of institutional support, i.e. for those that are in managerial and leadership positions (Elton 1996a).

The need for change to extend to those in managerial and leadership positions is in fact apparent at all three levels of quality enhancement. At the third level, inspired leadership and competent management are needed to meet the challenges of the changing external world, while at the first level, the skills required by middle manage-ment to deal with staff are new to most. Hence staff development and training is needed for both top and middle management—Vice-Chancellors and Heads of Department in the language of the time before the Jarratt Report (1985)—in their roles both as managers and as leaders (Middlehurst and Elton 1992; Stewart 1992). At present, such training is effected solely through the 'fragmented' approach; however, only the 'focused' approach is likely to lead to success in the longer run. The whole subject of staff development has been reviewed recently by Brew (1995).

The case of medical education

While all that has been said so far is quite generally applicable to higher education, it is particularly important in the field of medical education, where the external environment is changing in two ways: the first, to achieve more with less, is common to all higher education, but the second, to meet the changing health care needs of the population, including the shift towards the community is particular to medicine. At the same time, medical education is probably saddled with a greater proportion of powerful and conservative teaching staff than average for all of higher education. The effort of the St Bartholomew's and Royal London School of Medicine and Dentistry (QMW), with the help of the EHE Initiative which appointed me as Higher Education Adviser to this project, to create a medical and dental curriculum to meet the needs of future society was therefore an interesting one to watch. The staff development aspect of this project hovered somewhere between levels two and three in quality enhancement, with level one largely neglected, while the approach to staff development was still largely of the 'fragmented' kind and there was effectively no staff development of the managerial variety. If the arguments presented above are right, then there is a need (now that the EHE Initiative has finished) for changing the approach to one that on the one hand is much more institutionally integrated and on the other tackles the problem associated with 'improving what is bad.' However, for medical education, as for all other aspects of higher education, there are dangers ahead.

Dangers ahead

The most obvious danger lies in the gross under-resourcing of staff development, particularly when considered in the light of what is beginning to look like a gross over-resourcing of quality assessment. This is not confined to financial aspects; perhaps the most serious aspect of it is that quality assessment is likely to remove a sizeable proportion of the best academic teachers from the productive task of teaching, curriculum design, and staff development. In this way, the assessment process may actually indirectly reduce the quality which it aims to enhance. It may even achieve this more directly, for it is well known that those who are assessed, whether they are teachers or students, tend to work towards the assessment to the extent of 'playing the system', rather than work through the intrinsic motivation of wanting to do a job professionally and well (Elton 1996b). External assessment implicitly assumes that university teachers cannot be trusted to act professionally and to some extent this is true, for if it were not, there would be no need to make a case for staff training and development. But the assessment with all its pressures is taking place in a rapidly changing situation where universities are beginning to realize that a true professionalism may be in their own best interests. As is so often the case with externally engendered change, there comes a moment when the balance between stick and carrot must change. That this point may be close, comes out of the evidence of the EHE Initiative (Elton 1992; Elton and Cryer 1994), which has from the start favoured the carrot, in contrast to the Funding Councils which continue to appear to favour the stick (Joint Planning Group 1996). At least this seems to be the case for teaching; the situation is quite different for research, where the research selectivity exercise constitutes a huge carrot, not only for those who benefit most from it, but even more for those who are marginally at risk of not benefiting from it. The playing field between research and teaching is not level, and if this situation does not change, the high hopes of those who are enthusiastic in their commitment to teaching are likely to remain unfulfilled.

References

Academic Audit Unit (1991). *Annual report of the Director.* CVCP Academic Audit Unit, Birmingham.

Brew, A, (ed.) (1995). *Directions in staff development.* Society for Research in Higher Education and Open University Press, Buckingham.

Brown, H. and Sommerlad, E. (1992). Staff development in higher education—Towards the learning organisation? *Higher Education Quarterly,* **46**, 174–90.

Cryer, P. (ed.) (1992). *Effective learning and teaching in higher education.* Universities' Staff Development Unit, Sheffield.

Elton, L. (1991). Enterprise in higher education: work in progress. *Education and Training,* **33**(2), 5–9.

Elton, L. (1992). Quality enhancement and academic professionalism. *The New Academic,* 1(2), 3–5.

Elton, L. (1996a). Task differentiation in universities: towards a new collegiality. *Tertiary Education and Management,* **2**, 138–45.

Elton, L. (1996b). Partnership, quality and standards in higher education. *Quality in Higher Education,* **2**, 95–104.

Elton, L. and Cryer, P. (1994). Quality and change in higher education. *Innovation in Higher Education,* **18**, 205–20.

Elton, L. and Partington, P. (1993). *Teaching standards and excellence in higher education : developing a culture for quality.* Green Paper No 1, 2nd edition. Committee of Vice-Chancellors and Principals, London.

HEFCE (1992). *Quality assessment.* Higher Education Funding Council for England, Bristol.

Jarratt (1985). *Effective studies in universities.* Committee of Vice-Chancellors and Principals, London.

Joint Planning Group (1996). Joint planning group for quality assurance in higher education: Draft final report, Unpublished.

Middlehurst, R. and Elton, L. (1992). Leadership and management in higher education. *Studies in Higher Education,* **17**, 251–64.

Schön, D.A. (1983). *The reflective practitioner.* Temple Smith, London.

Stewart, R. (1992). Management in the public and private sector. *Higher Educational Quarterly,* **46**, 157–65.

Warren Piper, D. (1992). Are professors professional? *Higher Education Quarterly,* **46**, 145–56.

Wright, P. (1992). Learning through enterprise: the Enterprise in Higher Education Initiative. In *Learning to effect,* (ed. R. Barnett), pp. 204–23. The Society for Research into Higher Education and Open University Press, Buckingham.

7.5 Staff development in UK medical schools

Angela Towle

A conference held a few years ago brought together medical teachers, educationists, and staff developers from UK medical schools to highlight key issues in effecting change through staff development based on the presentation of case studies and the sharing of ideas and experience (Towle 1993). Using information from the conference report and personal experience in three medical schools, I have attempted to summarize below the main issues in staff development in medical education in the UK, some key experiences so far and the lessons which have been learned.

The new emphasis on teaching

Staff development is a relatively new idea for most UK medical schools. Until recently, few medical teachers were required to undergo any educational training. It was widely believed that their professional qualifications and own experience of education were sufficient to guarantee that they would be at least adequate teachers. In addition, since medical students are amongst the brightest in the country there was the expectation that they would still be able to cope with any parts of the course that were less than satisfactorily taught.

This view is now being challenged not just in medical education but in higher education across all disciplines. Recent moves towards accountability and standard setting in the public sector are raising concerns about the cost effectiveness and quality of higher education, and hence the quality of teaching. They are highlighting the lack of incentives and opportunities for academics to develop the necessary personal skills not only to be effective teachers, but also curriculum designers. In this way staff development has been linked to the quality of teaching.

British institutions of higher education, under pressure to justify the public money which they receive, now face two processes of scrutiny in relation to their procedures and practices of quality assurance and control: academic audit and quality assurance. However questionable the effectiveness of these exercises in improving the quality of teaching (see Chapter 7.4), it is clear that medical schools have embraced the new emphasis on teaching and the need to introduce staff appraisal and training.

Furthermore, the introduction of managed competition in the National Health Service, based on contracting between purchasers and providers of health care, has raised the possibility of establishing explicit contracts for teaching between medical schools and health care providers (hospitals, general practices, etc.). As a first step in this direction, most schools have begun to monitor the quantity of clinical teaching provided by different providers for the purpose of monitoring allocation of the Service Increment for Teaching and Research (money provided by the Department of Health to compensate hospitals for the excess costs associated with teaching and research). Measuring quality in addition to quantity is a natural progression. All these initiatives have implications for staff development.

In addition, medical schools are in the process of reviewing their undergraduate curriculum in the light of recent recommendations from the General Medical Council. There is dawning recognition that changing the curriculum is unlikely to be effective without staff development to ensure that teachers are willing and able to change their teaching practice. Unless staff are provided with new skills, for example in supporting student-centred learning, and assisted towards new attitudes which will motivate them to embrace the change, the curricula which are being so carefully planned will not be implemented successfully.

The purposes of staff development

Staff development can be used to effect change at the level of the individual, the curriculum, or the organization (medical school). In relation to the individual, staff development can be used to improve the skills of inexperienced or poor teachers, to continue to improve the performance of good teachers or to provide new skills in order to facilitate new ways of teaching. Thus the emphasis moves from changing the behaviour of the individual teacher to changing the behaviour of groups in order to implement curriculum change, where teachers require different skills or attitudes in order to teach differently. Such efforts may, through incremental change, lead to cultural change within the institution and a reorientation of the entire faculty. On the other hand, organizational change on this scale may require a more radical approach, such as the development of a 'learning organization' in which learning is linked both to organizational strategy and individual goals.

Elton (page 000) refers to the paper by Brown and Sommerlad (1992) that identified three main approaches to staff development: the fragmented, the formalized, and the focused. Hatton and Bullimore (1993), from their experience at Leeds, provide a similar model which depicts staff development as an evolving process with four stages: a random stage where there is no recognition of staff development as a necessary function at either the individual or organizational level; a fragmented stage where staff development does exist but is related to individual needs only, not to organizational goals; a formalized stage where individual needs are met in a systematic way through individual performance review/appraisal, linked to departmental and ultimately university aims and needs; and a strategic stage where each individual has a personal development plan, linking their development needs with those of the department and the university. They place their staff development programme between stages three and four, but most medical schools in the UK have probably not progressed far beyond stage two, where staff development is largely a series of isolated events, often provided or taken by motivated individuals on their own initiative, rather than as a part of a planned strategy for bringing about the kind of changes which the school requires.

Staff development activities

Below are short case studies (based on a composite of experiences in several different places) which typify the current state of staff development in UK medical education in relation to three approaches: i) improving individual skills; ii) improving departmental teaching; iii) introducing curriculum change. These studies describe what happened and the lessons that were learned.

i) Improving individual skills

Medical school A, which had never provided or required any training for its teachers received a small external grant to introduce staff development. A keen member of staff and an administrative assistant devised a questionnaire which was sent to all staff, with a covering letter from the dean, in order to find out what experience or formal training members of the teaching staff had received, and what they perceived their needs to be. Approximately 600 questionnaires were sent out to all clinical teachers in the main teaching hospitals, basic scientists, and general practitioner tutors, although it was extremely difficult to obtain an up to date staff list (in fact one spin off from the exercise was that for the first time a reasonably complete list of teaching staff was compiled). The initial response rate was 40%, rising to 50% after a reminder letter; only twelve respondents had received any training in education. The responses showed a great demand for staff development and strong feelings that the profile of teaching needed to be raised within the school. Particular areas such as teaching in communication skills and small groups were frequently highlighted as desirable.

Medical school B, which had provided a variety of courses in medical education for a number of years, sent out a questionnaire to approximately 450 teaching staff to discover what existing expertise was present and to identify future training needs in relation to ten major topics, such as small group teaching, computer-assisted learning. Ninety people responded to the questionnaire; between 19 and 40 people expressed interest in attending workshops on each of the identified topics. A programme of seven different half-day workshops, each repeated twice on different days of the week, was planned based on the expressed needs of the staff. A brochure containing information about the years' programme of workshops was sent to all staff, who were invited to sign up. Attendance at the workshops ranged from one to eight, with an average of five; there were frequent last minute cancellations. Workshops held later in the year were progressively poorly attended. Those who attended the workshops found them valuable, although they wished more people had been there.

In comparison with the poor numbers at these workshops (even when designed to meet expressed needs), activities which were more specifically linked in with curriculum changes (e.g. on the role of tutoring for new course tutors) were better attended. Teaching skills courses were usually well attended because it was a condition of employment that new staff should attend one of these courses. It was concluded that because there had been a long history of staff development at this medical school, those most likely to come to educational events had already done so, and that a more targeted approach was needed to reach those who did not place a priority on such training. Sending out blanket publicity was time consuming and costly for very little return.

ii) Improving departmental teaching

The Department of General Practice in medical school C, like most similar departments in other medical schools in the UK, relies on about forty GP tutors to assist members of the academic staff in teaching about general practice, and has been organizing training for all its teachers for a number of years. There is an individualized induction course for new lecturers in the department and a faculty development programme for established lecturers based on a co-tutoring system. General practitioners in the teaching practices are encouraged to attend a variety of workshops to improve their teaching skills. These events are accredited for the Postgraduate Education Allowance (PGEA—an amount of money on offer to GPs who can provide evidence of continuing education in certain fields) and therefore there is some financial incentive for GPs to attend. There are also regular meetings of tutors: the programme for the meetings was based on a needs assessment exercise. These meetings are very well attended despite being in the evening and some tutors having to make a journey of forty miles. Each year there is an annual residential weekend at a pleasant out-of-town location. These activities are regarded as being good fun and very productive, but depend on a tremendous amount of hard work by one member of academic staff. One of the most valued aspects is the opportunity to learn from each other and share ideas, problems, and experiences. The result has been a more cohesive course for the students and more cohesive teaching by the tutors in a course they had assisted in developing.

iii) Introducing curriculum change

The most significant wide-scale change to have occurred in the UK recently has been the total reorganization, beginning in 1996, of postgraduate specialized medical training, popularly referred to as 'Calmanization', after the UK's chief medical officer Sir Kenneth Calman who championed the changes. Essentially this involves shorter, and more structured and formally supervised periods of training than hitherto, with an emphasis on appraisal and assessment and a need for liaison between Department of Health representatives (postgraduate deans) and the Royal Colleges (the arbiters, until now, of specialty training). Although postgraduate, this example offers a microcosm of how staff development can enhance such developments. The Royal College of Surgeons instituted a formal two-day introductory course 'Training the trainers' in 1995 as a precursor to these changes. College tutors were encouraged to attend, and indeed in one region the postgraduate dean identified funds and regulations to attempt to ensure that all surgical trainers took part in such training. The programme initially started with about five surgeons and five educational specialists giving about ten days (or more) per year, working in pairs, on the two-day event. However its success has prompted the recruitment of up to twenty-five further trainers from each camp with a view to expanding and regionalizing the course provision. At the same time a number of other College-based initiatives have utilized the increased educational expertise developed by the surgeons. The courses have a turnover of several hundred thousand pounds per year which has helped underwrite further developments. A course handbook has been produced, specifically aimed at surgeon educators (Harris, et al. 1996) and further volumes are planned. Although the implementation of Calman's proposals cannot conceivably be covered by a short two-day course, the sustained programme, aimed at a limited objective and with managerial and academic backing, has produced a considerable force for change in surgical education. The Royal College is no longer merely an exclusive club entered through ritualistic assessment procedures, but a thriving and expanding educational institution with its finger on the pulse of medical education in the UK today.

Problems and constraints

How much of current staff development is effective or achieves desired change are questions which are difficult to answer at an institutional level because rarely is the actual purpose of staff development considered in relation to the overall goals of the organization. The promotion of change at the level of the medical school (see Chapter 8.2) calls for a statement of the purpose and goals of staff development and a planned strategy for their achievement.

Such a strategy should take cognisance of the most effective and efficient means of achieving the purposes intended, especially since there are limited resources of time, money, and expertise. It should consider what kinds of activities are most likely to change behaviour and recognize that formal training courses of the type with which most people are familiar are not the only, nor even the best, way of effecting change.

Some academic staff still feel little need for staff development; others are willing but do not perceive it as a priority given all the other calls on their time. Teachers need to be convinced that participation in staff development activities will bring them benefits. Staff may be motivated in a number of ways, for example through specification in contracts, appraisal and promotion procedures, or by linking training to curriculum change. The aim must be to produce a culture within the medical school which values learning and expects participation in staff development activities. It is therefore vital that these are supported by key individuals within the medical school (deans, heads of departments, curriculum managers).

Shortages of funding and expertise place real constraints on delivering effective staff development. Few places have an identified central budget for staff development, either to support individual activities or to set up the infrastructure to support a staff development strategy. In relation to the latter, an urgent need in most medical schools is to improve communication between the dispersed and disparate people involved in teaching medical students. The increased emphasis on staff development has highlighted the shortage of expertise available to medical schools wishing to provide such activities. Two types of expertise are required: 'educational experts' who can provide skills training and 'independent facilitators' who can help the sharing and development of expertise which already exists within a staff group. Some schools have begun to identify what expertise exists already within their institution, and build up a critical mass of staff who raise awareness, act as role models or educational consultants, or run workshops. Others have begun to link in with their university staff training/development units or departments of education.

Another route is to form consortia between medical schools for the purposes of staff development. There are several reasons for this. First medical education is unique and complex; it does not share some of the attributes of other higher education areas and has others peculiar to itself: clinical teaching, social and emotional pressure, professional cultures and hierarchies to contend with, an unusually high workload, etc. One school will not have the human or financial resources to deal with all its problems; between them different schools are much more likely to house the appropriate expertise. Many more events can be mounted and with a higher and hence more cost effective attendance. The diversity of school approaches, now that accrediting bodies (GMC, National Boards and Associations) have demanded more attention to individual students, needs and choices, have also thrown up issues which need to be discussed collectively—assessments, problem-based learning, community approaches. National and pan-national associations (ASME, AMEE, AAMC) also need to become more involved and more proactive as major providers of cross institutional staff development. A focus is needed for some activities that individual schools are nervous or incapable of providing.

References

Brown, H. and Sommerlad, E. (1992). Staff development in higher education—towards the learning organisation? *Higher Education Quarterly* **46**, 174–90.

Harris, N.D.C., Peyton, R., and Walker, M. (ed.) (1996). *Training the trainers: learning and teaching*. Royal College of Surgeons of England, London.

Hatton, P. and Bullimore, D. (1993). The role of staff development in a changing environment: experience from the University of Leeds. 1A. *Effecting change through staff development*. Sharing Ideas 2 (ed. A. Towle), pp.33–38. King's Fund Centre, London.

Towle, A. (ed.) (1993). *Effecting change through staff development*. Sharing Ideas 2. King's Fund Centre, London.

8 Curriculum implementation

8.1 Managing change

Rodney Gale and Janet Grant

Introduction

There is an extensive and rapidly growing literature on the management of change. There is, growing in parallel, a realization that the context of change is important to its process and its outcome (Pettigrew 1985). Beneath all writings on change lie theories and views about the ways organizations function and the ways people operate within them. Spurgeon and Barwell (1991) have reviewed many of these in the context of the National Health Service.

Context is the theme word of the current (1990s) decade in relation to change. It has gradually become clear that, whilst there may be universal theories of change, they are only given meaning when adapted to the precise context in which they need to be used. Pettigrew *et al.* (1988) illuminated the role of context and indeed of local history in determining the change process. Pettigrew *et al.* (1992) have also tried to tackle the question of why different health authorities respond to the same stimulus in different ways and at different speeds. It is here that one has to face the detail of the local context.

Pettigrew *et al.* (1992) introduces the concept of receptive and non-receptive contexts for change. The receptive contexts are just the factors that tend to promote or enable change. They cover the environmental pressure, the clarity of goals and leadership, the intra-organizational relationships, the history of change locally, and the nature of the current change. A harmony among the set of variables enables change. This description has the virtue of highlighting the complexity of the change process and the number of variables that need to be considered, but it still remains more descriptive rather than prescriptive. The concern of this chapter is for those who wish to promote, encourage, stimulate, or lead change in their own institutions or organizations.

Turrill (1986) produced a booklet on change in the NHS that was firmly based on previous experiences in ICI. Much of the thinking on change in the industrial context of ICI was conditioned by that company's success in innovation and expansion. It was constrained only by its imagination and strategic capability; money was available and human resources could be found for good ideas. Change is seen as a process of taking stock of the current situation, imagining or deciding where you want to be, and planning how to get there. Resource constraints are not a major issue because new investment can be justified if there is a reasonable prospect of a return. The book is lacking on the messy interpersonal details that in our experience tend to dominate most change processes. A recent book by O'Connor (1993) is much stronger on such details and deals with the resolution of conflicts.

To probe further into the process of change and to anchor our thoughts in medical education at the undergraduate and postgraduate levels, we have to differentiate between the stimulus and response, between the sources of pressure for change and the organizational response. All change can be viewed as a process whereby influences from the environment become internalized and become part of the new organization (Plant 1987). A person, or persons, a representative group or structure, these can all be the agency through which the environmental influence enters the organization.

The environment can take many forms and can impinge in many ways and through many external agencies. The legislative environment can change, Government policy can change, resource distributions, attitudes, opinions, technologies, and knowledge can change. Ideas can emerge from research or from direct experience, from individuals inside or outside the organization, from groups affected or excited by the environmental stimulus.

Change can be perceived as an organizational response to an environmental stimulus that seeks to improve along a particular critical dimension, or it can be a response to remove something bad from the organization. This distinction between taking action to overcome a known organizational deficiency and changing just to improve for the longer term, becomes important in the management process we describe later.

It is easy for the organization and its members to recognize the presence of something bad. They may not all agree on the causes and cures of such problems as falling applicants, high failure rates on a course, overall student dissatisfaction with teaching methods, or potential losses of funding income, but they can agree on their existence.

The end result of the change process is also relatively uncomplicated and readily identifiable in increasing applications, exam success, new teaching methods, or more funding secured. There is a neatness and simplicity arising from a bounded problem, albeit a complex problem whose solution may well touch the whole organization.

However, it is much more difficult to promote change that will improve the health of an organization or its future competitive strength, when there are no obvious present problems. This is often the challenge faced by those seeking to reform a medical curriculum when there are no overt problems with the current arrangements and no shortage of applicants for places. A similar challenge is faced by those aiming to introduce novel teaching methods or to bring the community closer to the medical education process.

The challenge for change leaders is to communicate a vision of where the changes could lead and the potential advantages of pursuing such a route, without any real current reason for setting off on a difficult path, or any ability to assure those who will need to take risks to implement the novel idea, that it will definitely work. Major curriculum change is an act of faith that the new system will have significant advantages over the old in terms of the things that matter to the organization. The things that matter to one Medical School need not matter to another. The responses of all other relevant medical schools to the new curriculum in one school, cannot easily be predicted or planned for in advance. This adds another dimension of uncertainty. It is much easier to continue to live with the old curriculum rather than risk a painful journey to the new.

Change for future benefit needs to be promoted and led very carefully. By its very nature, it will involve visionaries who have the ability to foresee a new order of things and a strong motivation to take their organizations with them. Such acts of faith are inherently dangerous to organizations. Visionaries can be wrong and can often be narrowly focused, they can also see the shape of the future in ways that most other people can not. The actions of the change leaders shape the change process and influence the ultimate success criteria by which the impact of the change will be judged.

On the other hand, it is difficult to generate the momentum needed for changes with future benefits from an artificially assembled group who, perhaps, lack the personal drive to see changes through and cannot formulate a clear vision at which to aim. Charismatic leadership has a central role in the type of change that is future orientated.

The development of a community-based track at the University of New Mexico has been well documented (Mennin and Kaufman 1989; see Chapter 2.2). It is an interesting change because it lies somewhere between the two boundary cases that we have described. One of the driving forces for the change was the inability to attract doctors to work in the rural community served by the hospital and medical school. The solution was to produce more doctors locally and a community bias to the education process was a helpful design consideration.

The group leading the change process were driven by their own educational experiences which had been less than satisfactory. The group wished to change the way graduates were produced in order to prevent anyone suffering their fate in the future. The use of student-centred methods and problem-based learning arose from that motivation. The change was still radical and threatening to the majority of the faculty and was operated as a parallel stream with self-selected entry. The production costs of a graduate were higher and were sustained by a generous grant from a charitable foundation. The change helped to overcome the original problem and to satisfy its promoters, but failed to spread throughout the medical school.

Orders of change

Some change is small and incremental. Such change affects a few people or a few processes in the organization and is hardly noticed elsewhere. An example might be a small change to the content of a course or the introduction of a new teaching style in part of a course. Gradually such changes add up to a significant shift of position, organizational attitude, or behaviour. Such first order change is the normal way of life in families and in organizations. We may grumble on occasions, but we generally learn to live with new things; the walkman, camcorders, satellite communication, performance related pay, flexible hours, part-time students, etc. Each change is small enough not to disturb the normal equilibrium much.

Second order changes are more profound and affect more people and processes. The complexity arises from the way that parts of an organization are coupled together. It is difficult to change one part without having a profound effect on other parts. Curriculum change (see Chapter 2.1) and alterations to preregistration training are typical examples of this effect. The parts of a curriculum link together in a coherent way. What is learned at one stage will be used as a basis for a further stage. It is usually difficult to do other than maintain a curriculum and make modest, first order changes, until a complete revision emerges as the favoured course of action.

A complete curriculum revision is a major change. There will usually be several disparate groups or individuals who are stakeholders and whose views need to be addressed. Each stakeholder is also a holder of power or influence over the final outcome and can act positively or negatively. Medical graduates are not produced in isolation; there is a market for them. The market has a stake and will have expectations of the graduates, their skill and knowledge. This acts as a constraint on radical innovation for fear of disadvantaging the students in a competitive job market.

There has been relatively little major innovation, or second order change in existing medical schools in developed countries. There have been a number of changes, introduced as separate tracks or streams, which have allowed innovatory methods and traditional methods to coexist in an experimental framework (Moore *et al.* 1990). Those innovations that have succeeded often need a major effort to sustain and maintain them; their success relying on the continued efforts of supporters and promoters. This makes their success difficult to analyse and difficult to replicate, because the local context and local leadership issues are so important to the process of change.

Second order change can often have profound implications outside the host organization. We have discussed the need to produce graduates who can succeed in competitive job markets, but there are other implications. The current desire for a more community-based approach to medical education is hampered by supply side difficulties, particularly in inner London. There are too few suitable practices with the optimal mix of staff and facilities to accommodate the desired growth. It is not possible to create available resources in the short term.

Gradualism, or a series of small second order changes and first order changes, is the mode of change management most likely to succeed. This approach has the merit of allowing the organization to learn to change, to learn from its own success in tackling a small change. Tackling change more gradually diminishes the centrality of visionary leadership and increases the emphasis on managed processes. The vision needs to be part of the process and needs to be the guiding light in which more pragmatic management processes are able to move the organization towards its visionary goal. The same pragmatic approach helps to manage the changes needed to overcome a short-term difficulty in an organization. We describe a practical approach to managing change in medical education in the next section.

A model of change in medical education

The model we describe below was derived from the practice of medical education through properly designed experimental methods and has been returned to medical education in the form of several demonstration projects which have served to refine the model (Gale and Grant 1990 a, b, c; Nicholls *et al.* 1992). It is thus distinctive in its anchorage.

Most authors on change management rely on the distillation of their own experiences to derive theories or frameworks. This is a perfectly valid approach which may, however, produce theories that lack broad applicability. It is important to understand the experience base that is being systematized to be able to judge the applicability of the model. Much of the literature has a distinctly private sector feel to it, where profit imperatives drive the change processes. The public sector, and medical education in particular, merits its own theories of change management because the power and influence structures are not like those of the private sector.

Our primary research was conducted in 1989 at a time of rapid change in Government policy. We dealt with a broad section of medical educators, from general practitioners and medical school teachers to consultants, postgraduate deans, statutory and regulatory bodies, and government representatives. We interviewed a total sample of fifty five. Their thoughts and views were content analysed to reveal fifty four categories, which were further refined to produce the model outlined below.

There were three strands to the model: professional characteristics or culture, strategic stages, or core steps, and tactical choices or styles.

The professional characteristics are:

◆ Consultation
◆ Demonstration
◆ Evolution
◆ Ownership
◆ Power to hinder
◆ Commitment
◆ Energy and enthusiasm
◆ Motives.

These represent some of the cultural values of medicine. All doctors like and expect to be consulted and this usually means personally and not by post. The scientific basis of medicine places high value upon demonstration projects and requires an evolutionary approach of small changes. The issue of ownership is critical in that people need to feel that they are in charge of the change process and that it is providing answers to their questions and needs. The nature of consultant power is still a relevant consideration despite inroads made into it by general managers. Consultants have the power of veto by simply not participating and this means that due care needs to be exercised to avoid invoking this power.

The last three professional characteristics relate to the change leader or leaders. They are expected to show commitment to the project and not merely to pursue it as a hobby. They are required to exhibit energy and enthusiasm and not to display half-heartedness. They are required to have honest motives in putting themselves forward as change leaders. Any suspicion of a personal gain or personal advantage accruing from the change will cause the power to hinder, or worse, the power of indifference, to be invoked.

This set of professional characteristics helps to limit the speed of any change initiative and the scope of any intended change, mainly because of the need for extensive and repeated direct consultation.

The core activities and tactical choices are:

Core activity	Tactical choices
Establish the need or benefit	Do not sell solutions; lobbying; consultation; conjunction of local or national circumstances
Power to act	Ownership; key people; using committees; borrowed power; positional power; political or external power; expertise, charisma; information; resource control; indebtedness; prior agreement to act
Design the innovation	Feasibility; resources needed; starting time and duration; scale and degree; avoid losers; predict barriers and pathways
Consult	Leadership; teamwork; talking and explaining; listening
Publicize	Vision; presentation; amending proposals; communication
Agree detailed plans	Produce plans
Implement	Demonstration projects; have an implementation strategy; avoid scheming and bypassing; key people; opportunism; pathways and barriers are activated
Provide support	Overcome difficulties; encourage new behaviour; expect resistance; deal with objections
Modify plans	Accommodate small alterations; compensate losers
Evaluate outcomes	Needs met; benefits realized, modifications needed, evaluation strategy

Establish the need or benefit

Managing change to meet perceived needs is probably more common than changing to reap benefits, but it is necessary to represent opportunity as an equally powerful starting point to need.

In terms of the tactical choices open to the change leader, the major lesson derived from our research and demonstration projects has been the realization that many change initiatives fail because the change leader is attempting to impose ready worked out solutions. This contradicts the fundamental principle of achieving a wide ownership for the change initiative. The change leader has to chart a narrow course between explaining the change idea and prescribing it precisely. For people to join in with a change idea, they have to feel that they can influence it and become part of it. On the other hand, they need to have a reasonable description of what is proposed before they can decide to become supporters.

We experienced a graphic example of trying to sell solutions among a group of keen and active medical students at the Free University of Berlin. They had been enthused with the idea of problem-based learning and had organized their faculty to help them. They worked hard, fostered other groups to start, and eventually convinced the Vice Chancellor of the merits of the idea. They worked out a scheme and presented it to the authorities who controlled the examination process and the awarding of degrees. This body rejected the solution and even failed to recognize an opportunity or need.

In considering how the problem could have been better tackled, it became apparent that effort should have been put into winning the support of the regulators and securing their agreement to run a pilot project, rather than in preparing a well worked out solution without their knowledge or involvement.

Our model is about the process of change and we think it is possible to decouple the change itself and the process of managing it. This of course is not completely tenable since the type of change attempted will have a bearing on the change strategy adopted. The alternative is to analyse all the factors that do, and could, influence the environment of medical education and all the factors that motivate or define potential change leaders. A recent WHO publication (WHO 1991) attempted to identify different strategies for initiating change locally, but even this document assumed the desire for change already existed somewhere in the system.

Power

Use of the change model has reinforced our thinking on power issues. It is worth repeating that the change leader needs to assemble sufficient power or influence at the outset to see the changes through to their conclusion. In the sense that change alters the balance of powers in an organization, it is thus a political process. In our formulation of the change model, we identified a large number of power sources. Our development work has revealed even more ways in which the change leader can influence colleagues, committees, and others with a stake in the change. There should be no difficulty in finding the required amount of power to see through the desired changes.

The example of the Berlin students is a good negative one. They failed to appreciate that the regulatory body had the power to approve or block any proposed initiative. The regulatory body therefore needed to be involved at the outset.

Borrowed power has emerged as the favourite power to ensure sufficient weight behind change initiatives in postgraduate medical education. The power of the post-graduate dean was borrowed. The dean has become very much more powerful as a result of the recent reforms of postgraduate medical and dental education and can be 'borrowed' for even more complex change projects.

We have detected a wide range of personal influencing styles that have been used to encourage fellow consultants to participate in the induction and counselling initiatives that we have managed. The following personal influencing styles were used:

- Expertise
- Position and authority
- Information

- Charisma
- Resource control
- Indebtedness.

The power of expertise in one's own field often carries over into all other fields of endeavour that are entered. An expert is given greater credibility in all matters, even outside the range of expertise.

The power of position depends upon the importance or influence of the role. The role of clinical tutor has grown considerably in recent times, along with increasing recognition of the need to develop a series of curricula for doctors in training. The reforms of postgraduate education have caused a better definition of the job of clinical tutor and increased contact with unit management and financial functions. There is often a specific contract covering the duties and responsibilities of the role and, above all else, the role has much higher visibility within the hospital. These factors all combine to increase the positional power and authority of the clinical tutor.

Information power is that most often deployed in negotiations, it is the power of knowing something someone else does not know, or having better access to those that do. This power can be deployed to influence colleagues.

Charismatic power is somewhat more difficult to define, it is the ability to influence people because of the way you are, because of your personal qualities or personal characteristics. This power is either obvious or inaccessible. It is difficult to train someone to be charismatic and it is a power that works to differing degrees with different colleagues.

The power to control resources or access to resources is another potent source of influence. It is the material analogue of information power. It can be used destructively to block initiatives or constructively to encourage new developments.

The last widely used influencing device was indebtedness. This is the principle whereby an act of consideration to a colleague initiates a future reciprocal favour. Vast positive spirals of cooperation and helpfulness can be built on such a simple device. Equally, vast negative spirals result if it breaks down.

In medical education, it is necessary to recognize the dispersed nature of power. Every teacher in every classroom, every consultant on every wardround is virtually sovereign. The contribution of individuals to any collective endeavour must be by informed willingness and not by any threatened coercion. Individuals can undermine the change initiative if they so choose. This means that change must only proceed with wide support or interested neutrality. A powerful method to undermine is to agree to the changes in public and yet act counter to them in private.

All our considerations are of elected change, where the stakeholders exercise some freedom to participate. If sufficient power is available, coercive or dictatorial change is possible. A short term gain by coercive means may often lead to a long-term revolt among those affected. Resistance is the last bastion of the disenfranchised.

Design the innovation

At the design stage, it is necessary to sacrifice the purity of an idea in order to make progress. Wide consultation, keeping an open mind and involving all the key players in the process, lead to a dilution and broadening of the original concept in order to foster wide ownership. Wide consultation often improves an original idea, too.

In some circumstances, particularly when the change is moderately small and concerns a small number of people, the design task may be left to a small and trusted group. This is not the ideal recipe, however, for major curriculum reform. Task groups may prove helpful but they need to be controlled by a more representative body.

Doctors are very busy people and do not always have the spare capacity to invest in active participation in change. The concept of seeking general agreement of all involved and then licensing a small group to execute the design, may actually have wide validity. This is especially the case when moderately small changes are being attempted. The important issue is then one of communication between the design team and the wider group of stakeholders. This is discussed below.

Refine

The refinement stage can vary in length and complexity depending on the number of people or processes involved. The major need is to draw in as wide a body of opinion as possible and to communicate the emerging design to those who hold a stake in the outcome. The real danger in the design process relates back to the original section on establishing the need for change. It is generally fatal to a change initiative to design the solution behind closed doors only to spring it upon an unsuspecting world when they least expect it. There is a strong tendency to do this if the change idea is contentious or controversial. There is a feeling that all may be lost if news of the change gets out before the group has worked out what to do. It may be harder to work in the open, but the final product is better.

The refinement process is a way of further spreading ownership of a change idea and of canvassing the opinions and views of others in order to improve the quality of the solution. It is also a stage of communicating, of letting people know what is going on. Communication with a committee or with a person in authority who may have requested work on the change is essential. Failure to do so can lead to a loss of momentum in the project and it can lead to the change idea being forgotten. Failure to communicate with committees that may be involved could lead to withdrawal of their support and goodwill or its transfer elsewhere.

Communication can take many forms from the direct verbal transfer of information to the brief note, the committee paper, or an interim report. The form of communication must be adjusted to the local context and local expectations.

Publicize

Publicity is a way of communicating with a wider audience beyond the immediate stakeholders and of keeping everyone informed of the whole picture as it develops. The leaders of smaller projects that form part of a larger initiative are not always in possession of the overall picture of where the project is going, or who else is working on it. Such fragmentation can be efficient but can lead to isolated and self-contained units who do not appreciate the need for wider publicity. In this situation, it is vital for the overall change leader to take on the role of coordinator and publicist.

Another important aspect of publicity is to portray major changes as relatively minor affairs. Most people will readily accept first order changes but become worried by more major upheavals with less certain outcomes. This poses a particular challenge in curriculum reforms.

Detailed planning

Experience has not greatly altered our views on the need for detailed planning prior to implementation. Too many changes go wrong because of an impatience to see something actually in place before it has been properly designed and publicized. Others fail because of a 'travelling hopefully' philosophy that denies the need for anticipation and detailed planning of who does what, where, when, and to whom. Much of what has been attempted to reduce junior doctors hours has suffered from an urgency to implement before proper planning had taken place.

Implement

Implementation strategy depends on circumstances. Our demonstration projects have revealed a rapid implementation mode for change that has been undertaken with a mandate from a committee or other powerful body and is in a relatively accepted area of developmental need. In these circumstances the solution is so highly valued by all that they will tolerate a slightly less refined product. The change must be sufficiently developed to be taken seriously and can then be refined by the process of evaluation and modification.

The scientific basis of medicine leads to a high premium being placed on the demonstration project. If it is possible to operate such a demonstration, this is a powerful route to implementation. Running the demonstration project allows everyone to gain valuable experience and to improve upon the original design. This may indicate a staged approach to curriculum reform.

Provide support

The essence of this stage of the change process is to ensure that the new ways of behaviour become enshrined as the normal ways of behaviour, as quickly as possible. In this regard, providing support has aspects of continuing to smooth the pathway of change by removing obstacles that have arisen and it has aspects of communication and feedback to the key players on the progress of the reforms or changes.

In our demonstration projects, we introduced an evaluation step soon after a major implementation. This was designed to detect any actual or perceptual problems and to provide positive feedback to those who had been involved. We included the providers and recipients, consultants, PRHOs, and SHOs in the feedback, because creating a positive climate for the new ways of working was a high priority and the junior medical staff were important in this process.

The evaluation method included questionnaire data and data derived from semi-structured interviews. We also took note of, and encouraged, spontaneous feedback from anyone involved in the change or closely associated with it. It is important to have all information channels open for communication at this critical time. Failure at implementation is one of the most common failure modes for change initiatives. Even gossip can provide little insights that can help the change leader to apply scarce resources in the right place in order to reinforce the changes. The change is still a fragile object until it become established because it can easily be reversed.

As a result of our experiences, we have modified our original model (Gale and Grant 1990 *b,c*) to include 'provide support' in a loop with 'modify plans and evaluate'. Our thinking is that, if modifications are needed, then a suitable point at which to re-enter the process of change is at the level of 'provide support'. This argument assumes that the modifications are not so vast as to constitute a complete overhaul or a brand new design. Given their minor nature, it is not necessary to go back to the start of the process, because all existing agreements still hold. It is even possible to miss out on formulating new detailed plans and implementing anew.

In the process of providing support, it is possible to include minor alterations to the changes. This can be accomplished through more formal means, such as written documents or on the basis of personal communication and discussion. The latter method is to be preferred as the initial contact whenever possible. This mode of operation is possible in systems that have a reasonable repeat frequency so that previous experience is still fresh when the task or process is next repeated.

Modify plans

Our development work has revealed a fast-track method for implementing relatively small changes in relation to periodic events, such as induction processes or counselling schemes or repeated course modules. The method rests on the suitable frequency of the event which means that it is possible to adopt a rolling design philosophy. Rather than spending a long time in designing and refining the innovation, it is possible to set the broad outlines, produce the first detailed plan and try it out in practice, as a continuing series of demonstration projects. This constitutes an action research approach to development. The lessons from this experimental development approach can then be absorbed and built into the next event, using the concept of modifying plans each time.

Given that the starting plan is moderately robust, the developmental strategy can give rise to a philosophy of changing, continuous change, and development, rather than discrete and final changes. The first implementation is very important. It must be good enough to generate more successful features than features needing modification. This method is not a charter for badly worked out change, but a method to accelerate development upon a firm foundation.

If the initial plan is way off the mark, the developmental strategy harbours the danger of the whole initiative becoming discredited. It is also not recommended for changes to more continuous or frequently repeated processes, where there is no breathing space between events, nor for those repeated too infrequently. It may be possible to attempt curriculum reforms through tackling small areas at a time. The repeat frequency of the average course allows this approach.

Evaluate

We have already discussed the part played by evaluation in the progress from implementation onwards. We need to differentiate this type of evaluation, which is aimed at specific knowledge needs, from the more open and enquiring evaluation which needs to take place near the end of the change initiative.

The final evaluation seeks not just to know how well the parts are working, but whether they are helping to solve the original problem or acting to fulfil the potential of the original opportunity. It is all too easy, in the thick of the battle for change, to lose sight of why you started in the first place. The final evaluation should anchor you firmly back to your original intentions.

Interim evaluation is also important. A change leader needs a constant supply of information on how well each stage is progressing. The perceptive change leader tunes in to a variety of information sources and uses a variety of evaluation methods to gather information and make minor adjustments on the basis of what is discovered. Change management is much more a process of action learning than a static scientific experiment that has to run its course before we can know its result. Change management involves constant adjustments and shifts of direction based on the frequent evaluation of parts, or stages of the process.

References

Gale, R. and Grant, J.R. (1990*a*). Leading educational change. *Journal of Course Organisers*, **Spring**, 63–71.

Gale, R. and Grant, J.R. (1990*b*). *Guidelines for change in postgraduate and continuing medical education*. The Joint Centre, London.

Gale, R. and Grant, J.R. (1990*c*). *Managing change in a medical context: guidelines for action*. The Joint Centre, London.

Gale, R., Jackson, G., Nicholls, M. (1992). How to run an induction meeting for house officers. *British Medical Journal*, **304**, 1619–20.

Mennin, S. and Kaufman, A. (1989). The change process and medical education. *Medical Teacher*, **11**, 9–16.

Moore, G., Block, S. and Mitchell, R. (1990). *A randomised controlled trial evaluating the impact of the new pathway curriculum at Harvard Medical School*. Office of Sponsored Research, Harvard Medical School.

O'Connor, C. (1993). *The handbook for organisational change*. McGraw Hill, Maidenhead.

Pettigrew, A. (1985). Contextualist research a natural way to link theory and practice. In *Doing research that is useful in theory and practice* (ed. E. Lawler), pp.00–00. Jossey Bass, San Francisco.

Pettigrew, A.M., Ferlie, E., McKee, L. (1988). Understanding change in the NHS. *Public Administration*, **66**, 297–317.

Pettigrew, A.M., McKee L., Ferlie, E. (1992). *Shaping strategic change*. Sage, London.

Plant, R. (1987). *Managing change and making it stick*. Fontana/Collins, London.

Spurgeon, P. and Barwell, F. (1991). *Implementing change in the NHS. A practical guide for general managers*. Chapman and Hall, London.

Turrill, E.A. (1986). *Change and innovation a challenge for the NHS*. The Institute of Health Services Management, London.

WHO (1991). *Changing medical education: an agenda for action*. World Health Organisation, Geneva.

8.2 Overcoming the barriers to implementing change in medical education

Angela Towle

Barriers to change in medical education

Calls for reform of medical education are occurring in many countries throughout the world, and with increasing frequency (see Chapter 1). Within the USA alone, there have been at least twenty four major reports this century advocating reform, seven since the seminal *General Professional Education of the Physician* (GPEP) report of 1984. The rate of publication has increased to almost one per year. Typically, these reports identify similar problems with medical education, claim that previous reports have gone unheeded, argue that reform is essential and urgent, and prescribe corrections that are strikingly similar (Christakis 1995).

Despite the repeated calls for reform, and the support for change from medical educators (Cantor 1991), large-scale, coherent, and sustainable change has been consistently difficult to achieve in any country. Bloom (1988) has characterized past attempts to modify medical education as a 'history of reform without change, of repeated modifications of the medical school curriculum that alter only very slightly or not at all the experience of the critical participants, the students and teachers'. His explanation is that the scientific mission of academic medicine has crowded out its social responsibility to train for society's most basic health care delivery needs. Research is the major concern of the institution's social structure; education is secondary and essentially unchanging.

Other barriers to change have also been reported. In their latest set of recommendations on the undergraduate curriculum, the UK General Medical Council (General Medical Council 1993) examine reasons for 'the persistent gap between the good intentions of successive Councils and the implementation of their recommendations'. They relate the present problems to the historical development of medical education and attempts to accommodate within the curriculum a rapidly expanding and diverse knowledge base taught by quasi-autonomous departments. The Association of American Medical Colleges (1992) in trying to ascertain why most medical schools have done little to correct the major shortcomings in the ways they educate their students over the last sixty years, identified five specific barriers to change. These were:

- Faculty members' inertia;
- Lack of leadership;
- Lack of oversight for the educational programme;

- Limited resources and no defined budget for medical education;
- The perception that there is no evidence that implementing changes will make the necessary improvements.

A more detailed study of six selected US medical schools to identify factors that facilitate or obstruct innovation in medical education was carried out by Cohen *et al.* (1994). They found the most important barriers (out of a total of eight items) to be teacher resistance and promotion policies. One school mentioned interdepartmental competition and another cited lack of financial support for teaching, lack of leadership, and lack of dean's support. The most important facilitators of change (out of a total of twelve items) were: i) support of the dean; ii) department chair's support; and iii) students' concerns. At all the schools, similar conditions appeared to obstruct or discourage change. These included: minimal rewards for teaching; limited resources for education; a departmental structure which contributed to territorial management of the curriculum; and general resistance by teachers to change. Teacher resistance was uniformly linked to a perceived lack of rewards for teaching and a sense of the importance of research for promotion and tenure.

Their findings suggest the importance of translating culture into structures (for example organizational roles, decision-making groups, curriculum, etc.) that support and reflect the new goals. Critical to the institutionalization of a new culture was the centralization of curriculum governance. A combination of four interrelated factors are essential to a foundation for broad-based educational change: resources; leadership committed to change; a coherent set of educational objectives; effective decision-making structures.

Mennin and Kaufman (1989) identify a list of institutional barriers to change generic to medical schools all over the world. They include:

- Fear of loss of control by traditional educators;
- Failure of innovators to align their proposals with the values and goals of the institution;
- Predominance of the *status quo* (faculty members who were once students in the same system have been conditioned to believe in and support that system);
- Departmental allegiances;
- Unrealistic expectations that change can occur quickly;
- Faculty promotion based on research and service;
- Innovators not being influential leaders of opinion.

They identify institutional characteristics that favour change including: a criticism of courses; changing staff due to turnover and/or expansion; junior staff members influential in educational policy making; rotating departmental chairpersons; institutions that are financially dependent on attracting students and their tuition; student unrest; a history of change and responsiveness to the needs of the local community. They conclude that the institution likely to innovate is one that is flexible and/or one in which the environment is in crisis.

Factors which facilitate and obstruct change in UK medical schools

In 1995 a questionnaire was sent to each of the curriculum facilitators funded by the Department of Health through the Undergraduate Medical Curriculum Implementation

Support Scheme (UMCISS). Under the scheme about UK £50,000 per year was made available between 1994 and 1997 to each medical school to fund one or more people to help implement the GMC's recommendations as set out in *Tomorrow's doctors* (General Medical Council 1993). Most facilitators had been in post for about 18 months at the time of the survey. Since the facilitators are at the centre of curriculum change, information about their activities and perceptions provides a convenient overview of the state of educational developments in each school. Replies were received from 25 of the 26 schools in the scheme, and from 32 of the 34 facilitators.

Information was sought about the kinds of tasks the facilitators were doing; their main achievements; the tasks they had been unable to do; and their perception of factors which facilitated or hindered change. The questionnaire presented lists of some of the factors known to either act as barriers or to facilitate change in medical education as reported in the North American literature and summarized above. Respondents were asked to add any other factors which they had encountered in their institution, and then to select the five which they had found to be the most significant and list in rank order. Responses were received from thirty facilitators. The results are shown in Tables 8.1 and 8.2.

Table 8.1 Barriers to change

	Rank score[1]	Number reporting[2]
Low status/priority of teaching	75	21
Faculty inertia/complacency	39	11
No resources or defined budget	35	11
No evidence for changes	30	11
Senior staff fear loss of control	28	9
Departmental allegiances	27	12
Lack of staff development	25	10
Lack of oversight for educational programme	23	5
Poor communication	22	8
Effects of NHS pressures	22	7

[1]Rank score (max 5/report; total 150)
[2]Number reporting factor in top 5 (max=30)

Additional barriers identified by more than one facilitator included: lack of leadership; lack of protected time for innovators; innovators not influential leaders of opinion; and differences in attitudes of clinicians and basic scientists. Only one factor in the top ten ranking was not on the original list of thirteen provided. This was, 'Effects of NHS pressures' a rather specific concern to medical schools in the UK at present because of the enormous amount of concurrent reorganization in the health service. Two barriers from the original list of thirteen provided were not recognized as being important (only ranked as fifth choice by one respondent each). These were: quick results are an unrealistic expectation and innovators fail to align proposals with values and goals of staff and institution (both cited as barriers by Mennin and Kaufman 1989).

Clearly, by far the most significant perceived barrier to change is the low status and priority of teaching, ranked almost twice as important as the second barrier, faculty members' inertia or complacency about the need for change. The problem of lack of recognition of the need for change among faculty members has its counterpart in the fourth ranked factor: the perception that there is no evidence that the planned changes will lead to improvements. A different, practical rather than attitudinal, issue is the lack of resources or a defined budget for medical students' education, ranked third.

Table 8.2 Factors which facilitate change

	Rank score[1]	Number reporting[2]
Support of the dean	87	21
Commitment of key individuals	59	16
Project money for education (incl. UMCISS)	48	15
Students concerns	32	11
Changes in medical practice	24	9
External pressure (e.g. GMC, HEFCE)	24	7
Other schools' experiences	18	10
Like-minded innovators in key positions	15	4
Expertise of facilitator	13	3
Motivated teachers at grassroots	11	5

[1]Rank score (max 5/report; total 150)
[2]Number reporting factor in top 5 (max=30)

Additional factors identified by more than one facilitator included: support provided by the medical education unit; getting ownership; and an effective education committee.

Clearly the most significant facilitating factor is perceived to be the support of the dean, followed by the commitment to change of key individuals, such as the education/curriculum (sub)dean, heads of departments, senior staff, committee chairs. Project money for the educational change, especially UMCISS money was ranked third. Factors ranked 4–7 are all sources of 'external' pressure for change: dissatisfied students; changes in medical practice (such as the move from in-patient to out-patient care) requiring changes to traditional clinical teaching; pressure from external accrediting or funding bodies such as the GMC and Higher Education Funding Council; awareness of change in other medical schools, a source of both pressure and encouragement.

Understanding the barriers to change

In order to explain better the barriers to curriculum change which have been repeatedly cited, possible strategies for change are discussed within the context of three different arenas in which change occurs: organizations and the change process; change in universities and medical schools; change and the individual.

Organizations and the change process

The logical approach to change is to:

1. Devise an overall strategy
2. Turn the strategy into a plan
3. Seek sanction from those in authority
4. Implement the plan.

Experience shows that such a rationalistic model does not work because of the speed of change, the world is more complex, and there is little emphasis on the human side—politics and motivation—which block change. In their research on innovations and innovation processes in higher education based on seven case studies, Berg and Ostergren (1979) note that the innovation process is either consistent with or divergent from the main characteristics of the system. In the former case the innovation process is one of dissemination, in the latter of a political battle.

Major change which challenges the system is a political process and political processes are not wholly rational. As a political process, the introduction of change involves considerations of key players, opinion leaders, stakeholders, external forces, and equilibria. All of these have been brought together in a model developed by Lewin (1951) which Berg and Ostergren found an appropriate framework for their analysis of curricular developments in higher education. Lewin identified three stages in the change process:

- Unfreezing (change is initiated when a stable situation is 'unfrozen' so as to make it ready to move).
- Moving (change is produced as forces re-align themselves around a new centre of equilibrium).
- Refreezing (change is made permanent and becomes the new orthodoxy until it is challenged again).

Stable systems are maintained by an equal distribution of forces on each side of a quasi-stationary equilibrium. Change is initiated when the equilibrium is disturbed by driving forces gaining dominance over opposing forces, which naturally first react to the change by resisting it. Innovation becomes a political process in the sense that there are opposing forces fighting for dominance around the equilibrium.

Based on their analysis of Lewin's model, Berg and Ostergren argued that most aspects of innovation in higher education may be accounted for by the four concepts of power, leadership, ownership, and gain/loss (needs and interests). They identify two broad types of need: physical need for survival and security (including status and recognition of competence) and ideological need. From the standpoint of the system, the ideology of the system must be maintained; from an individual standpoint the most valuable gain is one of having created something that gives satisfaction. It is these two broad types of need and the gains and losses associated with them that most noticeably place systems and individuals into the category of driving or restraining forces.

One reason why Lewin's approach is difficult to apply in practice is that it requires us to study a social system as a whole, since the forces in it are strongly coupled to each other, so that changes applied to one force will result in changes to all the forces. If Lewin is right then simplistic models which are based on changes in one force in a system are unlikely to produce a permanent change in the system, or at least not the desired change. What are needed are strategies for change acting across a wide front.

Strategies for change

Chin and Benne (1976) identified three kinds of strategies:

- Empirical/rational—persuades through reasoned argument and reference to fact and research findings.

+ Normative/re-educative—achieves change through education—often informal or due to group pressure which leads to acceptance of changed norms. Two approaches are problem solving and personal growth.
+ Power/coercive—use of political and economic sanctions and rewards.

It is inherent in the idea of stability that stable systems at first react to change by resisting it. The unfreezing stage therefore requires an external pressure which overcomes this resistance. Pressure can be applied, usually overtly, from outside the institution (e.g. by accrediting or funding authorities). Or it can be done, usually covertly, from within the institution at a higher level of the hierarchy. Best of all, it could arise from peer pressure. All of these are power strategies which have the potential to change the environment of a department or institution to a position where it is open to change. At this point, the second 'moving' stage can begin and it is here that those in academic teacher training play a major role, usually through a mixture of rational and normative strategies. The final 'refreezing' stage is also likely to require a power strategy, but while the balance between sanctions and rewards is more usually tilted towards sanctions in the unfreezing stage, it should be biased more towards rewards in the refreezing stage. Sanctions and rewards are needed in both the first and third stages.

In each of the three stages there is what Lewin calls a force field of driving and opposing forces, and change requires that the driving forces exceed the opposing forces. Forces may include forces of argument and social pressures corresponding to rational or normative strategies, as well as the more obvious power forces. There is evidence to show that change proceeds more smoothly and easily if the imbalance between the two sets of forces is achieved by lowering the opposing forces rather than by increasing the driving forces, since an increase in the driving forces typically results in a corresponding increase in the opposing forces. Berg and Ostergren (1979) found that managerial forces, whether due to vice chancellors or government, were more effective when they reduced opposition than when they increased support. Unfortunately, those who desire change are more likely to be able to influence the driving forces directly; attempting to lower the opposing forces may be more effective but more difficult (since in general the change agents have little control over these forces).

Elton (1987) highlights that changes in curricula generally require academics to learn new educational knowledge, skills, and attitudes and these often conflict with those held previously. Under the circumstances, planned change initially involves a process of unlearning, which is an aspect of Lewin's unfreezing, without which new learning cannot take place. Such unlearning is almost invariably a threat to the personality, individual or collective, and as such will be resisted. In direct contradiction of Lewin's principle to reduce the degree of conflict, what usually happens is the unfortunate subject is made to feel uncomfortable or even guilty about their traditional attitudes, while no attempt is made to make them feel safe to give up the old and learn the new. The result is a massive defensiveness and resistance to change (Dwyer 1977).

A crucial part of the unfreezing process concerns attitudes. Elton quotes an example in which a programme designed to change attitudes failed or even provoked serious adverse reactions because only the threatening part of the unfreezing process was fulfilled before moving on to the changing process. What was missing was the reassuring part of the unfreezing process which Lewin considers so essential and which should come from the security of the group of which the individual is a member.

In the initial unfreezing stage, staff development can act as a supporting force, while preservice training could result in teachers entering the system already predisposed towards change so that they themselves provide the supporting force. During the change stage some form of staff development is almost certainly required if the change is to result in something worthwhile. If it does not happen change may still occur but lead to seriously defective programmes.

Change in universities and medical schools

The literature on change suggests that innovation is more likely to occur in some types of organizations than in others. Elton (1981) postulates that as institutions universities are essentially traditionalist to an extent that makes them inherently almost incapable of internally generated change. The basic reason for this lies in what academics actually do. As teachers they perform the important but traditional task of preserving what is best in the received knowledge and wisdom of the past and transmitting it to the next generation. Even as researchers, most concentrate on solving routine problems in which a dominant theory is applied, that is an activity which preserves and strengthens the past rather than changes the future.

Moreover, the basic departmental structure of traditional universities is likely to inhibit change. Departmental autonomy gives every university a 'federal' structure rather than a strongly centralized system; the head of department remains a key figure in their own department and largely as a result a key figure throughout the university government. If change is to succeed in a university or a faculty as a whole it is necessary to convince the heads of departments and their senior colleagues of its value.

Hefferlin (1969) identifies several other barriers to innovation in universities. Within higher education, institutional reputation is not based on innovation which is therefore considered a rather unprofitable endeavour. Faculty members have observed their vocation for years as students before joining it, therefore socialization runs deep within the university and innovation that runs against the grain is more likely to be thought of as deviant. Academic institutions are deliberately structured to resist precipitant change and procedures for approving change are elaborate and slow.

Bloom (1989) has analysed the medical school as a social organization and identified some of the features which account for the fact that innovation is so taxing that innovators prefer to set up new schools. He argues that research and education, despite the sincere manifest intention to be partners have become rivals and even, at times, enemies. He believes the crisis of medical education today arises from the clash between ideology and social structure. Thus the medical school is forced to maintain itself indirectly on resources that are allocated to support the goals of either research or patient care; educational values become subordinate to the requisites of the organizational structure of the medical school. The protection of territorial domains supersedes the achievement of educational goals as the driving force of the institution. Certain new schools have been able to synchronize organizational structure more closely with educational values but the challenge for more traditional schools embarking on curriculum reform is to address the structural problems of what is in effect a modern corporate bureaucracy.

Strategies for change

Bloom (1992) highlights that it is essential when conceiving strategies for innovation to understand the resistance to change in the medical school in terms of function as well as motivation. The widespread consensus for educational change cannot succeed if it replaces or undermines the parallel importance of research and service in the medical centre. Educational change involves the same organizational structures which frame research and service. Therefore when departmental autonomy is targeted for educational reform, the effect on research as a vital parallel function must be assessed. Such assessment reveals conflicting interests. Departmental autonomy has not been a barrier to the research development of scientific knowledge. At the same time, division of effort becomes a barrier to an educational effort like the organ-systems curriculum which is specifically intended to integrate rather than focus learning in reductionist scientific thinking. The drive toward centralizing authority for education in some structure within the medical school that supersedes the autonomous control of individual departments adds a new player in the competition for a scarce pool of resources. If educational authority is to compete it will need to contribute new resources to the pool. Each medical school must plan its own programme. However, it will not succeed unless it addresses the structural problems of organization, the sources of authority and allocation of resources, and the power centres of decision making.

From their study of innovation processes in four US medical schools, Bussigel *et al.* (1988) concluded that no one factor alone is responsible or even most important for innovation outcome: much more important is how organizational factors relate to each other. Thus, which set of change strategies to adopt will be dictated by the specific institutional situation. For example, departmental autonomy combined with broad participation may achieve results similar to a structure with weak departments and limited participation in educational planning.

On the basis of their study, it is advisable that the leader of the change incorporates into the planning process an awareness of the relationship between existing organizational structures and the needs of the innovation. It is reasonable to assume that an attempt to introduce change will conflict with at least some of the established organizational structures.

There is usually more than one way to address incompatibilities between the innovation and existing organizational structures. A radical method is to do away with structures or replace them with ones more compatible with the innovation, but this method may be impossible or inefficient. A more moderate approach that influences the nature of the problematic organizational structures or introduces a balance to them may be more successful. Bussigel *et al.* (1988) conclude that because of context dependency it is impossible to offer concrete advice on what organizational alterations must occur in order to facilitate change at a medical school since both the nature of the innovation and the idiosyncratic school context must be considered. What is important is that the planning strategy is broad, that it examines how dominant organizational structures relate to innovation requirements, and that planners have sufficient power to make necessary adjustments.

Evidence from the literature of the way conflicts are resolved within organizations indicates that medical schools exhibit unique characteristics with respect to conflict resolution. Whereas high performing industrial organizations prefer open and constructive confrontation, medical schools tend to prefer bargaining, a mode in which each interest group tends to maximize its own interests. Another commonly employed technique is unilateral decision making in which individual groups ignore the impact of their decisions on other groups for as long as possible (Bussigel *et al.* 1988). They conclude that informal patterns of educational decision making may be more significant for the innovation than formal decision making.

From a study of teamwork among physicians, Delbecq and Gill (1985) draw several conclusions about decision making and leadership. Medical organizations are made up of very independent professionals with high needs for power and control. However, physicians also believe strongly in due process and majority rule. They recognize that at some point individual expression of strong points must cease and a decision must be formulated. They look within the organization for leadership that ensures appropriate due process which is achieved through: clearly perceived representative structures; visible processing of decisions; and clear decision rules.

Change and the individual

Organizational change often runs into some form of human resistance (Kotter and Schlesinger 1979). The four most common reasons why people resist change are: a desire not to lose something of value; a misunderstanding of the change and its implications; a belief that the change does not make sense for the organization; and a low tolerance for change. All human beings are limited in their ability to change, with some more limited than others. Five categories of adopters of change have been recognized: innovators, early adopters, early majority, late majority, and laggards, each category having their own particular personal characteristics, salient values and social relationships, and communication behaviour (Stocking 1992). The communication behaviour of the different groups is important because it begins to show why information is a necessary but not sufficient condition for change: the adopters in the early and late majority categories are much more influenced by other people than they are by publications.

A particular example of individual resistance to change within the context of medical curriculum change is highlighted in a study by Dharamsi (1996) of medical educators involved in a major change from a traditional to a problem-based learning curriculum. One of the main sources of their resistance to, or ambivalence towards, the change arose from the requirement to change their fundamental views about teaching and learning. Having taught in a university setting for at least twenty years, they were concerned that the new curriculum would cause them to lose their identity, their roles as experts, as teachers of something (i.e. their discipline) and not just teachers. The basic scientists judged their credibility and effectiveness by being able to transmit their knowledge to students and answer questions knowledgeably, which meant they had to know their content matter as experts. The clinicians saw their teaching role as helping students to understand the connections between basic science and clinical practice. Both groups' experiences of change were interpreted as having given up their espoused roles and responsibilities to adopt a new one, which in most cases was seen as conflicting. Reconciliation was difficult because the legitimacy of change was not recognized and the teachers' identity was seen as being compromised.

Since most of the studies on change are from the perspective of the change agent, those who resist change are usually seen in negative terms. Klein (1976) believes that what is usually thought to be irrational resistance to change is, in most instances, more likely to be either an attempt to maintain the integrity of the target system to real threat, or opposition to the agents of change themselves. He discusses the importance of the defender role. The defender, whoever they may be and however unscrupulously or irrationally they may appear to present themselves and their concerns, usually has something of great value to communicate about the nature of the system which the change agent is seeking to influence. If the change agent can view the situation with a sympathetic understanding of what the defenders are seeking to protect, it may prove desirable either to modify the change itself or the strategy being used to achieve it. In certain situations the participation of defenders in the change process may even lead to the development of more adequate plans and to the avoidance of some hitherto unforeseen consequences of the projected change.

Strategies for change

Strategies for overcoming individual resistance include education and communication, participation and involvement, facilitation and support, negotiation and agreement, manipulation and co-optation, and explicit and implicit coercion. Coercive strategies allow rapid implementation, a clear plan of action and little involvement of others. In contrast, techniques involving participation and involvement require a much slower change process and a less clear-cut plan (Kotter and Schlesinger 1979). The chances of successful change can be improved by:

1. Conducting an organizational analysis that identifies the current situation, problems, and the forces that are the cause of those problems.
2. Conducting an analysis of factors relevant to producing the needed changes, including who might resist the change, why and how much, and whose co-operation is essential.
3. Selecting a change strategy, based on the previous analysis, which specifies the speed of change, amount of preplanning and degree of involvement of others; that selects specific tactics for use with various individuals and groups; and that is internally consistent.
4. Monitoring the implementation process to identify the unexpected in a timely fashion and react to it intelligently.

Strategies for planned curriculum change in medical schools

Levine (1980) identifies five approaches to planned change: rational; human problems or human relations; power; and eclectic, which is a pragmatic rather than an ideological approach, based on what works. Levine characterizes the eclectic approach as a 12-ingredient recipe for successful change encompassing procedures, goals, postures, and innovation stages.

1. Create a climate, even a demand for change.
2. Diminish the threat associated with innovation and avoid hard-line approaches.

3. Avoid being timid.
4. Appreciate timing.
5. Gear the innovation to the organization.
6. Engage in information dissemination and evaluation.
7. Communicate freely.
8. Get organizational leaders behind the innovation.
9. Build an active base of support.
10. Establish rewards.
11. Plan for the post-adoption period.
12. Other (e.g. have an implementation plan).

Below, using three examples of curriculum change, some of these 'recipes for success' are illustrated at work in the real world.

The innovative track

The innovative curriculum track has been adopted as a strategy for change at many medical schools. At a conference in Albuquerque (Kantrowitz *et al.*, 1987), attended by eight such schools, seven reasons were identified why an innovative track can be used as an agent of change.

1. It minimizes threat.
2. It bypasses departmental control.
3. It provides a protected environment.
4. It allows extensive student involvement in the community.
5. It offers alternative approaches to learning.
6. It provides an ethical approach to educational innovation.
7. It permits experimental comparison.

In addition, based on the experience of the participating schools, a core set of 23 strategies were identified grouped in a format roughly approximating to the sequence of change: getting started; building support, overcoming resistance; evaluation; networking; options for the future of the track. Among the strategies for building support and overcoming resistance were the need to build broad-based sympathy early from both within the institution and from appropriate community and government constituencies; to avoid isolation by the core planners from the rest of the institution; and to show flexibility in compromising on specific educational methods while defending and protecting the basic values underlying the new track. Compromise should be understood as a willingness of the innovators to conform, to a degree, with the common goals of the institution and a sign of the openness to input from colleagues. An additional strategy identified by Mennin and Kaufman (1989) is to develop understanding of the new programme through participation by faculty and students.

The case of Harvard

One of the most extensively documented processes of carefully planned curriculum change is that which has occurred at Harvard Medical School over the past twenty years.

Based on their experience, a number of principles have emerged as being key to the implementation of the new curriculum (Moore 1991, 1994) which seem to be generalizable to any medical school (see also Chapter 2).

1. Take a 'do it and fix it' approach that limits discussion and moves towards action.
2. Develop a strategy to isolate and protect the initial development of an educational innovation.
3. Find a means to counterbalance the decentralized financial and operational organization of the medical school. To achieve comprehensive curricular change, leaders must create a centralized, interdisciplinary group to provide an overview and integration of the entire span of medical education.
4. Balance the freedom to experiment with faculty participation through evaluation, review, and comment. The creative energy and commitment of those relatively small numbers of faculty and students interested in the early adoption of new approaches must be fostered, and their efforts not derailed by forcing them to work with the resisters of change. The entire faculty need to agree to the overall goals and purposes of education while operational implementation can be confined to a relatively small group of planners and workers. While all faculty members are encouraged to review and comment, authority for important detailed decisions must be reserved to smaller groups or to individuals.
5. Identify methods of documenting excellence in teaching and using this information in the academic promotion process (see below).
6. Use management techniques to facilitate the design, development, and production of the curriculum.

Of all the strategies listed above, Moore identifies goal-directed management of the entire process to guide production and keep it on schedule as perhaps the most important. Strong central management was needed to balance the heavy commitment to discussion and review by the faculty and the decentralized development of the curricular blocks. Moore emphasizes that in a project as complex as curricular change, effective project management is critical. Business-related techniques such as programme budgeting, strategic planning, use of critical path methods to specify milestones and develop timetables, and project monitoring to assure progress, were valuable tools in managing people and projects.

The experience at Sherbrooke

Des Marchais *et al.* (1992) have documented the strategies employed to change from a traditional to a problem-based learning (PBL) curriculum at Sherbrooke, Quebec. Implementation over a seven-year period is described according to a four-stage framework: need for change; selection of the PBL solution; planning for implementation; full-scale adoption of the PBL method. Several strategies are highlighted as being important for the success of the innovation. Changing the undergraduate curriculum was an institutional project. The proposed curriculum was widely distributed throughout the institution in a planning document which linked the history and educational philosophy of the institution with the process and content of the change. It served as the basis for a series of departmental meetings in which the Vice-Dean Education and the Under-graduate Program Director were requested to debate the proposal. The Dean made it clear that changing the curriculum was a faculty priority to which all teachers were expected to contribute. A new reward system was instituted to take into account time and energy required for the curriculum development. Workshops on medical pedagogy and a one-year programme for teacher development were introduced in order to educate the teachers, as well as specific PBL training.

Specific strategies for overcoming barriers to curriculum change

Improving leadership

Good academic leadership is required in order to deal with the structural resistance to change inherent in the organization of medical schools. Lack of leadership has been identified as a major barrier to change; conversely, strong, politically adept leadership is one of the important prerequisites for major institutional reform. Leadership needs to occur at all levels of the institution. The dean is obviously a key figure, but there are others: associate or sub deans, curriculum chairs, department heads etc. who need good leadership and management skills. There is little training or staff development in academic leadership which is specifically geared towards the problems of medical schools. Good leaders largely develop by chance and people are frequently appointed to key academic positions for reasons other than their qualities and skills in leadership, management, least of all for their interest or competence in education. A study of senior faculty by Nelson et al. (1990) found virtually no knowledge of past or current educational research at either a practical or theoretical level.

Several attempts have been made to address the issue of academic leadership in North America. The Association of American Medical Colleges provides management work-shops for newly appointed deans and has recently recommended that it should develop a new management workshop 'to marry the administrative, political, and financial issues all deans address with the educational programme activities all deans should address' with follow-up activities at each institution by staff of the AAMC or consultants employed by them. McMaster University has run an invitational Executive Program for Academic Leaders since 1989. The Educating Physicians for the Future of Ontario (EFPO) project has 'Developing ongoing leadership' as one of its key objectives in order to influence the direction of medical education during its five-year mandate. The main strategy is a fellowship programme that provides opportunities for the training of clinicians whose desired academic focus is medical education.

Bryan (1994) reflecting on the role of the dean in the process of effecting curriculum change suggests several specific strategies, including: developing matrix positions between academic departments and an interdisciplinary education group in the medical school; offering faculty the opportunity to participate in education workshops and seminars at home and elsewhere; recognizing educational skills and leadership ability in faculty promotion and compensation; encouraging opportunities for mentor relation-ships to develop; reallocating resources; championing the cause of educational innova-tion. In addition, the dean has the role of maintaining the long term goal of providing a better learning environment for the students, refusing to be dissuaded by an occasional mistake or side-step. This visionary leadership role of the dean, its complexities and contradictions, has been discussed in a broader context of the medical school within the changing health environment by MacLeod (1996).

The following aspects of leadership were found to be the most important to the successful institution of innovative tracks (Kantrowitz *et al.* 1987). The ability to:

+ Influence others (charisma)
+ Be credible and convincing to a broad institutional audience
+ Be an advocate who believes strongly in the innovation
+ Be a risk taker with considerable self assurance
+ Be flexible and able to compromise.

Those who generate the initial ideas for the curricular innovation are not necessarily those most capable of leading a successful effort at translating those ideas into a programme acceptable to the institution.

Improving the status of teaching

It is clear that one of the major barriers to change cited repeatedly is the low status of teaching and lack of recognition and rewards for effort in educational activities. While the lack of incentives and reward for people to spend time and energy on medical education always threatens to compromise the quality of teaching and learning it becomes especially problematic at times of curriculum change when extra effort is required to be directed into education. The most obvious way to increase the status of teaching is through effective promotions policies which allow academic staff to be promoted on the basis of excellence in teaching. This may be through the normal career pathway in which excellence in teaching or research are equally valid, or a by establishing a separate career track for educators. An example of a teacher-clinician ladder which has resulted in a significant culture shift in the professional value system of the medical school has been described by Lovejoy and Clark (1995).

Whereas promotion is the most obvious and talked about reward, there may not be many promotions and other methods of valuing teaching will be required. For example, Stritter *et al.* (1994) describe a Teaching Scholars Program which provides faculty interested in education with an opportunity to improve teaching skills, network with similar individuals, a forum for scholarly discussion about teaching and recognition as a Teaching Scholar.

Moreover, there is good evidence that the most effective incentives are not the tangible, material rewards but intrinsic motivation generated, for instance, by interaction with students, and having the time and support to pursue one's interest in education. For example, at McMaster University, 269 full- and part-time staff were asked to identify and rank from a list of fourteen items the three 'tangible and intangible' rewards that might be most effective in inducing them to participate in educational activity. Two of the three rewards most frequently cited were intangible personal enjoyment items: contact with learners (first in both groups) and positive feedback from peers and learners (third ranked by both groups) (Keane 1994). Ramsden (1992 pp. 248–69) points out that promotions, salary increases, and prizes for teaching may have some symbolic value in that they communicate the values of the institution to its staff and to the world at large, but their direct effect on good teaching is negligible. He believes recognition of efforts to improve teaching must begin by providing academic staff with the time outside their normal teaching and research duties to plan, implement, and discuss the effects of their changes. Time may be made available by staff release schemes or through the contributions of an educational development adviser or unit. The institutional features which have been found to influence faculty members' willingness to experiment with their teaching include administrative support of teaching, help and time to think of alternatives, flexibility in scheduling and availability of money for instructional resources (Wilkerson and Hundert, 1991).

Effective faculty development

Medical teachers require new knowledge, skills, and attitudes in order to embrace, plan, implement, and teach any new curriculum. Effective faculty development will help teachers re-examine the assumptions they hold about teaching and to develop insights into their changed roles in the new curriculum, for example from transmitter of information to stimulator/guide of learning (Wilkerson and Hundert, 1991). Wilkerson (1994) describes how an institutional commitment to faculty development and carefully designed programmes were used to encourage the adoption of curricular change at Harvard. She describes seven principles on which faculty development was based which can be generally applied to any medical school.

1. Faculty need to understand the educational philosophy of the new curriculum.
2. Learning is more likely to occur when faculty perceives a need for new information, skills, or knowledge.
3. Faculty development is more powerful if it occurs in the context of the teachers' own courses.
4. Large group workshops are useful in raising consciousness and introducing teaching skills; but
5. Their most powerful contribution is the opportunity they provide for faculty to learn from each other.
6. Intensive teaching skill development comes from actual participation in the new curriculum accompanied by opportunities for feedback from students, peers, or educational consultants.
7. Smaller gatherings on multiple occasions at multiple sites increase the chance of involving those central to the programme, especially clinical faculty.
8. The participation of high status role models in planning and implementing faculty development enhances the credibility and usefulness of the programmes.

Summary

Major barriers to change in medical education are identified from the literature and a survey of British medical schools. Three ways of thinking about change are discussed and related to possible strategies for change: organizations and the change process; change in universities and medical schools; change and the individual. Strategies for planned curriculum change in medical schools are illustrated by three examples: the innovative track; the case of Harvard; the experience at Sherbrooke. Three specific strategies for overcoming barriers to change—improving leadership, improving the status of teaching and effective faculty development—are described.

References

Association of American Medical Colleges (1984). Physicians for the twenty-first century. Report of the Project Panel on the General Professional Education of the Physician and College Preparation for Medicine. *Journal of Medical Education* **59** (11), Supplement, part 2, 208 pp.

Association of American Medical Colleges (1992). Educating medical students. Assessing change in medical education: the road to implementation. (ACME-TRI report).

Berg, B. and Ostergren, B. (1979). Innovation processes in higher education. *Studies in Higher Education*, **4**, 261–7.

Bloom, S.W. (1988). Structure and ideology in medical education: an analysis of resistance to change. *Journal of Health and Social Behaviour*, **29**, 294–306.

Bloom, S.W. (1989). The medical school as a social organisation: the sources of resistance to change. *Medical Education*, **23**, 228–41.

Bloom, S.W. (1992). Medical education in transition: paradigm change and organisational stasis. In *medical education in transition: commission on medical education: the sciences of medical practice* (ed. R.Q. Marston, and R.M. Jones), pp. 15–25. The Robert Wood Johnson Foundation, Princeton, NJ.

Bryan, G.T. (1994). The role and responsibility of the dean in promoting curricular innovation. *Teaching and Learning in Medicine*, **6**, 221–3.

Bussigel, M.N., Barzansky, B. and Grenholm, G. (1988). Innovation processes in medical education.

Cantor, J.C., Cohen, A.B., Barker, D.C., Shuster, A.L. and Reynolds, R.C. (1991). Medical educators' views on medical education reform. *Journal of the American Medical Association*, **265**, 1002–6.

Chin, R. and Benne, K.D. (1976). General strategies for effecting changes in human systems. In *The planning of change* (eds W.G. Bennis, K.D. Benne, R. Chin, and K.E. Corey) 3rd edn., pp. 22–45. Holt, Rinehart and Winston, New York, USA.

Christakis, N.A. (1995). The similarity and frequency of proposals to reform US medical education. *Journal of the American Medical Association*, **274**, 706–11.

Cohen, J, Dannefer, E.F., Seidel, H.M., Weisman, C.S., Wexler, P., Brown, T.M., *et al.* (1994). Medical education change: a detailed study of six medical schools. *Medical Education*, **28**, 350–60.

Delbecq, A.L. and Gill, S.L. (1985). Justice as a prelude to teamwork in medical centres. *Health Care Management Review*, **10**, 53–9.

Des Marchais, J.E., Bureau, M.A., Dumais, B., and Pigeon, G. (1992). From traditional to problem-based learning: a case report of complete curriculum reform. *Medical Education*, **26**, 190–9.

Dharamsi, S. (1996). *Medical educators' experience of anticipated curricular change to case/problem-based learning and its relationship to identity and role as teacher.* MSc Thesis. University of British Columbia.

Dwyer, M.S. (1977). Mastering change in education: understanding the anxieties created by change. *Educational Technology*, **17**, 54–6.

Elton, L. (1981). Can universities change? *Studies in Higher Education*, **6**, 23–33.

Elton, L. (1987). *Teaching in higher education: appraisal and training.* Kogan Page, UK.

General Medical Council (1993). *Tomorrow's doctors*. GMC, London.

Hefferlin, J.B. (1969). *Dynamics of academic reform*. Jossey-Bass, San Francisco.

Kantrowitz, M., Kaufman, A., Mennin, S., Fulop, T. and Guilbert, J.-J. (1987). *Innovative tracks in established institutions for the education of health personnel*. WHO Offset Publication No. 101. World Health Organization, Geneva, Switzerland.

Keane, D. (1994). Most effective rewards for educational activity: one medical faculty's perceptions. Abstract. 6th Ottawa conference on Medical Education.

Klein, D. (1976). Some notes on the dynamics of resistance to change: the defender role. In *The planning of change*. (ed. W.G. Bennis, K.D. Benne, R. Chin, and K.E. Corey) 3rd edn, pp.117–24. Holt, Rinehart and Winston, New York, USA.

Kotter, J.P. and Schlesinger, L.A. (1979). Choosing strategies for change. *Harvard Business Review*, March–April, 106–14.

Levine, A. (1980). *Why innovation fails*. State University of New York Press, Albany, USA.

Lewin, K. (1951). *Field theory in social science*. Harper and Row Publishers, New York.

Lovejoy, F.H. Jr and Clark, M.B. (1995). A promotion ladder for teachers at Harvard Medical School: experience and challenges. *Academic Medicine*, **70**, 1079–86.

MacLeod, S.M. (1996). The future of medical schools. Transition and turmoil: the work of a medical school dean. *Education for Health*, **9**, 13–24.

Mennin, S. and Kaufman, A. (1989). The change process and medical education. *Medical Teacher*, **11**, 9–16.

Moore, G.T. (1991). Initiating problem-based learning at Harvard Medical School. In: *The challenge of problem-based learning*, (ed. D. Boud and G. Feletti), pp. 80–7. Kogan Page, UK.

Moore, G.T. (1994). Strategies for change. In *New pathways to medical education*, (ed. D., Tosteson, S.J., Adelstein, and S.T. Carver), pp.30–7. Harvard University Press, USA.

Nelson, M.S., Clayton, B.L., Moreno, R. (1990). How medical school faculty regard educational research and make pedagogical decisions. *Academic Medicine*, **65**, 122–6.

Ramsden, P. (1992). *Learning to teach in higher education*. Routledge, UK.

Stocking, B. (1992). Promoting change in clinical care. *Quality in Health Care*, **1**, 56–60.

Stritter, F.T., Herbert, W.N.P., Harward, D.H. (1994). The Teaching Scholars Program: promoting teaching as scholarship. *Teaching and Learning in Medicine*, **6**, 207–9.

Wilkerson, L. (1994). Faculty development. In *New pathways to medical education*, (ed. D. Tosteson, S.J. Adelstein, and S.T. Carver), pp. 79–99. Harvard University Press, USA.

Wilkerson, L. and Hundert, E.M. (1991). Becoming a problem-based tutor: increasing self-awareness through faculty development. In: *The challenge of problem-based learning*, (ed. D. Boud and G. Feletti), pp. 159–71. Kogan Page, London.

Conclusions

9 Medical education into the next century

Lesley Rees and Brian Jolly

Introduction

In Chapter 1 a rationale that will govern our vision of medical education in the next century was portrayed. In this chapter we summarize, using examples from our own experience, the most notable trends that have taken place in medical education. We will attempt to locate them in the context of other changes that have engulfed the medical world in general, and the UK in particular. The most notable of these, and the most pressing for many engaged in the continual process of curriculum change are the widespread developments associated with the publication by the GMC (1993) of the document *Tomorrow's doctors*. By 1999 most schools will have implemented new curricula, but it is sobering and even disenchanting to acknowledge that many of the young doctors produced by these new systems will not emerge until 2005 and, indeed, will have ceased practising before the century is halfway through. Hence, in a rapidly evolving environment, the challenge of the future will not be in how to manage change but in how to perpetuate it.

Curricula after 'Tomorrow's doctors'

One of the main features of the GMCs '*Tomorrow's doctors*' guidelines is the attempt to provide medical schools with the rationale for devising 'Core and options' curricula. The essential idea, buttressed by concerns over factual overloading, the rapidly changing knowledge base of medicine, the need for self-directed learners and the need to try to diversify UK curricula, is that a central kernel of competence in medicine should be defined, but the remaining knowledge and skills may be left to the discretion of individuals or medical schools. Although this approach has been tried in the past (Robbins 1977) it has not, until now, met with a great deal of success. The reasons may stem more from historical and political factors than from any inherent deficiency of the model. In the 1950s and 1960s there was a rapidly developing group of specialties, there was little or no interest from the general medical community in the idea of educational expertise being useful and relevant to the teaching of medicine, the concept of problem-based learning was in its infancy and the means to deliver 'core' curricula, in terms of quality assurance procedures applied to teaching, mostly embryonic.

As we approach the twenty-first century the impetus to define core skills seems to have resurfaced. Medical school committees sit to consider the 'core' elements of medicine; specialists and Colleges have taken up the challenge (Royal College of Physicians 1996). The advantages to busy clinicians of having a few students address their specialty, motivated by a special study module, rather than a whole moderately interested cohort, are becoming obvious.

In addition the revolution in attitudes towards the quality of education has been dramatic. About ten years ago evaluations of our (then) undergraduate medical course, by finalists and preregistration house officers, showed a huge variability in clinically based teaching, both in quantity and quality. The curriculum emphasized and assessed retention and regurgitation of factual knowledge and appeared to have no clearly defined objectives or philosophy. Learning of communication skills occurred only by the apprenticeship model and the concept of patient-centred care was virtually non-existent (Jolly and Rees 1984; Jolly and Macdonald 1989).

At the same time the Association of American Medical Colleges' report 'Physicians for the twenty-first century (AAMC 1984)' placed patients and their families at the heart of medical education and emphasized that communication, patient autonomy, and the doctor–patient relationship must underpin the whole educational process (see Chapters 1–3). The apprenticeship model, until recently so embedded in our own UK system was deemed obsolete, unworkable, undesirable, and inappropriate. The AAMC also clearly spelled out that the knowledge, skills, values, and attitudes that students must learn should be clearly defined, where they would learn them should be prescribed and teachers should be taught to teach and to evaluate performance objectively.

In the UK, the more recent GMC report also recognized that changes in clinical practice, technology, and the new environment of the NHS would mean that the settings in which learning took place would shift from hospital to general practice, primary care, and the community. It failed, however, to grasp the nettle of the inevitable move toward multiprofessional education.

In hospitals we now have an increasingly specialized, and often unpredictable clinical resource and patients who should not be exposed to 'unskilled' learners. The development of technical, communication and 'transferable' skills (such as computer literacy) has become a topic of interest across the educational spectrum.

Examples of curricular change: learning skills

Traditionally medical students learnt both clinical and communication skills in patient care areas with students observing and then practising in the 'apprentice' mode. Although this has been regarded as intrinsically more effective, than sitting in a lecture theatre (with students learning rapidly and gaining in confidence), the opportunities to learn these skills in this way in the future is, for reasons described above, no longer sustainable.

In addressing these problems the skills centre has increasingly become an important learning resource, not only for undergraduates but for postgraduate medical and nurse education. A skills centre is a facility in which students and qualified staff learn clinical, communication, and information technology skills to a specified level of competence prior to or co-ordinated with direct patient contact. Here, patients are not used as 'teaching aids' and students are not overwhelmed by the multi-dimensional problems of a sick person lying in a complex environment (Studdy *et al.* 1994) and will not perform the skill on the patient until a required level of competence is achieved.

The skills centre provides a realistic but less threatening environment in which models, simulations and simulated patients are employed and a structured approach to skills learning and assessment, with teacher supervision, ensures separate mastering of each skill. Independent access enables students to practice, refine, and maintain competence.

Postgraduate students can learn specialized skills such as minimal access surgery in centres such as that at the Royal College of Surgeons, England. Furthermore, video recording/playback facilities and, the use of two way mirrors, quite an old idea undergoing rejuvenation, facilitate teachers', learners', and peer feedback and analysis. Importantly, such centres can enable shared learning amongst different health professionals encouraging understanding of the different roles and skills belonging to different members of individual clinical teams. In this environment students can be prepared for work experience to a pre-specified level and skill acquisition organized on a longitudinal basis with different levels of competence assessed at each point.

The clinical skills laboratory, within St Bartholomew's and the Royal London School of Medicine and Dentistry, based on the Maastricht model (University of Limburg, Netherlands) was established as a joint venture with the College of Nursing and Midwifery. This new resource (Dacre *et al.* 1996a), the first within a medical college in the UK, enabled the emergent philosophies to be incorporated in the design. These included the concepts of shared multiprofessional learning and teamwork. The education resources employed within the centre include real patient volunteers, primed patient volunteers, simulated patients (actors), teaching rooms linked by two-way mirrors, videos, video/playbacks, mannequins and simulators, computer-assisted learning, interactive videos, and CD ROM. Fundamental communication skills as well as specific issues such as breaking bad news are learned in small groups.

It remains to make the degree of competence required by students explicit. A clinical 'skills matrix' was compiled that is a composite description of all the clinical and communication skills necessary for medical and nurse education and the level of competence required of each skill. A catalogue of 59 separate communication skills and 540 clinical skills was established and a clear consensus reached that communication is an essential and integral part of every skill (Dacre and Nicol 1996).

All skills, both clinical and communication, are assessed by an objective structured clinical examination (OSCE) which consists of a series of stations employing many of the resources mentioned above. The first OSCE is taken Eight months after joining the clinical course and no student can enter for the final MBBS examinations unless they have passed. Does it work? The difficulties inherent in the assessment of clinical competence are legion and well documented (Carnegy 1992; Hart 1992). None the less our experience of competence in one skill alone, intravenous drug administration, assessed by OSCE showed a 14% improvement after two years specific skills centre training (Dacre *et al.* 1993).

Until all communications between physician and patient are recognized as potentially therapeutic acts the profession will continue to 'fail' those that it serves (Mayerson 1976). Indeed, some say that it beggars belief that an understanding of the psychological sequelae and care of 'medical' patients is only recently deemed desirable for preregistration house officers (Royal College of Physicians (London) and Royal College of

Psychiatrists UK Joint Working Report 1995; Sharpe *et al.* 1996). Regrettably, this reflects the professional division between psychiatry and medicine, promoted by their separation in undergraduate curricula and into separate Royal Colleges at the postgraduate level. The publication of their joint report and subsequent debate is much to be welcomed.

Medical schools in the UK are making progress and in the main have at least acknowledged the issues as important. The postgraduate deans, those who commission and purchase education and clinical care and those who promote and monitor standards in continuing medical education, in particular the Royal Colleges, should do likewise and place communication between doctors and their patients at the heart of medicine.

Shared multiprofessional learning and team working

In the UK, '*The patients' charter*' (Department of Health 1996*a*) whilst commendable as a starter, does not address the issue of patient autonomy and informed consent in any real depth. In the USA, disclosure about risk and benefit, evidence-based therapies and outcomes, the place of clinical trials and audit, and how these are evaluated, are regarded as legitimate patient concerns and must be explicit. Indeed, if we do not embrace this within the UK how can we expect an intelligent public debate about difficult decision making in medicine and the allocation of scarce resources? Patients must enter the ethical debate as full partners and feel free to discuss quality of life, psychological, cultural and religious issues and the nature of suffering, to mention but a few factors (Faulder 1985; Kleinman 1987; Neuberger 1987, 1997; Fallowfield 1990).

In December 1994 in the UK the then Minister of Health asked the Standing Medical and Nursing and Midwifery Advisory Committees 'To consider how patient care can be enhanced by professionals from different disciplines co-operating and co-ordinating work across organizational boundaries'. A joint working group was appointed and convened four focus groups to consider specific interfaces *vis-à-vis* health and social care; general medical services and community medical services, primary and secondary health care and carers (DoH 1996*b*). Their main conclusion was that professional collaboration within and between health and social care services is more important than ever, given the number of administrative boundaries to be negotiated and the separate sources of funding. On education they said that all those responsible for the education and training of health professionals should encourage and support programmes which help them to operate as team members. Efforts should be made to increase the common elements in basic and post-basic education and training for related professions, to familiarize students with the attitudes, values and working practices of other professions. Furthermore, continuing professional development programmes should also emphasize commonality of purpose and, where appropriate, not be confined to a single profession. Local programmes of 'joint education and training should also be developed further'. Recent reviews (Barr 1994; Barr and Shae 1995) demonstrated that such initiatives are still relatively sparse.

The modern health professional must fulfil a complexity of different roles. These include healer, technician, counsellor (Downie and Calman 1987) but might also include educator, scientist, friend, politician, advocate, or campaigner. At times these roles may be confusing both to the patient and the professional and encompass conflicting values (see Chapter 2.3). Recent publicity in the national and medical press regarding issues surrounding multiple pregnancies, serves to highlight some of these dilemmas. From the patients' standpoint it dramatically illuminates the inherent conflicts between a doctor's commitment to an individual, the professional concern for ethical needs of 'society' and the cost-benefit analysis of a therapy delivered with a finite health care resource (Berkowitz 1996; Duncan 1996). The implication of all this is that a doctor must, to some extent become a multi-faceted professional; no longer 'in charge' but fulfilling a role as and when required. That role may not be easy to define (Davidson and Lucas, 1995). As well as changing roles frequently, doctors must also recognize that they will also be working as members of multiprofessional teams, and that communication with patients will occur within a wider therapeutic team.

Our own experience of shared learning of nurse and medical students in the St Bartholomew's Skills Centre reveals that this experience leads to a greater understanding and respect for each other's roles, through the identification of 'common values, knowledge, and skills across professions and work settings and creating a shared philosophy of care' (Carpenter 1995). Although in 1997 there is now growing literature supporting interprofessional education in the health sciences and descriptions of various initiatives in evaluation, as yet there is no evidence of improved patient care. But there has been evidence demonstrating a change in attitudes and stereotyping (Mazur *et al.* 1979; Carpenter 1995).

This intense interest in interprofessional education is driven by complex forces. The relatively recent restructuring of the NHS with increased community-based care and education, the care delivered jointly between health and social services, combined with the never-ending pressure on resources had led to a demand for a more flexible work-force and the blurring of professional boundaries. Furthermore, in the UK shortages of hospital-based doctors and GPs and the 'New deal' on working hours and other conditions for junior doctors has increasingly led both local NHS managers and the NHS executive (NHSE) to question historical professional boundaries. Nurses in particular are working across the traditional 'doctor boundaries' with nurse led clinics and wards where nurses control admission and discharge and manage all aspects of care. Nurse practitioners with advanced levels of knowledge and skill carry their own case load and make decisions about referral to doctors. Nurse prescribing is a frequently discussed issue (Bradley *et al.* 1997). In other roles, specialist nurses will work alongside physicians in hospital, follow up patients in the community and run their own clinics.

In the NHS of today the commissioning of non-medical education and training is now in the hands of consortia with a strong general management membership. This will lead to pressure for multiprofessional service-based education and training because purchasers want their personnel to be trained in the way that they will practice—interprofessionally. These consortia have been instructed by NHSE to 'actively explore opportunities to commission multidisciplinary education and training and programmes which provide opportunities for shared learning' (Shaw 1995). This is indeed facilitated by all health professionals being educated in universities, increasing the practical opportunities for multidisciplinary learning. In the UK all health sciences have been brought together in several Universities (Sheffield, Leeds, Southampton, Kings College London, Dundee, Nottingham, Kingston/St George's, London, and Manchester) and a number of organizations are actively working to promote interprofessional education.

These include the Centre for Advancement of Interprofessional Education (CAIPE), The Royal Colleges of Nursing (RCN) and General Practice (RCGP), and with a wider remit the European Network for Development of Multiprofessional Education in the Health Sciences (Gobb 1994).

Whilst many members of the 'medical' profession (i.e. the doctors) feel instinctively threatened by forces driving multiprofessional education and working, to us it seems an inevitability. However Belbin (1981), the team and team work 'guru' sounds a note of caution. However much we may prepare professionals to work as equal members of a team if we create expectations that cannot be translated into reality, the end result will be conflict and frustration. The workplace has to be restructured if team work is to flourish (Belbin 1981).

Continuing medical education

All professional bodies in the UK have introduced a system for ensuring continuing professional development. For physicians this was the result of the 1993 Conference of Medical Royal Colleges and their faculties in the UK who agreed general principles supporting formal continuing medical education programmes for the profession.

The overwhelming majority of physicians recognize that it is not possible for a physician, having gained a career appointment, to become buried in clinical practice and to rely solely on what is learnt by experience for the ensuing twenty-five years or more. To maintain their high standards of medical care, many physicians keep on acquiring and disseminating new knowledge by reading journals, writing articles, and teaching medical students. They undertake research and audit, participate in clinical meetings and attend specialist society conferences. Given the rapid advances in medical science, the greater expectations of an increasingly informed public and the growing tendency towards litigation it is inevitable that doctors must not only keep abreast of the latest developments, but also be seen to do so. The necessity to create time for continuing medical education (CME) is now acknowledged by the profession and by government.

The Colleges of Physicians (UK) have devised a simple system for internal and external CME and have wisely rejected the notion of weighting different activities. After all, how does one compare giving a lecture with attending the same lecture? It is envisaged that the Colleges will maintain a register of all the physicians who have satisfactorily participated in CME and expect that all physicians will ultimately possess a College CME certificate. A target of fifty hours CME per annum was set and a recent audit (P.Toghill, personal communication 1997) demonstrated a 90% questionnaire return with many physicians undertaking 50 to 100 hours per annum. A target of 100 hours may eventually become the norm.

Performance assessment

One of the changes identified in Chapter 1 is the trend towards public accountability of professions. An important factor in this development in the UK has been the publication by the GMC of *The duties of a doctor* (GMC 1995). This is a comprehensive set of guidance rules or notes for any individual doctor on good medical practice, ethical problems of HIV infection, advertising and other topics. The GMC hopes that these guidelines will provide a means to improve standards. They might be used by institutions in a number of ways, but certainly as a basis for undergraduate training and staff development as they form a considerable advance on *Tomorrow's doctors* (GMC 1993). For example the guidelines cover not only the need to be professionally competent in the technical sense, but also, for example to 'develop the skills of a competent teacher', 'work constructively within . . . teams', and 'recognize the limits of (their) professional competence'.

The GMC and the government have attempted to ensure that these guidelines are enforceable by enabling regulating bodies to investigate the performance of practitioners about whom complaints have been received. Until recently, in medicine, proven impaired health or negligence were the only factors that could result in removal from the medical register or restrictions on practice. However in the UK during 1997 new legislation came into force which will allow the General Medical Council to scrutinize in detail the clinical performance of a medical practitioner and make recommendations on remedial activity, which may include removal from the register.

The GMC performance procedure uses a framework based on the current state of knowledge about the assessment of clinical competence (GMC 1996; Newble *et al.* 1994). It will usually involve observation, by trained assessors, of doctors in action with real or simulated patients, of the technical and procedural skills of those doctors, and of their record keeping. The procedure will include extensive discussion with the practitioner about decisions taken in real clinical situations sampled from the profile of cases dealt with by that doctor. Notably, the doctor's attitudes to his/her patients will be one facet of performance under scrutiny along with their clinical acumen. In addition each assessment panel will include a trained lay assessor to incorporate, amongst other things, the patient's perspective. The assessments will be standardized in format, but based on the individual's practice profile (Southgate and Jolly 1994). Any such assessment will be preceded by in depth investigation and screening of the complaints, from patients or others, that invoked the procedures. The outcomes could entail retraining in some aspects of medicine, restricted or supervised practice or, if patient safety is in jeopardy, removal from the register.

Performance assessment and CME

The GMC performance procedures will no doubt have an effect on medical education, especially at postgraduate level. For example CME activities in the future will be taking place in a slightly different milieu—one in which the performance procedures will have the potential to act as a definition of minimal competence. Since the procedures will be invoked by complaints, and since the vast majority of complaints stem, at least initially, from poor interpersonal or interprofessional communication, this aspect of practice is liable to come increasingly under the microscope. Opportunities for retraining, in this and other areas, will need to be offered by trusts, postgraduate deans and universities. Thus CME, especially for general practitioners, is likely to need reorientation towards the analysis and improvement of everyday practice, rather than the latest tertiary or technological breakthrough (see Shires *et al.* 1995). If the performance procedures provoke a searching and methodical review of continuing education systems they may have done the profession a service that is long overdue.

Another possible manifestation of the constant spectre of performance monitoring may be that Royal Colleges might be more willing, or be forced, to discuss reaccreditation (recertification) based on assessment of practice activity, as is the option in some Australian colleges (Newble and Paget 1996). This will be in contrast to the current vogue for accumulating continuing education points or hours as a means of demonstrating continuing competence. The definition of core objectives for College membership and professional viability (see Newble and Paget 1996) may take on a more prominent function in the definition of competence.

It is true that current continuing education systems offer a certain amount of flexibility in educational delivery and choice. But one of the drawbacks to this education-only approach is that it does not provide critical, but supportive, appraisal to the individual practitioner. Nor, it must be said, did postgraduate training activities up until 1996 offer much in the way of this type of feedback to the individual practitioner. This is, however, one of the goals of the reforms of postgraduate education—the 'Calman' reforms (DoH 1997), to which we now turn.

Post Calmanism and the definition of curricula

The last few years of the nineties have seen the development of new approaches to postgraduate education in the UK—the so-called 'Calman reforms'. These have emanated from an attempt to make the route to specialty accreditation much more streamlined. The hallmarks of this trend, which has its roots in the North American system, are a shortened, more structured, approach to the acquisition of clinical expertise, a strict assessment and appraisal system through which junior doctors must progress satisfactorily, the award of a certificate of specialty training accrediting trainees to practice their branch of medicine and, currently, a certain degree of uncertainty about what happens to 'unsuccessful' trainees. In addition the GMC has recently described the professional and educational requirements of the preregistration post, the precursor to specialty training, in *The new doctor* (GMC 1997).

Most professional bodies or Royal Colleges have published core curricula for their members to underpin their general professional training. The most recently published at the time of writing was the *Core curricula for senior house officers* (Royal College of Physicians 1996). This outlines what is to be learnt and delivered, the environment in which it should take place, and the support, supervision, and assessment to be expected by individual doctors. A network of regional tutors, college and associate college tutors was established to enable implementation and regular feedback is obtained and support given by college visits to listen and learn. With the implementation of the recommendations of the Calman report, general professional training is now accomplished in two years and entry into higher specialist training possible in medicine and surgery only by the attainment of the MRCP or the new FRCS respectively. Specialist training now occupies five years with physicians obtaining the Certificate of Completion of Specialist Training CCST and surgeons passing the specialist level FRCS.

One of the major differences between the new and the old systems is the amount of explicit responsibility consultants must take for training, supervising, appraising, and assessing juniors. Training programmes should be more carefully defined, and there should be closer links between professional activities and educational ones.

The extent to which these activities will affect undergraduate education is hard to gauge. There are many factors at work. First, seniors may need to concentrate effort on their postgraduate trainees and this may reduce their capacity to educate undergraduates. Second more basic training will be came out in the community or with general practitioners, by virtue of the reasons discussed in Chapters 1 and 4. Hence students progressing to hospital specialties will have experienced much of their medicine in the primary care setting. In addition, concentration on the 'core' in both basic and clinical undergraduate levels may produce postgraduate trainees with radically different experiences from those of their predecessors, possibly perceived as lower standards. This confluence of events may cause a number of difficulties.

For example trainees in many GP vocational training schemes currently undergo a complex series of rotations and other vocational activities designed specifically to hone their basic human attributes: sensitivity to racial and gender issues, communication skills; practice management and organization, and so on. Moreover, for many years all GP trainers have undergone training themselves, and the ethos of these courses is very much geared towards preparation for everyday patient-centred problems in general practice. The incoming trainee of the future will be much more acclimatized to the nature of general practice and much less so to hospital medicine. Many existing strategies in GP VTSs may be redundant, while those for hospital specialties may make a number of assumptions about technical expertise and background knowledge that turn out to be unwarranted. New specialist trainees may appear to the hospital specialist to have been de-skilled by their general or primary care perspectives. Rather than generating complementary or synergistic systems of hospital based and primary care specialty training we may be heading for a simple reversal of the trends operating in the seventies and eighties.

One of the solutions may lie in the 'special study' part of the undergraduate curriculum. These are currently envisaged as opportunities for students to specialize in topics excluded from the new curricular cores. These are likely to be the hospital specialties such as paediatric cardiology, plastics, intensive care, urology, neurosurgery, etc. These attachments may well be much longer than they were in old style curricula. If such attachments are to serve a purpose in assisting to develop clinical skills, it is important that such options include high fidelity clinical opportunities for students, with appropriate levels of responsibility, rather than academic, esoteric, or library-based projects of only marginal practical relevance to the specialty. The latter is likely to ensue if students are seen as presenting a higher workload, or as irrelevant or non-contributory. The library project might become a simple device to process them through a department.

There is a popular but unsubstantiated belief amongst consultants that attachment of students to their specialty is important for later recruitment. In their view students opting later for a career in a hospital specialty depend, almost uniquely, on their undergraduate experiences to make informed choices about their future roles. However, many specialties will no longer be automatically involved in undergraduate rotations. It would be sensible for some specialists to design activities at undergraduate level as an initiation into the vocational requirements of the job. This may put even greater pressure on teaching resources. Ways must be found to alleviate this strain on the system.

Some specialties have spent time considering, somewhat paradoxically, what might be considered 'core' for their specialty (Dacre *et al.* 1996*b*). Such approaches may result in unwieldy or overcrowded lists of objectives or they could contribute a sensible way forward of sharing expertise and rationalization of content. Specialty groups tend to maintain a stronger network of interchange and collaboration than medical schools: for example specialty society meetings frequently attract larger numbers of attendees than medical school events—the national perspective is important. By combining resources pertaining to specialties across institutions, students may be enabled to learn more effectively at the same time as reducing the workload on staff and the pressure on a single institution. For example SSMs could be run in one institution for students from several medical schools. This would also then be working in the same direction as rationalization of patient services, although it would lead to a rather fragmented or devolved status for the medical school; at least for the SSM delivery.

Skill mix

A further issue about to explode onto the medical scene, especially in primary care, is the debate about the appropriateness of the skill mix in medicine. The basic question is should the medical professional—the doctor—have a monopoly on the diagnosis and management of the patient? In many ways this debate is similar to that which guided the virtual destruction of the restrictive practice or 'closed shop' of the 1960s and 1970s. Both confrontations have been fuelled by employers striving to reduce labour costs and the increased availability of technological approaches. But in the current discussion customers (patients) as well as employers are also having some influence. Increasingly, the patient has more power as alternative means to health care proliferate, for example in the widening spectrum and increasing number of both regulated or deregulated independent practitioners including the rise of complementary medicine (e.g. The Osteopaths Act 1993) and more opportunities for privately financed health care. This trend is happening against a background of progression towards evidence based health care that can hardly keep pace with scientific and socio-economic developments.

Taking primary care as an example, Jenkins-Clarke and Carr-Hill (1996), cite three reasons for the challenge to doctors' supremacy:

- the sharing of care needed in an ageing, home-based, patient population
- difficulties of recruiting adequate numbers of GPs
- the enhanced professional scope of practice and specialist nurses.

This approach is backed up by other documents. The NHS executive document on '*Primary care: the future*' (1996) refers to nurses developing their role in primary care and leading primary health care teams in some instances.

The immediate implications of this for undergraduate education are far reaching. First, there will need to be a co-ordinated interdisciplinary approach to health care training in the future. Second there will be some skills and techniques that all health care professionals must be capable of undertaking and which could be learnt much more effectively (possibly even *cost-effectively*) in an interprofessional forum (Robinson *et al.* 1993).

There will be a major problem in the interim. Newly qualified doctors will be coming onto the employment market with the warnings of senior consultants about the de-skilling of the profession still ringing in their ears. They may be ill equipped for shared working and, importantly, shared decision making. Their postgraduate training will still be geared to Royal College curricula that, although developing rapidly are not yet coming to terms with interprofessional training in any meaningful way Hence the major breakthrough **must** come in the undergraduate or early postgraduate years. It is here that the opportunities exist for contiguous, well planned, efficiently managed joint education and they far outnumber those occurring at any other stage of training.

Furthermore with the move to modularity in higher education, other opportunities will present themselves. It is not uncommon to find students doing combined honours in French and German, Economics and History, Management and Accounting. But where are the Medicine and Physiotherapy courses, or Nursing with Radiography? The nearest we have currently are MB–PhD tracks, where the argument seems to be that research is an appropriate and natural extension of the medical field. Although the agenda for professional isolation has been set elsewhere and will be increasingly challenged, such *joint* professional approaches may be more sensible than attempting to define the '*generic* health care professional' (e.g. see Schatz *et al.* 1996). At the same time they may also help to clarify the true nature of transferable skills (if they exist) in health care professionalism and allow course designers to experiment with the definition of medical (health care) expertise. It is already easy to argue that the basic knowledge about the human body and its mechanisms required, for example by doctors, nurses, dentists, and osteopaths overlaps considerably, but education rarely proceeds conjointly. The reasons for this are not always clear or are historical rather than rational. Perhaps that step needs to be taken.

The virtual medical school

As we have seen, medical education is being drawn towards an environment that extends beyond the controlling influences of the medical school and the teaching hospital. As it focuses more on patient autonomy, basic skills, and community-oriented practice, the question of the need for organization and control of curricular quality becomes paramount. The major drawbacks of the apprenticeship model were its inflexibility (one person communicated his or her knowledge to the learner) and its unfeasibility in modern health care. Its preeminence as a supervisory model was rarely in doubt. Although the potential for operating an apprenticeship model has receded in the hospital it may not be so elusive in primary care and to some extent continues to be used successfully there. Indeed, if education is to follow the provision of care, as in the primary care-led NHS, the development of good general undergraduate education based in general practice is essential.

The intensive, long term relationship between physician and pupil has been realized in general practice vocational training schemes. For it to be educationally productive at undergraduate level, its quality—the delivery of aims, objectives, highly effective educational material and assessments—needs to be assured. One model has been tried by Oswald *et al.* (1995) at Cambridge. Alternatively, the capacity for such management and delivery lies in the existence of the Internet or World Wide Web (see Chapter 4.2). Friedman (1996) has described the potential uses of the Web for creating the 'virtual medical school'. In this 'school' clinical activity and problem solving with patients forms the general thrust or educational direction, while 'knowledge' and other academic content is delivered via the Web through a collegiate definition and monitoring process. It is difficult to argue against the economic and clinical viability of this process. The Web is recognized as the only means of keeping in touch with the changing knowledge base. It is also cited as a potential instrument of rapid diagnosis and information transfer in medicine—so-called *telemedicine*. It is but a short distance from this to the realization that almost all the required attributes of the future health care professional—self direction, sensitivity to rapid changes in the need for updating, IT literacy, clinical problem solving ability, as well as a sound and well tested knowledge base—are achievable by coupling centrally co-ordinated academic programmes delivered on Internet, to constant and closely supervised clinical activity. In this environment teachers as well as learners would receive guidance via the same medium, meeting as a cohort only infrequently as and when the need, for example for global clinical assessments, arose.

In the virtual medical school all clinical teachers would require mandatory elementary training, both in the use of IT and in basic teaching skills. However there are problems: currently many GPs seem reluctant to engage in academic activity unless specifically recompensed. By contrast the hospital milieu has always welcomed students. Hence for this type of education to succeed, the funding arrangements for undergraduate educational activity in general practice must be reappraised. Perhaps part of the solution relies on the creation of salaried GP posts with specific responsibility for academic input, encouraged by Academic Units of General Practice to devote time to teaching in the same way that professorial units of medicine and surgery encouraged the development of hospital academic medicine in the 1960s. The service increment for teaching (SIFT), allocated by regions to teaching hospitals will need redistribution for this to succeed.

Educating the educators

Finally, several important reports have recently indicated that it is important for those who teach medicine at the undergraduate or postgraduate levels to be appropriately trained so to do (Irby 1996; SCOPME 1994; Department of Health 1996*b*). Non-clinically qualified staff who teach parts of the curriculum, such as basic sciences, ethics, law, and communication skills also need such training. Ideally all doctors should be professional in their approach to teaching, and systems will have to be put in place for doctors to acquire the relevant teaching skills. Contracts should include provision for acquiring, updating or developing such skills, and academic and professional promotion criteria should formally include and encourage teaching. These skills need also to span curriculum development, project supervision and assessment as well as 'contact' skills. Although an increasing number of clinical staff are attending masters and other shorter courses on teaching, the proportion of all-teaching active doctors who have done so is still only about 6% according to two recent surveys done at Kings and Manchester (Lawson *et al.* 1996; Lawson 1997). For too long this has been an area of relative neglect within the UK and it is far too important to remain undervalued in the next century.

References

AAMC (Association of American Medical Colleges) (1984). *Physicians for the twenty-first century*. Report of the Panel on the General Professional Education of the Physician (GPEP Report) AAMC, Washington.

Barr, H. (1994). *In perspectus on shared learning*. CAIPE, London.

Barr, H. and Shae, I. (1995). *In shared learning* CAIPE, London.

Belbin, M. (1981). *Management teams*. Heinmann, London.

Berkowitz, R.L. (1996). From twin to singleton. *British Medical Journal*, **313**, pp.373–4.

Bradley, C.P., Taylor, R.J., Blenkinsopp, A. (1997). Primary care-opportunities and threats. Developing prescribing in primary care. *British Medical Journal*, **314**, 744–7.

Carnegy, Baroness (1992). Opening address in *Approaches to the assessment of clinical competence* R.M. Harden, I.R. Hart, and H. Mulholland, Part 1, pp.1–2. Dundee Centre for Medical Education, Dundee.

Carpenter, J. (1995). Doctors and nurses: stereotypes and stereotype change in interprofessional education. *Journal of Interprofessional Care*, **9**, (2), 151–61.

Continuing Medical Education (1994). Report of the Royal Colleges of Physicians of Edinburgh, Glasgow and London.

Dacre, J.E. and Nicol, M. (1996). Clinical skills: The learning matrix for students of medicine and nursing. Ratcliffe Medical Press, Oxford.

Dacre, J.E., Jolly, B., Griffiths, S., Noble, G. (1993). Giving intravenous drugs—students should be trained and tested. *British Medical Journal*, **307**, 1142.

Dacre, J., Nicol, M., Holroyd, D., Ingram, D. (1996*a*). The development of a clinical skills centre. *Journal of the Royal College of Physicians of London*, **30**, 18–24.

Dacre, J.E., Jolly, B.C., and Griffiths, S. (1996*b*). Medical education and rheumatology. *British Journal of Rheumatology*, **35**, 269–74.

Davidson, L. and Lucas, J. (1995). Multiprofessional education in the undergraduate health profession curriculum: observations for Adelaide, Linkoping and Salford. *Journal of Interprofessional Care*, **9**, 163–76.

Department of Health (1996*a*). *In the patient's interest, multiprofessional working across organisation boundaries*. DOH, London.

Department of Health (1996*b*) Government White paper: *A service with ambitions*. Department of Health, London.

Department of Health (1997). *A guide to specialist registrar training* (2nd edn). DoH, London.

Downie, R.S. and Calman, K.C. (1987). Healthy respect—ethics in health care, London 159–60.

Duncan, N. (1996). Light the blue touch paper and stand well clear. *British Medical Journal*, **313**, 432.

Fallowfield, L. (1990). *The quality of life—the missing measurement in health care*. Souvenir Press, London.

Faulder, C. (1985). *Whose body is it? The troubling issue of informed consent*. Virago, London.

Friedman, C.P. (1996). The virtual clinical campus. *Academic Medicine*, **71**, 647–51.

GMC (1993). *Tomorrow's doctors: recommendations on undergraduate medical education*. General Medical Council, London.

GMC (1995). *The duties of a doctor*. General Medical Council, London.

GMC (1996). *The performance procedures: position paper No.3*. General Medical Council, London.

GMC (1997). *The new doctor: recommendations on the preregistration year*. General Medical Council, London.

Gobb, R. (1994). Multiprofessional education, European network for development of multi-professional education in health science (EMPE). *Journal of Interprofessional Care*, **8**, pp.85–92.

Hart, I.R. (1992). Trends in clinical assessment In *Approaches to the assessment of clinical competence*, (ed. R.M. Harden, I.R. Hart, and H. Mulholland) Part 1, pp.17–23. Dundee Centre for Medical Education, Dundee,

Hopkins, A., Solomon, J., and Avelson, J. (1996). Shifting boundaries in professional care. *Journal of the Royal Society of Medicine*, **89**, 364–70.

Horder, J. (1994). Interprofessional education for primary health and community care: present state and future needs. In *Interprofessional Relations in Health Care*, (ed.) (Soothill, K. *et al.*), pp.00–00. Edward Arnold, London.

Irby, D.M. (1996). Models of faculty development for problem-based learning. *Advances in Health Sciences Education*, **1**, 69–81.

Jenkins-Clarke, S. and Carr-Hill, R. *Measuring skill mix in primary care: dilemmas of delegation and diversification*. Discussion paper No 144. Centre for Health Economics, York.

Jolly, B.C. and Rees, L.H. (1984). Room for improvement: an evaluation of the undergraduate curriculum at St Bartholomew's Hospital Medical College, Mimeo, SBHMC.

Jolly, B.C. and Macdonald, M.M. (1989) Education for practice: the role of practical experience in undergraduate and general clinical training. *Medical Education*. **23**, 189–95

Klass, P. (1987) *A not entirely benign procedure—four years as a medical student*. Signet, New York.

Kleinman, A. (1987). *The illness narratives: suffering, healing and the human condition*. Basic Books, New York.

Lawson, M., Seabrook, M., Jolly, B.C., and Pettingale, K.W. (1996) Teachers at King's: who teaches and how? Paper presented at the annual conference of the Association for the Study of Medical Education. *Medical Education*, **30**, 71–2.

Lawson, M. (1997). Unpublished data—personal communication to the authors.

Mayerson, E.W. (1976). *Putting the ill at ease*. Harper and Row, Maryland, USA.

Mazur, H., Beeston, J.J., and Yerxa, E.J. (1979). Clinical interdisciplinary health team care; an educational experiment. *Journal of Medical Education*, **54**, 703–13.

Neuberger, J. (1987). *Caring for dying people of different faiths*. Lisa Sainsbury Foundation, London.

Neuberger, J. (1997). Personal communication.

Newble, D.I., Jolly, B.C., and Wakeford, R.E. (ed.) (1994). *Certification and recertification in medicine: issues in the assessment of clinical competence*. Cambridge University Press, Cambridge.

Newble, D.I. and Paget, N. (1996). The maintenance of professional standards programme of the Royal Australasian College of Physicians. *Journal of the Royal College of Physicians of London*, **30**, 418–20.

Odegaard, C. (1988). *Dear doctor*. Henry Kaiser Foundation,

Osteopaths Act (1993). HMSO, London.

Oswald, N. Jones, S., Hinds, D. and Dale, J. (1995). The Cambridge community-based clinical course. *Medical Education*, **29**, 72–6.

Robbins F. (1977). Curriculum innovations at Case Western Reserve University School of Medicine. *Ohio State Medical Journal*, **73**, 41–2.

Robinson, G., Beaton, S., and White, P. (1993). Attitudes towards practice nurses: survey of a sample of general practitioners in England and Wales. *British Journal of General Practice*, **43**, 25–9.

Royal College of Physicians (1996). *A core curriculum for senior house officers in general (internal) medicine and the medical specialties*. RCP, London.

Royal Colleges of Physicians and Psychiatrists (1995). Joint Working Report: *The psychological care of medical patients: recognition of need and service provision.* London.

Salvage, J. (1995). What's happening to nursing? *British Medical Journal*, **311**, 274–5.

Schatz, I.J., Realini, J.P., and Charney, E. (1996). Family practice, internal medicine, and paediatrics as partners in the education of generalists. *Academic Medicine*, **71**, 35–9.

SCOPME (1994). *Teaching hospital doctors and dentists to teach.* (ed. J. Oxley) Standing Committee on Postgraduate Medical Education (SCOPME), London

Sharpe, M., Guthrie, E., Peveler, R., and Feldman, E. (1996). The psychological care of medical patients: a challenge for undergraduate medical education, *Journal of the Royal College Physicians of London*, **30**, 202–4.

Shaw, I. (1995). *Evaluating interprofessional training—planning guidance for 1996/7* educational commissioning, EL(95) 96. Department of Health, Leeds.

Shires, L., Jolly, B.C., and Wakeford, R.E. (1995). Evaluation of postgraduate education allowance events: a pilot project. *Education for General Practice*, **6**, 297–307.

Southgate, L. and Jolly, B.C. (1994). Determining the Content of Recertification Procedures. In (ed. D.I. Newble, B.C. Jolly, and R.E. Wakeford) *Certification and recertification in medicine: issues in the assessment of clinical competence*, pp.00–00. Cambridge University Press, Cambridge

Studdy, S.J., Nicol, M.J., Fox-Hiley, A. (1994) Teaching and learning clinical skills, Part 2— Development of a teaching model and schedule of skills development. *Nurse Education Today*, **14**, 186–93.

Towle, A. (1991). *Critical thinking: the future of undergraduate medical education.* King's Fund Centre, London.

Index

*(NB. Page numbers in **bold** denote a more significant section of text)*